Hospital Surgery

D0589843

Hospital Surgery

Foundations in Surgical Practice

Edited by
OMER AZIZ
SANJAY PURKAYASTHA
PARASKEVAS PARASKEVA

Foreword by
PROFESSOR THE LORD ARA DARZI OF DENHAM KBE

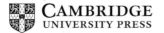

CAMBRIDGE UNIVERSITY PRESS
Cambridge, New York, Melbourne, Madrid, Cape Town, Singapore, São Paulo, Delhi

Cambridge University Press
The Edinburgh Building, Cambridge CB2 8RU, UK

Published in the United States of America by Cambridge University Press, New York

www.cambridge.org
Information on this title: www.cambridge.org/9780521682053

First published 2009

Printed in the United States

A catalogue record for this publication is available from the British Library

Library of Congress Cataloguing in Publication data
Hospital surgery : foundations in surgical practice / edited by
Omer Aziz, Sanjay Purkayastha, Paraskevas Paraskeva ; forward by Ara Darzi.
     p. ; cm.
Includes index.
ISBN 978-0-521-68205-3
1. Surgery, Operative. I. Aziz, Omer, 1976–   II. Purkayastha, Sanjay.
III. Paraskeva, Paraskevas.   IV. Title.
[DNLM: 1. Surgical Procedures, Operative.   2. Hospitalization.
3. Perioperative Care. WO 500 H828   2008]
RD32.H77   2008
617′.91–dc22   2008041690

ISBN 978-0-521-68205-3 paperback

To our parents: Kishwer, Aslam, Sheela, Sudipta, Pezouna and Antonios, for inspiring us and giving us the opportunity to achieve

Contents

Contents

Contributors

Abosede Ajayi
Medicine, Chelsea and Westminster
Hospital, London, UK

Emma J. Alexander MBBS MRCP FRCR
Specialist Registrar in Clinical Oncology,
Charing Cross Hospital, London, UK

Ziad Alyan
Department of Emergency Medicine,
Chelsea and Westminster Hospital,
London, UK

Ann Anstee
St Mary's Hospital, Imperial Healthcare
NHS Trust, London, UK

James Arbuckle
Endocrine Surgery Unit, Hammersmith
Hospital, London, UK

Ben Ardehali MSc MRCS
Specialist Registrar in Plastic Surgery,
Pan Thames Rotation, London, UK

Thanos Athanasiou
Senior Lecturer and Consultant of
Cardiothoracic Surgery, Department of
Bio Surgery and Surgical Technology,
Faculty of Medicine, Imperial College
and St Mary's Hospital, London,
UK

Omer Aziz
Department of Bio Surgery and
Surgical Technology, Faculty of
Medicine, Imperial College and
St Mary's Hospital, London,
UK

Priya Bhangoo
Specialist Registrar in Emergency
Medicine, St Thomas' Hospital, London,
UK

Robert Brightwell
Department of Bio Surgery and
Surgical Technology, Faculty of
Medicine, Imperial College and
St Mary's Hospital, London, UK

Tim Brown MRCS
Specialist Registrar in Surgery and
Honorary Clinical Fellow, St Mark's
Hospital, London, UK

Peter Butler
Consultant Plastic Surgeon, Royal Free
Hospital, London, UK

Tess Cann
Department of Bio Surgery and
Surgical Technology, Faculty of
Medicine, Imperial College and St
Mary's Hospital, London, UK

Avril Chang
General Surgery, King's College
Hospital, London, UK

Nicholas Cheshire
Professor of Vascular Surgery,
St Mary's Hospital Campus, Imperial
College Healthcare NHS Trust, London,
UK

Andre Chow
Department of Bio Surgery and
Surgical Technology, Faculty of
Medicine, Imperial College and
St Mary's Hospital, London, UK

Susan Cleator
Consultant in Clinical Oncology and
Radiology, St Mary's Hospital, London,
UK

Elaine Cronin
Stoma Care Department, St Mary's
Hospital, London, UK

Ara Darzi
Department of Bio Surgery and
Surgical Technology, Faculty of
Medicine, Imperial College and
St Mary's Hospital, London,
UK

Andreas Demetriades
The National Hospital for Neurology
and Neurosurgery, London, UK

Johann Emmanuel
Anaesthetic Specialist Registrar,
Central London School of Anaesthesia
Rotation, London, UK

Veni Ezhil
Specialist Registrar, Department of
Oncology, Imperial College and
St Mary's Hospital, London, UK

Bill Fleming
Consultant Endocrine Surgeon,
Hammersmith Hospital, London, UK

David Floyd
Consultant Plastic Surgeon, Royal Free
Hospital, London, UK

Piers A. C. Gatenby
Specialist Registrar in General Surgery,
Academic Surgical Unit, Imperial
College NHS Trust, London, UK

Richard Gibbs
Consultant Vascular Surgeon, St Mary's
Hospital, London, UK

Joan Grieve
Consultant Neurosurgeon, The National
Hospital for Neurology and
Neurosurgery, London, UK

Munther Haddad
Consultant Paediatric Surgeon, Chelsea
and Westminster and St Mary's
Hospital, London, UK

Imran Hamid
Specialist Trainee, Trauma and
Orthopaedic Surgery, Chelsea and
Westminster Hospital, London, UK

George Hanna
Department of Bio Surgery and
Surgical Technology, Faculty of

Medicine, Imperial College and
St Mary's Hospital, London,
UK

Andrew Hartle
Consultant Anaesthetist, St Mary's
Hospital, London, UK

Andrew J. Healey
Department of Surgical Oncology and
Technology, Hammersmith Hospital,
London, UK

Michele Hendricks
Specialist Registrar, Imperial School of
Anaesthesia, London, UK

Alexander G. Heriot
Consultant Colorectal Surgeon, Peter
MacCallum Cancer Centre and
St Vincent's Hospital, Melbourne,
Australia

Jonathan Hoare
Consultant Gastroenterologist,
St Mary's Hospital, London, UK

Ros Jacklin
Department of Bio Surgery and
Surgical Technology, Faculty of
Medicine, Imperial College and
St Mary's Hospital, London,
UK

David James
Department of Bio Surgery and
Surgical Technology, Faculty of
Medicine, Imperial College and
St Mary's Hospital, London,
UK

Matt Jarrett
Locum Consultant Anaesthetist,
Basingstoke Hospital, Hants, UK

Michael Jenkins
Consultant Vascular Surgeon, Regional
Vascular Unit, St Mary's Hospital,
London, UK

Long R. Jiao
Department of Surgical Oncology and
Technology, Hammersmith Hospital,
London, UK

Ravul Jindal
Senior Registrar, Regional Vascular
Unit, St Mary's Hospital, London, UK

Shahid A. Khan
Clinical Senior Lecturer and Consultant
Physician, Department of Hepatology
and Gastroenterology, St Mary's
Hospital and Hammersmith Hospital,
Imperial College London, London, UK

Umraz Khan
Consultant Plastic and Reconstructive
Surgeon, Charing Cross Hospital,
London, UK

James Kinross
Department of Bio Surgery and
Surgical Technology, Faculty of
Medicine, Imperial College and
St Mary's Hospital, London, UK

George Krasopoulos
Specialist Registrar in Cardiothoracic
Surgery, London Chest Hospital,
London, UK

Alex C. H. Lee
Department of Paediatric Surgery,
Leeds Teaching Hospitals NHS Trust,
Leeds, UK

Daniel Leff
Department of Bio Surgery and
Surgical Technology, Faculty of
Medicine, Imperial College and
St Mary's Hospital, London, UK

Richard Leonard
Consultant in Critical Care and ICU
Director, St Mary's Hospital, London, UK

David Lomax
Consultant Anaesthetist, St Mary's
Hospital, London, UK

Richard Lovegrove
Department of Bio Surgery and
Surgical Technology, Faculty of
Medicine, Imperial College and
St Mary's Hospital, London, UK

Helen Mandefield
Organ Donation Service Manager,
South Thames Transplant Coordination
Service, London, UK

Sharleet Mahal
Specialist Trainee, Imperial College
NHS Trust, London, UK

Rachel Massey
Department of Bio Surgery and
Surgical Technology, Faculty of
Medicine, Imperial College and
St Mary's Hospital, London,
UK

Pawan Mathur
Consultant General and Colorectal
Surgeon, Department of
Gastrointestinal Surgery, Barnet
Hospital, Barnet, UK

Erik Mayer
Specialist Registrar, Department of
Urology, St Mary's Hospital Campus,
Imperial College Healthcare NHS Trust,
London and Department of Bio Surgery
and Surgical Technology, Imperial
College London, London, UK

Reza Mirnezami
King's College London, London, UK

Rupert Negus
Consultant Physician and
Gastroenterologist, St Mary's Hospital,
London, UK

Marios Nicolaou
Department of Bio Surgery and
Surgical Technology, Faculty of
Medicine, Imperial College and
St Mary's Hospital, London, UK

Mei Nortley
St Mary's Hospital, London, UK

Sukhmeet S. Panesar
Department of Bio Surgery and
Surgical Technology, Faculty of
Medicine, Imperial College and
St Mary's Hospital, London, UK

Paraskevas Paraskeva
Department of Bio Surgery and
Surgical Technology, Faculty of

Medicine, Imperial College and
St Mary's Hospital, London, UK

Anurag Patel
Specialist Trainee, King's College
Hospital, London, UK

Marc Pelling
Consultant Radiologist, St Mary's
Hospital, London, UK

Mike Platt
Consultant Anaesthetist, St Mary's
Hospital, London, UK

Danielle Power
Consultant Oncologist, Imperial College
and St Mary's Hospital, London, UK

Sanjay Purkayastha
Specialist Registrar, Academic Surgical
Unit, St Mary's Hospital, London, UK

Sudipta Purkayastha
Consultant Orthopaedic Surgeon,
Medway Maritime Hospital,
Gillingham, Kent, and Visiting
Professor, Department of Bio Surgery
and Surgical Technology, Faculty of
Medicine, Imperial College and
St Mary's Hospital, London, UK

Mohammed Shamim Rahman
Specialist Trainee, Imperial College
NHS Trust, London, UK

Steven Reid
Consultant in Liaison Psychiatry,
Department of Liaison Psychiatry,

St Mary's Hospital, London,
UK

Jai Relwani
Shoulder Fellow, Reading Shoulder
Unit, Reading, UK

Caroline D. Rodd
Consultant Vascular Surgeon,
Gloucestershire Hospitals NHS
Foundation Trust, Gloucester, UK

Mathew Rollin
Endocrine Surgery Unit, Hammersmith
Hospital, London, UK

Ed Rowe
Department of Urology, Southmead
Hospital, Bristol, UK

Angharad Ruttley
Specialist Registrar in Psychiatry,
Department of Psychological
Medicine, St Bartholomew's Hospital,
London, UK

Ravi Sastry
Emergency Medicine, Kent and Sussex
Hospital, Tunbridge Wells, UK

Serene Shashaa
Fellow, Pulmonary and Critical Care
Medicine, Rush University Medical
Center, Chicago, Illinois, USA

Abdul Shlebak
Imperial College Healthcare NHS
Trust, St Mary's Hospital, London,
UK

Nakul Talwar
Specialist Registrar, Department of
Forensic Psychiatry, Langdon Hospital,
Dawlish, Devon, UK

Anisha Tanna
Specialist Registrar in Renal Medicine,
Hillingdon Hospital NHS trust,
Uxbridge, UK

Julian Teare
Consultant Gastroenterologist,
St Mary's Hospital, London, UK

Paris Tekkis
Department of Bio Surgery and
Surgical Technology, Faculty of
Medicine, Imperial College and
St Mary's Hospital, London, UK

Teo Teo
Consultant Obstetrician, St Mary's
Hospital, London, UK

Huw J. W. Thomas
Consultant Gastroenterologist and
Professor of Intestinal Genetics, St
Mary's Hospital and Imperial College,
London, UK

Mark Thursz
Department of Hepatology and
Gastroenterology, Imperial College and
St Mary's Hospital, London, UK

Henry Tillney
Department of Bio Surgery and
Surgical Technology, Faculty of
Medicine, Imperial College and
St Mary's Hospital, London, UK

Neil S. Tolley
Consultant ENT-Thyroid Surgeon,
St Mary's Hospital, London,
UK

Lai Pun Tong
General Surgery, Central Middlesex
Hospital, London, UK

James Uprichard
Faculty of Medicine, Imperial College
London, London, UK

Justin Vale MS FRCS (Urol)
Consultant Urological Surgeon,
Department of Urology,
St Mary's Hospital Campus, Imperial
College Healthcare NHS Trust, London,
UK

David Walker
Specialist Registrar in
Gastroenterology, Department of
Gastroenterology, St Mary's Hospital,
London, UK

Neil Walker
Specialist Registrar in Endocrinology,
Oxford Centre for Diabetes,
Endocrinology and Metabolism,
Churchill Hospital, Oxford, UK

Susanna Walker
Specialist Registrar, Imperial School of
Anaesthesia, London, UK

Patricia Ward
Consultant in Emergency Medicine,
St Mary's Hospital, London,
UK

Stephen Ward
General Surgical Registrar, Department
of Surgery, St Helier Hospital,
Carshalton, Surrey, UK

Greg Williams
Consultant Burns, Plastic and
Reconstructive Surgeon, Chelsea and
Westminster Hospital, London, UK

Danny Yakoub
Clinical Research Fellow and Honorary
Surgical Registrar, Department of Bio
Surgery and Surgical Technology,
Faculty of Medicine, Imperial
College and St Mary's Hospital, London,
UK

Paul Ziprin
Senior Lecturer and Consultant
Surgeon, Department of Bio
Surgery and Surgical Technology,
Faculty of Medicine, Imperial
College and St Mary's Hospital, London,
UK

Foreword

Surgical practice has witnessed some dramatic changes over the past decade. The advent of new imaging technologies has revolutionized the way that surgical disease is diagnosed, managed and followed up. Minimally invasive surgery and goal-directed recovery have tangibly improved the quality of postoperative care and reduced hospital stay. Advances in fields such as bioengineering and nanotechnology now offer the prospect of further huge leaps. What this has meant is that surgery has evolved into a truly multidisciplinary specialty, relying heavily on the input of a host of healthcare professionals. Throughout this there remains a real need for core knowledge of surgical management to be put into a modern perspective, particularly for the junior doctor who needs this information at his or her fingertips.

In parallel to technological advances, Western World healthcare systems have also been going through major restructuring programmes in order to cope with the increasing demands of modern medicine. In the UK, medical training has changed through the Modernising Medical Careers (MMC) programme and surgical teaching has had to cope with the changes to both medical school and postgraduate exams. Medical students and junior doctors being produced by these new systems have the same duty of care towards their patients as those of years gone by. This has to be provided to the highest standard.

There is now a real responsibility to provide easily accessible and up-to-date knowledge of surgical management to those who need it the most. Hospital Surgery is a text that can be used by medical students and junior doctors alike to hone their knowledge of surgery for both the clinical and exam setting. Those involved in composing this text are truly enthused by the specialty and have devoted large portions of their

personal time to teaching the subject. In this book, their aim has been
to combine traditional approaches with a modern view point, making
Hospital Surgery an invaluable asset in the armoury of any individual
involved in surgical practice.

Professor the Lord Ara Darzi of Denham KBE HonFREng FMedSci

Preface

> Knowing is not enough; we must apply. Willing is not enough; we must do
>
> Johann Wolfgang von Goethe

Our journey to acquire knowledge towards a surgical career began at St. Mary's Hospital Medical School. The first time we all met, two of us (Omer Aziz and Sanjay Purkayastha) were medical students being taught by a senior house officer called 'Barry' (Paraskevas Paraskeva). His teaching was clear to follow, enthusiastically delivered, and extremely practical. It instilled in us all a responsibility towards our patients, and pride in the way that we managed them. A close friendship and collaboration subsequently ensued, and has lead to us teaching and examining hundreds of medical students together every year in the UK.

The three of us have been fortunate to have been influenced by some excellent texts and inspiring clinicians during our training, which has been a key part of us developing and forming our surgical judgement. In recent times however, we have felt the increasing need to combine key surgical principles with modern practical knowledge, for the medical student or junior doctor to use on a daily basis on the wards. *Hospital Surgery* aims to provide this up-to-date knowledge in a clear and concise format. We hope that this handbook provides those who are learning to manage surgical patients with the strong foundation they need.

Consent and medico-legal considerations

NAKUL TALWAR, ANGHARAD RUTTLEY AND STEVEN REID

Individuals have a fundamental right to determine what happens to their own bodies. It is unlawful and unethical to carry out a medical procedure without first obtaining valid consent. Legal aspects of medical practice are subject to continuous change and it is necessary for health professionals to keep abreast of developments in medical law. In particular the Mental Capacity Act 2005 is likely to have a profound influence on current practice.

■ What is consent?

While there are various definitions of consent, essentially it identifies the agreement between patients and health professionals to provide care. For consent to be valid one must appreciate the essential principles of valid consent. This requires that the patient must be adequately informed, have the capacity to make the decision for him/her self and make the decision voluntarily. Nobody can give or withhold consent on behalf of a competent adult.

■ Capacity

Capacity is the decision-making ability of an individual in relation to a specific matter at the material time, which is not impaired due to a disturbance in functioning of the mind or the brain either temporarily or permanently.

All registered medical practitioners are eligible to assess capacity. Adults are always assumed to have capacity unless demonstrated

Hospital Surgery: Foundations in Surgical Practice, ed. Omer Aziz, Sanjay Purkayastha and Paraskevas Paraskeva. Published by Cambridge University Press. © Cambridge University Press 2009.

otherwise. Capacity assessments are decision-specific and may fluctuate over time. Patients with mental illness may have capacity to consent to treatment for physical illness even when psychiatrically unwell or vice versa.

Prior to a capacity assessment an individual must be provided with all the relevant information including the nature and purpose of the proposed intervention, the risks associated with accepting or refusing the intervention and other available options. Any adult has capacity to consent (or refuse) medical treatment if he/she can satisfy the four legal criteria:

1. Understand and retain the information relevant to the decision
2. Believe the information
3. Use the information and weigh it in the balance to arrive at a decision
4. Communicate their decision (does not have to be verbal).

■ Case example

Mr C was a patient suffering from paranoid schizophrenia and was being detained in a psychiatric hospital when he developed gangrene in his right foot. He held a delusional belief that he was an eminent surgeon and refused to consent to a below-knee amputation. He sought an injunction to prevent surgeons from carrying out the amputation. Justice Thorpe granted the injunction and held that Mr C understood the nature, purpose, and effects of the proposed amputation. Hence he retained the capacity to make a decision regarding his treatment. This has subsequently been cited in various cases and is known as the 'Re C Test'.

■ Refusal of a medical procedure

Any adult patient of sound understanding has the right to accept or refuse treatment, even if the choice appears irrational, insensible or ill considered. If a patient has refused to consent to treatment, doctors must make a careful assessment of the patient's capacity at the material time. The more serious the decision the greater the capacity required. In cases of uncertainty advice should be obtained from senior colleagues. It may be necessary to consult Trust solicitors or seek a declaration from the court.

If the patient lacks capacity to consent to treatment, doctors have a duty of care to act in the best interests of the patient. Under the common law doctrine of 'necessity', treatment can be given to save life, ensure improvement or prevent deterioration of physical or mental health and should be accepted by a responsible body of medical opinion. It is good practice to seek a second opinion in such cases.

When determining the best interests of the patient, the responsible clinician should consider not only the most appropriate clinical care, but also other factors such as the wishes and beliefs of the patient when competent, and their current wishes. It is wise to involve people close to the patient in the decision-making process to gain additional information about the patient's wishes and values.

■ Jehovah's Witnesses

Jehovah's Witnesses are entitled to accept or refuse any proposed treatment and have the right to change their mind at any stage. Detailed advance directives are often prepared and doctors may be found guilty of assault if they knowingly breach the directive. In life-threatening situations where consent cannot be obtained and the individual's views are not known, blood transfusion should not be withheld. The views of relatives and friends may be sought but they cannot refuse transfusion on the patient's behalf.

■ Detention under the Mental Health Act 1983

The Mental Health Act may only be used to assess or treat mental illness. Physical disorders cannot be treated under the provisions of the Act.

Inpatients requiring detention in hospital when a mental illness is suspected can be detained under Section 5(2) of the Mental Health Act 1983. The Responsible Medical Officer or his/her nominated deputy is responsible for applying the section. In Acute Trusts this will usually be the Surgical Consultant or Registrar, although the psychiatric team should be notified immediately. Section 5(2) is not applicable in Accident and Emergency (A&E) or Outpatient (OPD) Departments.

■ Documentation

The professional seeking consent must be competent to do so. In practice this is usually the person carrying out the procedure. However it may be appropriate for professionals who have received specialist training in advising patients about a procedure to do so. Responsibility for gaining informed consent in law lies with the professional carrying out the procedure.

It is essential to document clearly the patient's agreement to the intervention and the discussions that led up to the same. A consent form may be used or oral consent may be documented in the patient's notes. It is good practice to seek written consent, although it is rarely a legal requirement. While it is not necessary to document a patient's consent for routine and low-risk procedures, it is good practice.

■ Children and adolescents

The competency criteria for valid consent are similar to those for adults. Professionals need to be extra vigilant so as to ensure that information is provided in an appropriate pace and form, in a non-coercive environment that respects privacy and dignity. This may include discussion in the absence of the parents.

In England and Wales, individuals above the age of 18 are presumed competent. Young people between the ages of 16 and 18 and deemed to be competent may consent to treatment, but unlike adults cannot refuse life-saving treatment. Individuals under the age of 16 can legally consent provided they satisfy the competency criteria (*Gillick* v. *West Norfolk and Wisbech Area Health Authority* [1985]: legal reference: 3 All ER 402 HL). Additionally parents, individuals or local authorities with parental responsibility, or courts can give consent for treatment on behalf of the individual.

If a competent young person refuses treatment or if parents dispute the treatment, resolution should be sought through discussion and compromise. If the issues cannot be resolved then the courts can be involved in the best interests of the individual.

The following are common questions that patients expect to have answered during the process of consent for a surgical procedure (taken from www.doh.gov.uk/consent):

What are the main treatment options?

What are the benefits of each of the options?

What are the risks, if any, of each option?

What are the success rates for different options – nationally, for this unit or for you (the surgeon)?

What are the complication rates for the procedure in question – nationally, for this unit or for you (the surgeon)?

Why do you think an operation (if suggested) is necessary?

What are the risks if nothing is done for the time being?

How can the patient expect to feel after the procedure?

When should the patient expect to be discharged and be able to get back to work?

Questions may also be about how the treatment might affect the patient's state of health or quality of life, for example:

Will they need long-term care?

Will their mobility be affected?

Will they still be able to drive – if so, when?

Will the procedure affect the kind of work the patient does?

Will it affect their personal/sexual relationships?

Will they be able to take part in their favourite sport/exercises?

Will they be able to follow their usual diet?

■ Further information

The Department of Health and General Medical Council have issued a number of documents on consent. These can be found at www.dh.gov.uk./consent and www.gmc-uk.org/guidance/library/consent.asp.

Elective surgery

SUSANNA WALKER AND DAVID LOMAX

■ Aims

To assess and optimize co-existing medical conditions prior to surgery

To anticipate potential problems, inform the relevant people, and address these prior to admission, e.g. requires ICU (Intensive Care Unit) bed.

■ History

1. CARDIOVASCULAR (CVS)

History of hypertension? On antihypertensive medications?

MI: when? What treatment? Cardiology follow-up? If less than six months ago postpone elective surgery

Angina: stable/unstable? How frequently requires GTN spray? Exercise tolerance

Any symptoms of PND (paroxysmal noctural dyspnoea) or orthopnoea? How many pillows does patient sleep on at night?

Past history of rheumatic fever: has patient ever been diagnosed with 'leaky valve'?

Any symptoms of palpitations, syncope, dizziness, blackouts, unexplained falls?

2. RESPIRATORY

History of asthma or COPD?

Episodes of bronchitis? If so, how frequently? Sputum production and colour of sputum

Hospital Surgery: Foundations in Surgical Practice, ed. Omer Aziz, Sanjay Purkayastha and Paraskevas Paraskeva. Published by Cambridge University Press.
© Cambridge University Press 2009.

Inhalers? Home nebulisers? Home oxygen therapy?

Any hospital admissions with respiratory problems? If so, any ICU admissions?

Severity of dyspnoea, exercise tolerance

Current or past history of smoking? How many per day for how many years?

3. ABDOMINAL

History of indigestion or reflux?

Any past episodes of jaundice? Does patient have a diagnosis of chronic hepatitis?

Is there a history of renal disease? What is the cause?

Does patient require dialysis? If so, liaise with renal team prior to setting date for surgery

Does patient have a fluid restriction regime?

4. NEUROLOGICAL

History of CVA?

Epilepsy: how well controlled? When was last seizure?

If frequent seizures, refer to neurology team for optimization preoperatively

Rare conditions, e.g. myasthenia gravis, Duchenne's muscular dystrophy, myotonic dystrophy, multiple sclerosis – take full history of progression of disease.

5. ENDOCRINE

Thyroid problems: is function regularly checked? Does patient have symptoms of stridor, dysphagia, dyspnoea?

Diabetes: enquire about details of current regime and systemic implications of diabetes

Steroid replacement: reason for steroids, length of course, current dose.

6. HAEMATOLOGY

Coagulopathies

Sickle cell disease: enquire about systemic complications, e.g. splenic
infarct, sickle cell chest, CVAs, cholecystitis

Thromboembolic tendency

Chronic anaemia: cause?

7. MUSCULOSKELETAL

Rheumatoid arthritis: is the neck affected? Symptoms of cervical cord
compression? Any associated symptoms, e.g. dyspnoea? Drug treatment?

8. ANAESTHETIC

Any previous anaesthetics?

Any problems, e.g. unexpected admission to ICU?

Any family history of problems with anaesthetics?

9. DRUGS

Full history of all current medications

History of any allergies to medications

Is there a history of latex allergy? An increasing problem, inform theatres
if necessary

Does patient use recreational drugs? Has patient used cocaine in previous 48 hours? If so, advise strongly against using prior to surgery.

10. SOCIAL

Does patient mobilize independently or need aids?

Smoker: how much, what and for how many years?

Alcohol: what exactly and how much?

■ Examination

CVS: BP, pulse, peripheral stigmata of cardiac disease, apex beat, heart sounds, evidence of oedema, carotid bruits, all peripheral pulses

Respiratory: rate, oxygen saturations, peripheral stigmata of respiratory disease, chest expansion. Percussion note, wheeze/crackles/consolidation on auscultation

Abdomen: previous scars from surgery, peripheral stigmata of liver disease, hepato- or spleno-megaly, aortic pulsation

Neurological: full neurological examination for any patient with neurological disease to document preoperative condition.

■ Investigations

The investigations required depend to a large degree on the findings from History and Examination, and the type of surgery planned. American Society of Anaesthesiologists Grades (ASA Grades) describe the fitness of a patient undergoing an anaesthetic.

ASA Grade	Surgery grade
I – Normal, healthy patient	1 – Minor, e.g. skin lesion, drainage of abscess
II – Mild/moderate systemic disease not limiting function	2 – Intermediate, e.g. inguinal hernia repair
III – Moderate/severe systemic disease limiting function	3 – Major, e.g. TAH, prostatectomy
IV – Severe systemic disease that is a constant threat to life	4 – Major +, e.g. THR, colonic resection
V – Not expected to survive 24 hours	—

From http//www.asahq.org/clinical/physicalstatus.htm with permission from the American Society of Anaesthesiologists.

■ General tests

Urine	Often performed on every patient, although NICE guidelines do not recommend in asymptomatic patients
FBC	All female patients All male patients >50 yrs

U&Es   All patients >65 yrs
LFTs   Any patient with liver disease, history of alcoholism
Clotting   Any patient on oral anticoagulants
           Any patient with liver disease or alcohol excess
           Any patient with known clotting disorder
ECG   All patients >50 yrs
           Male smokers >45 yrs
CXR   Any patient with cardiorespiratory disease
           All patients >50 yrs.

■ Specific tests

Crossmatch	Discuss with blood bank for local protocol
Sickle cell	All Afro-Caribbeans, also consider in Middle Eastern and Mediterranean patients
Pregnancy test	Any female of reproductive age who is uncertain of pregnancy status
ECHO	Any patient with cardiovascular disease with evidence of valve murmurs on examination. Signs of congestive cardiac failure, evidence of recent or old MI but no recent ECHO
Cervical spine	X-ray (flexion and extension views) any patient with significantly limited neck movement or signs of vertebral instability: especially rheumatoid patients
Thoracic inlet	X-ray for any patient with thyroid enlargement
Exercise testing and angiogram	Consider for any patient with symptoms of frequent or unstable angina. Will require discussion with cardiology team.

Summary table

Surgery grade	Grade 1			Grade 2			Grade 3			Grade 4		
ASA grade	I	II	III	I	II	III	I	II	III	I	II	III
FBC		CRRe	CRRe	?	CRRe	All	All	All	All	All	All	All
Clotting			Re	?	Re	Re	?	Re	CRe	All	All	All
Renal		CRRe	CRRe	?	CRRe	All	All	All	All	All	All	All
EGG		CR	CRRe	?	CRRe	All	?	All	All	?	All	All
CXR		CR	CRRe		CRRe	CRRe	?	CRRe	CRRe	?	All	All
Urine	?	CRRe	CRRe	?	CRRe	CRRe	?	CRRe	CRRe	?	CRRe	CRRe
ABG		R	CRRe		R	CRRe		CRRe	CRRe		CRRe	CRRe
Lung function						R		R	R	R	R	R
ECHO						C			C		C	C
Glucose		?	Re	?	?	Re	?	Re	R Re	?	Re	R Re

Re – Renal disease
C – Cardiovascular disease
R – Respiratory disease
All – All patients
? – Consider doing this test

■ Other considerations

1. MEDICATIONS: SPECIFIC RECOMMENDATIONS FOR SOME DRUGS REGULARLY ENCOUNTERED

Anticoagulants

Warfarin: check clotting and convert to heparin infusion

Aspirin: continue for minor case. Consult surgeon for major cases

Clopidogrel: stop seven days before surgery after consultation with cardiologist.

Anticonvulsants

Give all normal doses at normal times up until the time of surgery.

ACE inhibitors

May cause labile BP intraoperatively – withhold on morning of surgery.

Angiotensin 2 antagonists/inhibitors

Withhold for 24 hours preoperatively.

β blockers

Important to continue and take on day of surgery.

Ca Ch blockers

Continue and take on morning of surgery.

Digoxin

Take on day of surgery. Check K^+ as low level may precipitate toxicity and arrhythmia.

Diuretics

Consider withholding on morning of surgery – especially if surgery is planned for afternoon. Start iv fluids if diuretic given, to prevent severe dehydration pre-induction. Check U&Es night before or morning of surgery.

Hypoglycaemics

Tolbutamide: withhold 24 hours preoperatively. Withhold morning dose on morning of surgery

Insulin: convert patient to sliding scale before surgery if admitted as inpatient.

Monoamine oxidase inhibitors

Potential for severe interaction with ionotropes intraoperatively. Convert to alternative therapy two to three weeks preoperatively if possible.

Steroids

Patient should take normal morning dose on day of surgery. Additional supplementation will be given on induction.

2. UNUSUAL CONDITIONS

It is impossible to cover every circumstance, therefore if patients present with any unusual conditions that you are uncertain about, discuss the patient with an anaesthetist – preferably the Consultant Anaesthetist for the appropriate theatre list – prior to admitting the patient, so any extra investigations and arrangements can be organized.

3. REASONS FOR CONSIDERING AN ICU BED

If an ICU bed is required, the patient should have been discussed with the appropriate anaesthetist.

Some indications for an ICU bed would include:

a. Major surgery: e.g. AAA repair, gastro-oesophagectomy
b. Severe COPD: risk of not being able to extubate patient at end of surgery

c. Myotonic dystrophy
d. Muscular dystrophy
e. Myasthenia gravis.

4. NUTRITION

Nutritional status is important preoperatively as it has implications for the surgical outcome of the patient in terms of tissue healing and the general well-being of the patient.

Previously the assessment of a patient's nutritional status was performed from the end of the bed by looking at their general condition; this may still be useful but there are more objective parameters that can be used. Assessment can be considered in the following groups:

1. Clinical findings: history and examination, regular weights, body mass index
2. Anthropometric measurements
3. Skin fold thickness: e.g. triceps and iliac crest, arm circumference, grip strength
4. Blood tests: serum albumin, serum phosphate, serum transferrin, lymphocyte count.

If patients are undergoing major gastrointestinal surgery that may have long-term consequences on feeding regimes then this must be evaluated and sorted out prior to surgery, along with input from the dietician and the clinicians that will be involved in the patient's long-term care.

If the nutritional status of a patient is evaluated to be very poor prior to major elective surgery there may be a case for postponing the surgery until such time as this can be rectified.

Special situations in surgery: the diabetic patient

DANIEL LEFF AND PAUL ZIPRIN

■ Definition

Diabetes mellitus (DM) is a syndrome caused by the lack or diminished effectiveness of endogenous insulin and is characterized by hyperglycaemia and deranged metabolism

Type I, insulin dependent (IDDM): usually juvenile onset, associated with other autoimmune diseases, caused by insulin deficiency.

Type II, non-insulin dependent: older age group, often obese, insulin resistance and impaired secretion.

■ Preoperative assessment and precautions

Diabetic patients should whenever possible have their blood glucose control optimized prior to surgery. The reasons for good glycaemic control are as follows:

■ Prevention of ketosis and acidaemia
■ Prevent perioperative electrolyte imbalance and volume depletion secondary to osmotic diuresis
■ Increased risk of impaired wound strength/wound healing if control inadequate
■ Hyperglycaemia leads to an impaired immune response, and poor diabetic control, increases risk of infection.

Alert the team if:

■ HbA1c > 9 %
■ Fasting glucose > 10 mmol/l.

Hospital Surgery: Foundations in Surgical Practice, ed. Omer Aziz, Sanjay Purkayastha and Paraskevas Paraskeva. Published by Cambridge University Press. © Cambridge University Press 2009.

Take a full preoperative history and examination, and screen the diabetic patient for preoperative complications that might increase the risk of surgery:

1. Renal: nephropathy, renal failure, check urea and electrolytes, urinalysis
2. Cardiac: ischaemic heart disease, hypertension, arterial disease, ECG
3. Eyes: fundoscopy to exclude proliferative retinopathy
4. Infection: exclude preoperative focus, delay surgery until infections treated
5. Metabolic: confirm adequate glycaemic control, BM, HbA1C
6. CNS/PNS: exclude autonomic/peripheral neuropathy

■ Perioperative management of Type II diabetes

1. Place *first* on operating list if possible (reduces period of starvation/risk of hypoglycaemia).
2. Optimize control preoperatively and continue on normal oral hypoglycaemic medication until the morning of surgery.
3. Long acting sulfonylurea agents should be stopped 2 days prior to surgery (e.g. chlorpropamide, may need to be reduced or stopped 48 hours in advance).
4. Stop metformin the night before surgery to reduce the risk of lactic acidosis.
5. *Omit the morning oral hypoglycaemics.*
6. Avoid glucose-containing iv fluids.
7. Poorly controlled patients, or those undergoing major surgery should be started on a preoperative sliding scale regimen as for patients with Type I diabetes.
8. Restart the patient on normal oral hypoglycaemic regimen postoperatively when eating and drinking normally.

■ Perioperative management of Type I (insulin dependent) diabetes

1. Achieve good preoperative control.
2. Admit the patient the night before surgery.
3. If undergoing minor surgery, with preoperative BM < 10 mmol/l and patient first on operation list, it is possible to avoid iv insulin regimen.
4. If patient undergoing major surgery use a sliding scale of iv insulin infusion (see table below) along with 5 % dextrose (containing KCl)
   a. Alberti regimen (intravenous infusion of 5–10 g glucose/1–2 units of insulin/100 ml fluid/hr)
   b. PIG (potassium, insulin, glucose) regimen (10 % dextrose/10 units insulin/10 mmol KCl/10 hr).
5. Start the above regimen preoperatively and continue until eating normally.
6. Monitor blood glucose, before, during and after surgery, aiming for a blood glucose level of 6–10 mmol/l.
7. Restart the patient's routine s/c insulin regimen postoperatively when eating and drinking normally (only discharge the patient when their control is within recognized limits; insulin requirements can transiently increase after a stimulus such as surgery).

■ Recommended sliding scale regimen

Prescribe: 50 units of Actrapid insulin in 50 mls of normal saline to run according to sliding scale as shown in the table.

Blood glucose (mmol/l)	Insulin infusion rate (u/hr)
0–4	0.5
4.1–7	1
7.1–12	2
12.1–17.0	4
17.1–27.0	7
>27.0	10

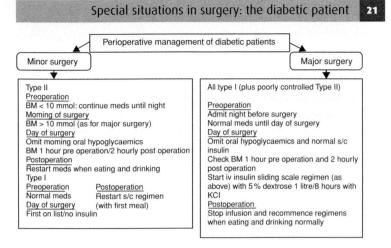

Algorithm: perioperative management of diabetic patients

Special situations in surgery: the jaundiced patient

DANIEL LEFF AND PAUL ZIPRIN

■ Preoperative management of the jaundiced patient

Adequate preoperative preparation is essential in the jaundiced patient. Preparation entails correction of metabolic derangement, optimizing the general condition of the patient, and specific measures that aim to reduce the incidence of complications associated with jaundice on systems such as:

1. Immune: increased risk of infections (cholangitis, septicaemia, wound infections)
2. Haematological: clotting abnormalities
3. Metabolic: electrolyte abnormality such as hypernatraemia and hypokalaemia
4. Renal: hepatorenal syndrome/acute renal failure
5. Hepatic: hepatitis, fulminant liver failure
6. CNS: delirium and hepatic encephalopathy
7. GI tract: gastrointestinal bleeding from varices
8. Endocrine: hypoglycaemia due to depletion of glycogen stores.

HISTORY

Duration of the jaundice (acute or chronic) and symptoms suggesting cause (e.g. dark urine, pale stools)

Family history of haemolytic illnesses e.g. spherocytosis, glucose-6-phosphate dehydrogenase deficiency

Hospital Surgery: Foundations in Surgical Practice, ed. Omer Aziz, Sanjay Purkayastha and Paraskevas Paraskeva. Published by Cambridge University Press. © Cambridge University Press 2009.

Drug history (many drugs including anaesthetic agents are metabolized by the liver and may therefore have a prolonged duration of action)

Detailed history of alcohol intake.

EXAMINATION

Full systematic examination

Exclude preoperative cholangitis/sepsis secondary to other causes

Exclude spontaneous bacterial peritonitis (SBP) in patients with chronic liver disease

Exclude preoperative hepatic failure (ascites, hepatic encephalopathy).

INVESTIGATIONS

FBC: exclude preoperative anaemia, and elevated WCC suggesting preoperative infection

Clotting screen: exclude prolonged prothrombin time (PT)

Urea and electrolytes: ensure normal renal function, exclude preoperative hypernatraemia and hypokalaemia

Liver Function tests: establish baseline bilirubin, transaminases and albumin

Blood glucose

Calculate the severity of chronic liver disease if present using *Child's classification* which helps quantify the perioperative risk (see table).

■ General perioperative interventions

Fluid balance: ensure adequate hydration to prevent *hepatorenal syndrome*; preoperative diuresis may reduce incidence (administer 5 % dextrose/saline for 12 hours preoperatively +/− loop diuretic at time of induction). Some report benefits of using low doses of the inotrope dopamine (causes renal vasodilation), though its use remains largely unproven.

Note: hypoalbuminaemia may lead to fluid retention in jaundice patients; manage the patient with a urinary catheter and accurately monitor fluid input/output charts.

Treat hypokalaemia: secondary hyperaldosteronism leads to Na$^+$ retention and K$^+$ depletion.

Clotting: decreased vitamin K absorption in cholestatic jaundice leads to reduced synthesis of factors II, VII, IX, and X, leading to a prolonged prothrombin time (PT). Intravenous injection of vitamin K (5–10 mg) will reverse the clotting deficiency within 1–3 days. If more urgent correction is required use fresh frozen plasma (FFP) within 1–2 hours of the surgical procedure.

Infection: (1) wound and (2) cholangitis. In general there is a greater risk of postoperative wound failure and wound infection associated with jaundice; use prophylactic broad-spectrum antibiotics to avoid risk of sepsis. Ciprofloxacin 500 mg po to prevent risk of cholangitis.

■ Specific perioperative interventions

Relieve jaundice prior to surgery if possible: endoscopic sphincterotomy to relieve CBD obstruction and remove common bile duct stones. Note: liver failure may be encountered in patients with prolonged CBD obstruction or with preoperative hepatocellular disease. If jaundice is severe (>150 mmol/l) and if concomitant sepsis evident, a period of decompression is required prior to surgery, via ERCP and endoscopic stenting +/− sphincterotomy.

Child's classification of the severity of chronic liver disease			
Category	A	B	C
Bilirubin	<35	35–50	>50
Albumin	>35	30–35	<30
Ascites	None	Mild to moderate	Severe
Encephalopathy	None	Mild	Moderate
Nutrition*	Good	Moderate	Poor
Risk of surgery	**Good**	**Fair**	**Poor**

*Pugh's modification replaces nutrition with prothrombin time

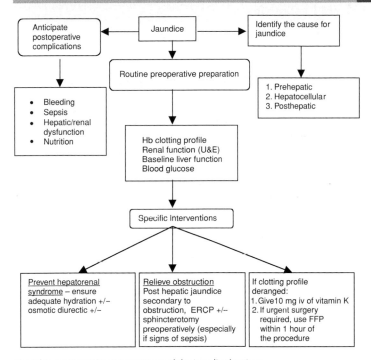

Algorithm: perioperative management of the jaundiced patient

Special situations in surgery: patients with thyroid disease

DANIEL LEFF AND PAUL ZIPRIN

■ Predict perioperative complications such as

1. Related to thyroid diseases
   a. Exacerbation of hyper or hypothyroidism, postoperative thyroiditis
   b. Airway management in patients with goitres or those undergoing thyroid surgery – anticipate difficult intubation and liaise with anaesthetist
   c. Thyroid storm (acute thyroid crisis)
   d. Specific postoperative complications related to thyroid surgery (see table).
2. Other systems
   a. CVS: tachyarrhythmias, exacerbation of preoperative atrial fibrillation, heart failure (thyrotoxic cardiomyopathy)
   b. Ophthalmic: thyroid eye disease in Graves' disease such as exophthalmos and ophthalmoplegia
   c. Preoperative anaemia: normochromic normocytic anaemia in hyper and hypothyroidism
   d. Liver disease: pre-existing deranged liver function in hyperthyroidism
   e. Musculoskeletal: pretibial myxoedema, thyroid acropachy
   f. CNS: delirium, psychosis
   g. Immune: increased risk of infection.

Hospital Surgery: Foundations in Surgical Practice, ed. Omer Aziz, Sanjay Purkayastha and Paraskevas Paraskeva. Published by Cambridge University Press. © Cambridge University Press 2009.

■ Preoperative management

HISTORY

Relating to both the presenting surgical condition (if not thyroid surgery)
Thyroid diseases
Family history of MEN syndromes in patients with thyroid carcinoma
Drug history (e.g. propanolol, carbimazole, radioiodine ^{131}I treatment, thyroxine).

EXAMINATION

General systematic examination
Examination of thyroid gland/goitre/assess for retrosternal expansion
Identify signs of preoperative thyrotoxicosis (restless, tremor, warm sweaty peripheries, thyroid acropachy, irregular pulse)
Exclude preoperative infection (may precipitate thyroid storm in hyperthyroid patients).

INVESTIGATIONS

Thyroid function tests: (TSH, free T4 and free T3) – exclude preoperative thyrotoxicosis
Thyroid autoantibody screen: if suspicious of preoperative Graves' disease
Thyroid US scan: if new onset goitre or localized nodule
Consider isotope scan: to determine extent of retrosternal goitre
FBC: exclude pre-existing anaemia associated with thyroid disease
Bone profile: establish preoperative Ca^{2+} level in patients undergoing thyroid surgery
CT scan: to exclude preoperative metastases in patients with thyroid carcinoma

Vocal cord check: to exclude pre-existing paresis, especially if there has been previous thyroid surgery.

■ Preoperative management of thyrotoxicosis

It is vital that patients are euthyroid prior to undergoing surgery. Preoperative control of hyperthyroidism is essential to prevent precipitating acute thyroid crisis. The speed with which restoration to euthyroidism is required will dictate the treatment choice.

The treatment options include:

1. Symptom control with β blockers, e.g. propanolol 40 mg/6 hr po
2. Thyroid suppression with carbimazole 15–40 mg/24 hr po for four weeks or propylthiouracil
3. Radioiodine (^{131}I), repeated until euthyroid
4. A combination of iopanoic acid (500 mg bd) and dexamethasone (1 mg bd) used in conjunction with propylthiouracil and β blockers, with which a rapid correction has been achieved.

■ Management of thyroid storm

Rare, severe form of hyperthyroidism. Life threatening condition occurring in patients inadequately controlled before surgery. Dyspnoea, tachycardia, hyperpyrexia, restlessness, confusion, delirium, vomiting and diarrhea occur. Examination may reveal goitre and a thyroid bruit. Liaise with the endocrinologists.

Treatment includes: (1) rehydration, 0.9 % saline 500 mls/4 hr; (2) NG tube if vomiting; (3) take blood for free T3/T4 and blood cultures; (4) cooling with tepid sponging; (5) paracetamol 1 g; (6) propanolol 40 mg/8 hr po (maximum iv dose: 1 mg over 1 minute, repeated nine times at >2 minute intervals; (7) start antithyroid medication:

carbimazole 15–25 mg/6 hr po; (8) dexamethasone 4 mg/6 hr po or hydrocortisone 100 mg/6 hr iv; (9) treat any suspected infective cause with broad spectrum antibiotics.

■ Preoperative correction of hypothyroidism

Thyroxine replacement therapy is the mainstay of treatment (start at low dose 25 μg and increase dose every fortnight to avoid precipitating tachyarrhythmias and cardiac failure). The normal long-term dose required is between 75 and 150 μg. Patients should remain on thyroxine until the morning of the surgery.

Specific complications of thyroid surgery	
Complication	Clinical features/treatment
Bleeding	Massive bleeding in 1/500 patients, can be life threatening, may require control in operating theatre. Haematoma more common
Airways obstruction	(1) Secondary to bleeding: open the wound to relieve obstruction. (2) Chondromalacia
Infection	Localized infection in 1-2 % of patients. Treat cellulitis with broad spectrum antibiotics, drain neck abscesses
Thyroid storm	See above for treatment
Nerve injury 1. Recurrent laryngeal nerve (RLN) 2. External laryngeal nerve (ELN)	RLN – if unilateral – hoarse voice (temporary in 4 %, permanent in 1 %), if bilateral airways obstruction ELN – affects pitch (opera singers)
Parathyroid injury/hypocalcaemia	Monitor serum calcium postoperatively
Swallowing difficulties	Common first few days postoperatively, rarely persistent
Failure to control hyperthyroidism	2–4 %, monitor T3/T4/TSH postoperatively/treated with radioactive iodine
Hypothyroidism	Especially if total thyroidectomy, check T3/T4/TSH. Thyroxine replacement
Unsightly scars	After wound infection, keloidosis, may cause tethering and affect swallowing

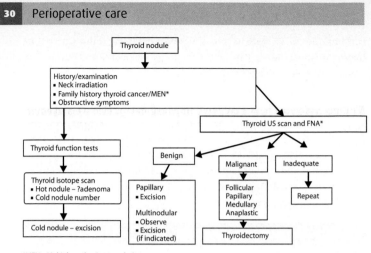

*MEN – Multiple endocrine neoplasia
FNA – Fine needle aspiration biopsy

Algorithm: perioperative management of the patient with thyroid disease

Special situations in surgery: steroids and surgery

DANIEL LEFF AND PAUL ZIPRIN

A number of patients that are attending hospital for elective and emergency surgery will be taking steroids for a number of different medical reasons including: asthma, inflammatory bowel disease, rheumatoid arthritis and sarcoidosis.

■ Effect of surgery

It is important to remember that there is an increase in ACTH and cortisol in response to injury and surgery. In response to minor surgery there is minimal increase in cortisol secretion (50 mg), and a 2–3 fold increase following major surgery (75–100 mg).

■ Why do patients require additional steroids?

Patients who are on long-term steroids tend to have a suppressed hypothalamic – pituitary – adrenal axis (see Figure 1). These patients are at risk of developing hypoadrenal crisis (circulatory collapse and shock), if supplementary cortisol is not provided. Not all patients who are treated with steroids will have this suppression, which depends on the dose and duration of steroid therapy.

Hospital Surgery: Foundations in Surgical Practice, ed. Omer Aziz, Sanjay Purkayastha and Paraskevas Paraskeva. Published by Cambridge University Press. © Cambridge University Press 2009.

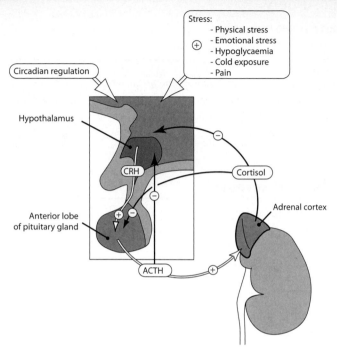

Figure 1

■ Which patients require supplementary steroids?

1. Pituitary – adrenal insufficiency on steroids
2. Pituitary or adrenal surgery
3. Patients on long-term corticosteroids at a dose of more than 10 mg prednisolone daily (or equivalent)
4. Patients who have received corticosteroids at a dose of more than 10 mg daily, in the last three months
5. Patients taking high dose inhalation corticosteroids (e.g. beclomethasone 1.5 mg a day).

■ Useful conversions

Prednisolone 5 mg is equivalent to:

Beclomethasone 750 µg
Cortisone acetate 25 mg
Dexamethasone 6 mg
Hydrocortisone 20 mg
Methylprednisolone 4 mg

■ How much steroid is needed?

Early regimens used high dose replacement therapy. Small studies have subsequently suggested that such regimens may actually impair wound healing, delay recovery and result in postoperative morbidity. The current guidelines recommend the use of much smaller doses.

Dose	Type of surgery	Recommended dose
Patients currently taking steroids		
<10 mg	Minor/moderate/major	Additional cover not required
>10 mg	Minor	25 mg hydrocortisone at induction, resume normal meds postoperation
>10 mg	Moderate	Usual dose of steroid preoperatively, 25 mg iv of hydrocortisone on induction, followed by 25 mg iv/8 hourly for 24 hours, then recommence preoperative dosage
>10 mg	Major	Usual dose of steroid preoperatively, then 50 mg of iv hydrocortisone at induction, followed by 50 mg iv/8 hourly for 48–72 hours, then recommence preoperative dosage
Patients who have *stopped* taking steroids		
>10 mg within three months of surgery	Treat as above	
> three months	No additional cover required	

■ Complications associated with steroid therapy in the perioperative period

1. Impaired wound healing
2. Increased risk of nosocomial infections
3. Addisonian crisis with cardiovascular collapse if under treated
4. Impaired glucose tolerance (monitor postoperative blood glucose)
5. Increased risk of peptic ulceration (consider use of PPI)
6. Mineralocorticoid effects, i.e. sodium and water retention, potassium loss and metabolic alkalosis (monitor fluid and electrolyte balance postoperatively).

Special situations in surgery: surgical considerations in the pregnant woman

SANJAY PURKAYASTHA

Pregnancy is responsible for many changes in women. With regards to surgery and surgical diagnoses these can be divided up into the following categories:

Anatomy
Physiology
Pharmacokinetics
Anaesthesia
Imaging
Social considerations

■ Anatomy

The gravid uterus is responsible for a shift in organs that are mobile and are usually sitting in the pelvis, e.g. small bowel, sigmoid colon, caecum and appendix. This leads to a different pattern of pain or symptomatology from pathology arising in such organs. A common example is the presentation of appendicitis which may present with diffuse right-sided pain or even right upper quadrant pain late in pregnancy. Tenderness/guarding is not usually over McBurney's point once the uterus is large enough for it not to be in the pelvis.

The gravid uterus later in pregnancy may compress the IVC, or even the aorta, when the patient is supine, and thereby reduce venous return and uterine blood flow, respectively. This can be avoided by positioning patients at an angle on the examination couch/operating table (e.g. with the use of a foam wedge).

Hospital Surgery: Foundations in Surgical Practice, ed. Omer Aziz, Sanjay Purkayastha and Paraskevas Paraskeva. Published by Cambridge University Press. © Cambridge University Press 2009.

■ Physiology

CARDIOVASCULAR

Increased: cardiac output, HR, stroke volume, blood volume, coagulable state

Decreased: colloid oncotic pressure (i.e. increased risk of pulmonary oedema), SBP and DBP, systemic vascular resistance.

RESPIRATORY

Respiratory alkalosis early in pregnancy with a compensated metabolic acidosis leads to less buffering capacity

Increased: oxygen consumption, minute ventilation, tidal volume

A large gravid uterus will also splint the diaphragm and lead to further potential respiratory compromise.

GASTROINTESTINAL

Increased: GORD; gastroparesis, cholestasis, cholelithiasis, haemorrhoids

Decreased: bowel motility.

RENAL

Increased: renal blood flow and GFR; risk of UTIs

Decreased: urea and creatinine levels.

HAEMATOLOGY

Always consult local reference values, however in general:

Increased: WCC, ALP, hypercoagulability

Decreased: Hb, Na, K, Ca, creatinine, urea, albumin, bilirubin

Unchanged: platelets, glucose, magnesium.

■ Pharmacokinetics

Many drugs may harm the fetus (especially in the first trimester) and the national formulary/pharmacist should be consulted if there is any doubt regarding the safe prescription of any medications during pregnancy.

■ Anaesthesia

For general anaesthesia: use aspiration prophylaxis and rapid sequence induction with cricoid pressure and intubation for women at >18–20 weeks gestation or any pregnant woman with symptomatic reflux.

Left uterine displacement is indicated for any pregnant woman >20 weeks gestation undergoing anaesthesia.

Continuous fetal heart-rate monitoring is recommended intraoperatively.

Measures to prevent perioperative thromboembolic events should be taken.

Consult the anaesthetic team early on and discuss the patient and case to allow potential problems to be identified early.

■ Imaging

Avoid X-rays where possible. Shielding of the fetus if necessary.

The use of ultrasound and MRI should be encouraged as alternatives if imaging is essential.

■ Social considerations

It is important to consider making arrangements for the other children of mothers if involved, and being able to be flexible with management if necessary, e.g. allowing patients to go home and come back in the morning if presenting at night (as long as it is clinically safe to do so). Be understanding about child-care issues and the psychological aspects of a difficult situation in pregnancy.

■ Non-obstetric surgery during pregnancy

Less than 1% of pregnant women require non-obstetric surgery during pregnancy, most commonly: appendicectomy, cholecystectomy and removal of an adnexal mass.

Laparoscopy is becoming a more popular method of surgery.

Timing and location of surgery is related to morbidity and preterm labour. First trimester surgery and surgery near the uterus are more commonly associated with such problems.

A delay in a diagnosis of peritonitis greatly worsens outcomes for the fetus.

■ Laparoscopy during pregnancy

Has the advantages of reduced pain, and hospital stay and immobility, therefore less analgesia, hospital stay-associated complications and thromboembolic events. However the major concern to the fetus is the pneumoperitoneum, therefore a limited pneumoperitoneum (maximum of 15 mmHg) should be used along with left-sided displacement of the uterus from the midline.

Ideally try to avoid elective surgery during pregnancy. Always think of the possibility of the patient being pregnant prior to surgery and perform a pregnancy test. If necessary then try to delay surgery till the second trimester (third trimester has an increased risk of preterm labour). Minimize fetal drug exposure and try to utilize local or regional anaesthesia if possible.

■ Trauma/emergency surgery

Always communicate early with the obstetric and neonatal teams to work together. Remember that you are essentially managing two patients in one: the mother and fetus, and BOTH need to be monitored if possible. Always assume female patients in emergency situations are pregnant until proven otherwise (by pregnancy tests). Follow ATLS guidelines for the management of a trauma patient.

■ Consent for surgery

Should be carried out by a senior, ideally the person who will be carrying out the procedure. The risks of the loss of the fetus and preterm labour should be discussed and the anaesthetic risk should be discussed by the anaesthetist. The risks of not operating and leaving the potential for peritonitis should also be discussed so that the patient is fully informed and understands the importance of performing non-obstetric surgery if necessary.

Haematological considerations: thrombosis in surgery

SANJAY PURKAYASTHA AND ABDUL SHLEBAK

■ Definitions

- **Thrombus:** an aggregation of platelets and fibrin with entrapped cells, mainly erythrocytes, in a blood vessel or a cardiac cavity.
- **Thrombosis:** the development of thrombi. This may be in the arterial or venous system.
- **Embolus:** a detached intravascular solid, liquid or gaseous mass that is carried by the blood to a site distant from its point of origin, thus obstructing the flow of blood. Most (99 %) arise from thrombi and are known as thromboemboli.
- **Ischaemia:** a period of insufficient blood flow (and therefore oxygen supply) to an organ or organ system.
- **Deep vein thrombosis (DVT):** thrombus formation in the deep veins, usually the deep pelvic system and/or the deep veins of the legs.

■ Aetiology

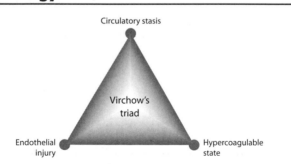

Figure 2 Virchow's triad

Hospital Surgery: Foundations in Surgical Practice, ed. Omer Aziz, Sanjay Purkayastha and Paraskevas Paraskeva. Published by Cambridge University Press. © Cambridge University Press 2009.

All three factors are increased during ill health and surgery, therefore patients are more predisposed to thrombosis.

There are patient factors, e.g. immobility, smoking, OCP (oral contraceptive pill)/HRT, hypercoagulable states (e.g. antithrombin, protein C and S deficiencies, APC resistance and factor V Leiden), malignancy, obesity and pregnancy.

There are disease factors, e.g. haematological conditions with a predisposition to clotting, acute illness causing hypercoagulability such as severe sepsis.

There are surgical factors, such as the length of surgery, the position of the patient and the type of surgery, e.g. increased thrombosis in orthopaedic surgery.

■ Where does thrombosis commonly occur?

The deep veins of the leg and pelvis commonly. For the majority of patients, initial thrombus formation occurs during surgery, but is only clinically apparent postoperatively.

Thrombosis can also occur in other sites, e.g. within cardiac chambers: commonly this is in the atria in patients with atrial fibrillation, where a large, dilated chamber that is not contracting synchronously with the rest of the cardiac structures results in increased turbulent flow. Prosthetic conduits such as aortic grafts and extra-anatomical bypasses in vascular patients are also at risk of thrombotic complications.

■ Common complications of thrombus formation

Occlusion of the vessel, conduit, or chamber.

Distal embolization in the lung (pulmonary), brain (resulting in transient ischaemic attacks or strokes, limbs (causing limb or digital/pedal ischaemia) are all relatively common clinical occurrences.

■ Common presentations

1. DVT: unilateral sudden onset limb swelling (usually the leg) and pain in a patient with risk factors for thrombosis.
2. Pulmonary embolus (PE): shortness of breath, haemoptysis, pleuritic chest pain, collapse.
3. Arterial thrombus: presentation depends on which vessel or conduit is occluded by thrombus or emboli, but classically, limb or digital ischaemia, with pain, pallor, pulselessness, cold limb, parasthaesia and paralysis.

■ Treatment

This can be broadly divided into prevention and therapy.

Perioperative prevention involves reducing the risks of the amenable factors, e.g. cessation of smoking and the OCP, weight reduction, early mobilization etc.

But also more active medical/surgical management, e.g. the use of thromboembolic deterrent stockings (TEDS), pneumatic compression devices during surgery, minimizing the length and trauma of surgery, and the use of heparin and low molecular weight heparin.

■ Heparin

A large polysaccharide molecule (mean molecular weight 15 000 Daltons), originally derived from bovine lung or porcine intestine, which acts as an anticoagulant by activating antithrombin. It therefore acts on the extrinsic coagulation pathway and can be monitored by measuring the activated partial thromboplastin time (APTT, or its ratio compared to normal, APTR). This used to be given as an intravenous infusion as thromboprophylaxis to all patients at risk; however, due to its complications of bleeding and adverse reactions such as heparin-induced thrombosis, and because of the need to closely monitor the function of the extrinsic system, low molecular weight heparins (LMWHs) have become used more widely for prophylaxis of DVT periopera-tively. These consist of only short chains of polysaccharide. LMWHs are defined as heparin salts having an average molecular weight of less than 8000 Da. All of the anticoagulant, pharmacokinetic, and other biologi-cal differences between unfractionated heparin (UFH) and LMWH can be explained by the relatively lower binding properties of LMWH. Com-pared with UFH, LMWHs have reduced ability to inactivate thrombin because the smaller fragments cannot bind simultaneously to AT and thrombin. In contrast, because bridging between AT and factor Xa is less critical for anti-factor Xa activity, the smaller fragments inactivate factor Xa almost as well as do larger molecules.

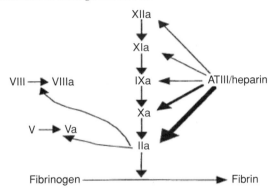

Figure 3 Mechanism of action of heparin

MONITORING IF INTRAVENOUS HEPARIN IS USED E.G. PREOPERATIVELY FOR A PATIENT WITH A PROSTHETIC HEART VALVE, RECURRENT PEs OR STROKES

Prophylactic dosing with intravenous heparin is usually guided by local protocols which should be sought out by the prescribing practitioner; however, usually an intravenous dose as a bolus and then an infu-sion (diluted up in either 5% dextrose or 0.9% sodium chloride) over

24 hours. FBC, APTT (or APTR) must be monitored regularly, and the rate of the infusion changed accordingly in order to keep the APTR at the desired range. Preoperatively the infusion is generally stopped 2–4 hours prior to surgery. If there is a doubt about the effect of heparin an APTR should be checked. Generally, if the APTR is <1.5 most surgery can go ahead. The complications of heparin include bleeding, heparin-induced thrombocytopaenia and occasionally hyperkalaemia.

If any of these complications or an adverse reaction is suspected, the infusion should be stopped and haematological advice sought (heparin overdose can be treated using protamine sulphate).

■ Prevention of thrombosis in surgery

Preoperative	Stop smoking Weight reduction Stop OCP/HRT TEDS Heparin/LMWH Use of IVC filter in severe/recurrent cases
Perioperative	Pneumatic compression boots/devices Reduce operative time and trauma Patient positioning Heparin/LMWH TEDS
Postoperative	Early mobilization TEDS Heparin/LMWH

Complex or recurrent cases should be discussed with the haematology team and the patient should be optimized for surgery prior to the procedure using a multidisciplinary approach, and the individual must be warned and counselled about the perioperative risks of thrombotic complications.

■ Warfarin

Warfarin acts by inhibiting vitamin K-dependent coagulation factors. Chemically, it is 3 H (α-acetonylbenzyl)-4-hydroxycoumarin, and therefore affects the intrinsic system.

Some patients are in need of long-term anticoagulation (e.g. those with atrial fibrillation, extra-anatomical vascular conduits, patients with prosthetic heart valves, occasionally CABG patients etc.). These patients need to stop their warfarin at least 48 hours prior to surgery and have their anticoagulation monitored haematologically with serial INR measurements (surgery can take place once this is <1.5).

However, if there is a severely increased risk of thrombotic complications subsequent to the cessation of warfarin, e.g. recurrent PEs, prosthetic mitral valve etc. then these patients must be admitted when their warfarin is stopped and started on intravenous heparin (see above). If in doubt the haematology team and/or the specialty team in question should be consulted. Postoperatively these patients should have their anticoagulation started back on their previous dose and be discharged once the INR is therapeutic again.

Warfarin dosing must be carefully prescribed. For patients that have never been on warfarin previously one daily dose of 5 mg, followed by 5 mg and then 10 mg is usually well tolerated. The INR is usually checked on day two and then 48 hours later.

The patient is discharged to the care of the anticoagulation clinic when the INR has stabilized in the desired range. Care should be taken with such a standard regime for patients taking medication such as NSAIDs, antiepileptics and antibiotics (for a comprehensive list please see the Appendix in the British National Formulary for interactions, section on coumarins).

Summary of INR ranges for different conditions

Condition	INR range
Above-knee DVT	2–3
Pulmonary embolus	2–3
Recurrent DVT PE	2.5–3.5
Prosthetic aortic valve	2–3
Prosthetic mitral valve	2.5–3.5
Tissue valves	2–3
Atrial fibrillation	2–3

Warfarin overdose should be treated by stopping the warfarin, and if the patient is actively bleeding, considering volume replacement, fresh frozen plasma and vitamin K replacement (see section on bleeding).

■ Perioperative management of thrombotic events

These may be either, commonly, venous or, less commonly, arterial. DVT and PE are treated by confirming the diagnosis and concurrently using short-term anticoagulation (with treatment dose LMWH and concurrently starting the patient on warfarin). This subcutaneous treatment of LMWH can be stopped once the INR is therapeutic (usually 2–3). For above-knee DVTs and PEs this treatment is continued for 3–6 months with regular anticoagulation clinic follow-up. The cause for the event must be investigated simultaneously.

Arterial thrombosis, although less common following most surgery, is more evident following vascular surgery. If this is clinically suspected the patient should be anticoagulated with intravenous UF heparin while the diagnosis is confirmed using imaging techniques such as contrast angiography. If an occlusive thrombus is confirmed then this can be treated with thrombolysis, angioplasty +/− stenting or surgical approaches such as endarterectomy or vascular bypass.

■ Antiplatelets and thrombosis in surgery

Antiplatelets such as aspirin and now more commonly clopidogrel are used to prevent arterial thrombotic events in coronary, cerebral and peripheral arteries in patients at risk of occlusive arterial disease and in patients with vascular bypass grafts and prosthetic extra-anatomical grafts. Such antiplatelets, especially used simultaneously, can cause excessive bleeding perioperatively. The risk/benefit ratio of such therapies must be considered preoperatively with discussion between the specialist teams concerned and if concerns are raised, platelet function tests can be carried out and perioperative platelet transfusions may be administered if appropriate.

Haematological considerations: bleeding

SANJAY PURKAYASTHA AND ABDUL SHLEBAK

■ Clinical features of bleeding disorders

In general terms bleeding may be caused by a platelet disorder or a clotting disorder. In some instances both elements are implicated (DIC and liver disease). It is very useful to dissect this based on history and clinical picture. The following features may help you to decide:

	Platelet disorders	Coagulation factor disorders
Site of bleeding	Skin and mucous membranes	Deep in soft tissues
Petechiae	Yes	No
Ecchymoses	('Bruises') small, superficial	Large, deep
Haemarthrosis/muscle bleeding	Rare	Common
Bleeding after cuts and scratches	Yes	No
Bleeding after surgery or trauma	Immediate, usually mild	Delayed (1–2 days) often severe

■ Platelet disorders

Classification: bleeding secondary to altered platelet quantity or quality

1. Quantitative disorders
    Increased destruction
    Dilutional effect (following massive transfusion)
    Decreased production (bone marrow failure and marrow infiltration)
    Abnormal distribution (in splenomegaly).

Hospital Surgery: Foundations in Surgical Practice, ed. Omer Aziz, Sanjay Purkayastha and Paraskevas Paraskeva. Published by Cambridge University Press. © Cambridge University Press 2009.

2. Qualitative disorders (commoner)

   Acquired disorders

   Drug induced (aspirin, ticlopidine, clopidogrel, GPIIb/IIIa inhibitors)

   End stage renal failure

   Cardiopulmonary bypass

   Paraproteinaemic conditions (plasma cell dyscrasias and amyloidosis)

   Myeloproliferative disorders

   Myelodysplastic disease

   Inherited disorders (rare).

These conditions require specialist investigations and work-up should be done in collaboration with a haematologist.

QUANTITATIVE DISORDERS, CAUSES OF THROMBOCYTOPAENIA

- Immune-mediated
- Idiopathic (Idiopathic thrombocytopaenic pupura, ITP), one of the commonest haematological conditions
- Drug-induced (heparin-induced thrombocytopaenia is the commonest; this is associated with paradoxical increased risk of thrombosis rather than bleeding)
- Collagen vascular disease (e.g. SLE)
- Lymphoproliferative disease including chronic lymphocytic leukaemia and lymphoma
- Sarcoidosis
- Non-immune mediated (consumptive)
- Disseminated intravascular coagulation (DIC, associated with coagulopathy)
- Microangiopathic haemolytic anaemia (MAHA) clotting studies are usually normal or mildly deranged. Examination of blood film shows abundant red cell fragmentation.

What are the differentiating features of acute vs. chronic ITP?		
Features	Acute ITP	Chronic ITP
Age	Children (2–6 yrs)	(Adults 20–40 yrs)
Female:male	1:1	3:1
Prodromal illness	Common	Rare
Onset of symptoms	Abrupt	Abrupt-indolent
Platelet count at presentation	<20 000	<50 000
Duration	2–6 weeks	Long term
Spontaneous remission	Common	Uncommon

TREATMENT OF ITP

The need for therapy is based on bleeding symptoms and platelet count. In general, patients with mucous membrane (mouth, nose, uterine) bleeding, 'wet purpura', may require therapy whereas lack of mucous membrane bleeding, 'dry purpura', may not require intervention. This table is a guide for the indication and the choice of therapeutic modalities in ITP patients.

Platelet count ($\times 10^{a}$)	Symptoms	Treatment
>50	None	None
20–50	No bleeding*	None
20–50	Bleeding**	Oral steroids (e.g. prednisolone 1 mg/kg)
		+/− iv immunoglobulin (1 mg/kg)
<20	No bleeding**	Oral steroids
<20	Bleeding**	Oral steroids +/− platelets

*inform a senior colleague ** inform senior; request haematology consultation
ITP not responsive to medical therapy may need a splenectomy

■ Acquired coagulation disorders

Acquired clotting factor disorders are commoner than inherited conditions. Laboratory investigation may help to diagnose and guide clinicians to the appropriate intervention. The following conditions are common examples:

VITAMIN K DEFICIENCY

Vitamin K is a fat-soluble vitamin. It plays an essential role in biologically activating factors II, VII, IX and X in the liver.

Source of vitamin K: green vegetables, synthesized by intestinal flora
Required for synthesis: factors II, VII, IX, X; protein C and S
Causes of deficiency: malnutrition, biliary obstruction, malabsorption, antibiotic therapy
Treatment: vitamin K +/− fresh frozen plasma.

DISSEMINATED INTRAVASCULAR COAGULATION

This represents a medical emergency; diagnosis and immediate management is paramount in order to save patient lives. It is associated with activation of both coagulation and fibrinolytic pathways. Laboratory indices include:

- Thrombocytopaenia
- Deranged clotting with prolonged PT
- APTT
- Elevated d-dimers
- Hypofibrinogenaemia.

The following are common clinical conditions associated with DIC: sepsis, trauma (head injury, fat embolism and multiple trauma especially), malignancy, obstetric complications, amniotic fluid embolism, abruptio placentae, vascular disorders, toxin (e.g. snake venom, drugs), immunological conditions, severe allergic reaction, transplant rejection, massive transfusion, acute promyelocytic leukaemia (FAB: M3).

Principles of management of DIC: NB this is an epiphenomenon and not a disease so:

1. Treatment of underlying disorder is the most important aspect
2. Supportive therapy:

   Platelet transfusion to correct the thrombocytopaenia
   Fresh frozen plasma and cryoprecipitate to rectify the coagulopathy
   Packed red cell transfusion to improve blood O_2 carrying capacity.

   Other therapy may be helpful but controversial:

   Activated protein C concentrate
   Coagulation inhibitor concentrates (ATIII)
   Anticoagulation with low dose heparin is controversial.

LIVER DISEASE

Several mechanisms may result in failure of haemostasis in liver disease, including:

1. Decreased synthesis of II, VII, IX, X, XI and fibrinogen
2. Patients with liver disease are prone to DIC
3. Thrombocytopaenia due to hypersplenism
4. Dietary vitamin K deficiency (inadequate intake or malabsorption)
5. Dysfibrinogenaemia
6. Enhanced fibrinolysis (decreased alpha-2-antiplasmin).

Management of haemostatic defects in liver disease

Treatment for prolonged PT/PTT
Vitamin K 10 mg once daily for 3 days – usually ineffective
Fresh-frozen plasma infusion (12–15 ml/kg, immediate but temporary effect).

Treatment for low fibrinogen
Cryoprecipitate (10 units per average adult will raise fibrinogen by 1 g/l).

Treatment for DIC (elevated d-dimer, low fibrinogen, thrombocytopaenia)
Replacement therapy with FFP, cryoprecipitate and platelets.

■ Inherited bleeding disorders

1. Haemophilia A and B
2. Von Willebrand disease
3. Other factor deficiencies

HAEMOPHILIA A AND B (CHRISTMAS DISEASE)

An x-linked recessive disease associated with a bleeding tendency. The degree of bleeding is related to the severity of the factor deficiency. This table lists the differences between haemophilia A and B.

	Haemophilia A	Haemophilia B
Coagulation factor deficient	VIII	IX
Incidence in males	1 in 10 000	1 in 50 000
Severity	Related to factor level < 1 % – severe – Spontaneous bleeding 1–5 % – moderate – Bleeding with mild injury 5–25 % – mild – Bleeding with surgery or trauma	Related to factor level
Complications	Soft tissue bleeding	Soft tissue bleeding

Haemophilia A and B are clinically indistinguishable

Symptoms: Haemarthrosis (most common). Fixed joints due to recurrent bleeding in a target joint. Soft tissue haematomas (e.g. muscle). Muscle atrophy. Shortened tendons.

Other sites of bleeding: urinary tract, CNS, neck (may be life-threatening). Prolonged bleeding after surgery or dental extractions. Skeletal deformity. School absenteeism. Viral illnesses associated with plasma factor replacement.

Treatment of haemophilia A

Depending on the severity of the condition and the site of bleeding. The choice of the type of factor also depends on age, previous exposure to

therapy and virological serology. Most children will be enrolled on a prophylaxis programme early in life to prevent bleeding complications.

Factor VIII (FVIII) concentrate

Recombinant factor VIII: Virus free/no apparent risk; no functional
von Willebrand factor; for children and newly diagnosed patients;
expensive

High purity (monoclonal) FVIII: virucidally treated; no functional von
Willebrand factor (VWF)

Intermediate purity FVIII: virucidally treated; may contain von Willebrand factor.

Dosing guidelines for haemophilia A

Mild bleeding
Target: 30 % dosing 2–3 daily for 1–2 days (15 U/kg)
Haemarthrosis, oropharyngeal or dental, epistaxis, haematuria.

Major bleeding
Target: 80–100 % 2–3 daily for 7–14 days (50 U/kg)
CNS trauma, haemorrhage, lumbar puncture
Neurosurgery and ophthalmic surgery
Retroperitoneal haemorrhage.

GI bleeding
Adjunctive therapy: tranexamic acid
DDAVP (for mild disease only)
Results in increase of FVIII by 2–5 fold
Tachyphylaxis may occur
Tranexamic acid should be used as it will inhibit fibrinolysis
First choice for minor procedures in mild cases of haemophilia.

Treatment of haemophilia B

Factor IX concentrate: recombinant human factor IX and high purity
factor IX
Initial dose: 100 U/kg. Subsequently 50 U/kg every 24 hours.

VON WILLEBRAND DISEASE

Probably the commonest inherited bleeding tendency affecting around 0.8 % of the population.

Clinical features

von Willebrand factor is an important clotting factor for primary platelet plug formation; it is synthesized in endothelium and megakaryocytes. It forms large multimers; functions include:

Carrier of factor VIII (prevents proteolysis of FVIII in the circulation)
Anchors platelets to damaged subendothelium
Inheritance – autosomal dominant
Incidence – 1/10 000
Clinical features – mucocutaneous bleeding including easy skin bruising, epistaxis, menorrhagia, post-dental extraction prolonged bleeding and post-surgical and post-trauma bleeding.

Classification

Type 1   Partial quantitative deficiency
Type 2   Qualitative deficiency
Type 3   Total quantitative deficiency.

Treatment of von Willebrand disease

DDAVP (deamino-8-arginine vasopressin)
Increases plasma VWF levels (2–5 fold) by stimulating secretion from endothelium
Duration of response is variable
Not generally used in Type 2 disease especially 2B, which is associated with thrombocytopaenia, as DDAVP may worsen the thrombocytopaenia
Dosage 0.3 μg/kg every 12 hours iv.

Factor VIII concentrate (intermediate purity): Haemate P is commonly used in UK
Virally inactivated product.

Cryoprecipitate
Source of fibrinogen, factor VIII and VWF
Not virally inactivated product
Only plasma fraction that consistently contains VWF multimers.

Haematological considerations: haemorrhage (massive-bleeding protocol)

SANJAY PURKAYASTHA, ABDUL SHLEBAK AND JAMES UPRICHARD

■ Definition

Loss of one blood volume (5 L in an adult) within a 24 hr period, or 50 % blood volume within 3 hours or a rate of loss of 150 ml per minute.

Most frequent cause of death is inadequate replacement of circulating volume and red cells.

■ Principles of management

Most blood banks have a clear-cut policy about managing transfusion in massive-bleeding patients.

TREAT SHOCK (SEE CHAPTER ON SHOCK)

Insert large bore peripheral cannulae.

Give crystalloid or colloid to achieve an acceptable systolic blood pressure and prevent tissue hypoxia.

Send blood samples for crossmatch, FBC, coagulation screen and renal function.

When blood is required immediately it may be necessary to issue Group O, Rh D negative un-crossmatched red cells if the patient's blood group is unknown.

ABO group-specific red cells should be given at the earliest possible opportunity. (ABO and Rh D grouping can be performed within five minutes.)

Intraoperative blood salvage may be of great value in reducing requirements for allogeneic blood.

Hospital Surgery: Foundations in Surgical Practice, ed. Omer Aziz, Sanjay Purkayastha and Paraskevas Paraskeva. Published by Cambridge University Press. © Cambridge University Press 2009.

MAINTAIN HAEMOSTASIS

Packed red cells do not contain coagulation factors or platelets, but the platelet count rarely falls below 50×10^9/l unless 1.5 blood volumes have been transfused.

Use platelet concentrates to maintain platelet count $> 50 \times 10^9$/l.
Use FFP to maintain PT ratio < 1.5 times the control value.
Use cryoprecipitate to maintain fibrinogen concentration at > 1.0 g/dl.

HOMEOSTASIS

Coagulation factors work best at physiological pH and temperature.

Beware of metabolic disturbances such as hypocalcaemia, hyper-kalaemia and acidosis.

When a fast rate of transfusion is required (>50 ml/kg per hour), a blood warmer should be used.

Samples to test FBC and coagulation must be monitored frequently; these may need interpretation by a haematologist.

Supplementary point of care testing may assist in managing massive haemorrhage. Haemostatic competence can be assessed by thromboelastography and platelet function using platelet function analyser with platelet mapping by defining residual platelet function.

Haematological considerations: blood products and transfusion

SANJAY PURKAYASTHA AND ABDUL SHLEBAK

■ Blood products

PACKED RED CELLS

One unit contains 250–350 ml unless there is cardiorespiratory compromise; most patients can tolerate a haemoglobin concentration of 8 g/dl comfortably and do not need transfusion.

PLATELET CONCENTRATE

One pool of platelets contains 250–300 ml. A normal adult pool would be expected to raise the platelet count by $20–40 \times 10^9$/l.

The cause of thrombocytopaenia should be established before platelets are given. For example platelets are absolutely contraindicated in thrombotic thrombocytopaenic purpura (TTP) unless the patient is bleeding or undergoing invasive procedures prior to plasmapheresis.

Many patients remain haemostatically competent with a platelet count as low as 10×10^9/l before suffering haemorrhagic complications. However, for most surgery the platelet count should be above 50×10^9/l. In high risk surgery (e.g. brain or eye), aim for above 100×10^9/l, whereas for epidural analgesia aim for 80×10^9/l.

FFP (FRESH FROZEN PLASMA)

One bag contains 250–300 ml. The usual dose is 12–15 ml/kg.

Indications:

Replace multiple coagulation factor deficiencies (e.g. liver disease, DIC). To correct coagulopathy associated with massive blood transfusion.

Hospital Surgery: Foundations in Surgical Practice, ed. Omer Aziz, Sanjay Purkayastha and Paraskevas Paraskeva. Published by Cambridge University Press. © Cambridge University Press 2009.

Urgent reversal of warfarin overdose-induced bleeding in association with vitamin K, but only in the absence of prothrombin complex concentrate (PCC).

Replacement of single factor deficiencies (e.g. Factor V) in situations when factor concentrate is unavailable.

CRYOPRECIPITATE

This is now pooled from five donations. One bag contains 100–200 ml. This contains FVIII, von Willebrand factor and fibrinogen. The usual dose is two pooled bags. It is used in hypofibrinogenaemia (fibrinogen <1 g/l) associated with massive blood transfusion, DIC and in unexplained bleeding in end-stage renal disease.

PCC (PROTHROMBIN COMPLEX CONCENTRATE)

Contains factors II, IX, X +/− VII. Principally, used for reversal of life-threatening warfarin overdose-induced haemorrhage.

rVIIa (RECOMBINANT FACTOR VIIa OR 'NOVOSEVEN')

Currently used as a 'last-ditch' treatment in situations of uncontrolled haemorrhage. It is also used in patients with FVIII inhibitors and in CNS bleeding with or without warfarin. Use must be discussed with a haematologist.

■ Pharmacological agents to reduce blood loss

APROTININ

Anti-fibrinolytic agent. Often used in cardiac surgery pre-sternotomy (e.g. dose 50 000 units) and then given as bolus injections intraoperatively (e.g. 500 000 units hourly). Its use is associated with reduced bleeding and reduced need for allogeneic red cell transfusion.

TRANEXAMIC ACID

Anti-fibrinolytic agent. Particularly useful in mucosal bleeding such as dental extraction, primary menorrhagia, bleeding associated with thrombocytopaenia and in blood loss associated with cardiopulmonary bypass surgery. It is also used in adjunct with DDAVP in bleeding-tendency patients (mild haemophilia and von Willebrand disease). Usual dose 15–25 mg/kg tds orally.

PROTAMINE SULPHATE

Used to reverse overdosage of heparin. (It is of limited benefit in the presence of low molecular weight heparins.) 1 mg neutralizes 80–100 units of heparin.

■ How to avoid errors with transfusions

Most deaths from blood transfusion are due to errors either in the collection or labelling of the sample for blood grouping, or in the laboratory or at the bedside prior to the administration of transfusion due to failure in checking patient identity.

In order to minimize these errors, it is imperative that the request form contains all relevant information on the patient's identification, location for transfusion, number and type of blood components, past obstetric and transfusion history, patient's diagnosis and the reason for the request. The sample tube must be labelled and signed immediately with full patient identification details. Pre-labelling is prohibited. The prescription of the blood components should specify the component type, including any special requirement (e.g. gamma-irradiated), the quantity given and the duration of transfusion.

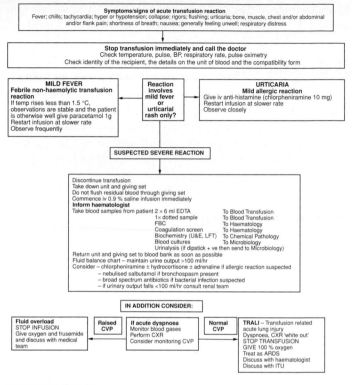

Management algorithm

■ Monitoring blood transfusion

Transfusion should occur in areas where patients can be readily observed by clinical staff.

Patients should be asked to report adverse effects immediately (such as shivering, rash, flushing, loin pain and shortness of breath). Vital signs (temperature, pulse and blood pressure) should be monitored before and after the start of each blood component. They should also be monitored after 15 minutes and then one hourly with each unit.

■ Infections acquired from transfusions

Which agents transmit?

Viruses: HBV, HCV, HIV, HTLV, CMV, EBV, *Parvovirus*
Parasites: *Plasmodium* (malaria), *Trypanosoma cruzi* (sleeping sickness)
Bacteria: *Treponema pallidum* (syphilis), others causing septicaemia
Others: e.g. prions.

   It is mandatory to test all donations for: HBV, HCV, HIV, HTLV and syphilis. In some donations testing for CMV, *Plasmodium*, *T. cruzi*, West Nile Virus is also performed. There is no readily available test for prions at present.

■ Suspected acute transfusion reaction

If a transfusion reaction is suspected follow the flow chart for further assessment and management.

Shock

RACHEL MASSEY AND PARASKEVAS PARASKEVA

■ Definition

The clinical condition resulting from insufficient blood flow to the tissues to meet demand.

■ Classification

1. Hypovolaemic
2. Cardiogenic
3. Obstructive:
   - Tamponade
   - Tension pneumothorax
   - Pulmonary embolism.
4. Distributive:
   - Septic
   - Anaphylaxis
   - Neurogenic.

■ Hypovolaemic shock

Secondary to a reduced intravascular volume.

Common causes:

Blood loss: haemorrhage, trauma, aneurysm

Third space fluid sequestration: burns, pancreatitis, peritonitis, bowel obstruction

GI losses: vomiting, diarrhoea, enterocutaneous fistulae

Hospital Surgery: Foundations in Surgical Practice, ed. Omer Aziz, Sanjay Purkayastha and Paraskevas Paraskeva. Published by Cambridge University Press. © Cambridge University Press 2009.

Renal losses: diabetic ketoacidosis, diabetes insipidus
Skin losses: sweating, burns.

Symptoms and signs				
Blood loss	0–15 %	15–30 %	30–40 %	>40 %
SBP (mmHg)	>110	>100	< 90	<90
Respiratory rate	16	16–20	21–26	>26
Capillary refill time	N	↑	↑	↑
Urine output	N	N	↓	↓
Mental state	Anxious	Agitated	Confused	Lethargic

■ Cardiogenic shock

Cardiac pump failure.

Diagnosed as the persistence of shock after correction of non-cardiac factors:

- Hypovolaemia
- Hypoxia
- Acidosis
- Arrhythmias.

Commonest cause is myocardial infarction. Other causes include:

- Cardiomyopathy
- Myocardial contusions following trauma
- Infections – myocarditis.

■ Obstructive causes of shock

Characterized by the triad of:

Low cardiac output
Tachycardia
Raised jugular venous pressure with peripheral vasoconstriction.

Causes:

- Cardiac tamponade (Figure 4)
- Tension pneumothorax
- Pulmonary embolus.

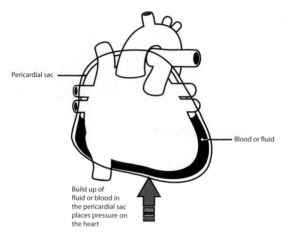

Figure 4 Cardiac tamponade

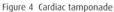
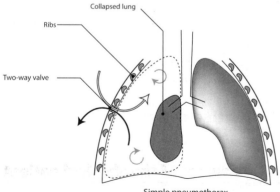

Simple pneumothorax

Figure 5 Massive pneumothorax

■ Distributive

Definition: occurs when peripheral vascular dilation leads to a fall in peripheral vascular resistance.

Causes:

Sepsis
Anaphylaxis
Neurogenic
Acute adrenal insufficiency.

■ Assessment of the shocked patient

When assessing a patient it is important to find both the underlying cause and to make an assessment of the degree of shock. Although shock and hypotension often coexist it is not necessary for the patient to be hypotensive to make a diagnosis of shock, and it is more important to assess the patient for evidence of hypoperfusion. Evidence of hypoperfusion can be obtained by examining:

- Temperature of the peripheries
- Capillary refill
- Conscious state
- Urine output – a healthy adult should have a urine output of at least 0.5 ml kg/hr.

Additional information may be obtained by performing an arterial blood gas and identifying acidosis (metabolic).

All patients should also have heart rate and blood pressure measured and ideally central venous pressure monitored formally via a central venous line.

■ Management of the shocked patient

Make an assessment of the patient looking at the parameters discussed above.

Airway: a patient's airway is likely to be patent in shock but may be compromised in anaphylactic shock or in a trauma setting in a patient with a tension pneumothorax and obstructive shock.

- All patients should be initially managed with high-flow oxygen (15 l/min) via a reservoir face mask.

Airway adjuncts such as Guedel airways and nasopharyngeal tubes may be used.

Breathing: marked tachypnoea is a very good indication that a patient is severely ill, but may not be the result of respiratory failure. Patients with a tension pneumothorax, tamponade or pulmonary embolus will obviously have respiratory failure, but a breathless patient with normal oxygenation indicates a non-respiratory cause such as acidosis or sepsis.

Circulation: assessment of circulatory status should include both blood pressure and perhaps more importantly tissue perfusion, which can be assessed by looking at capillary refill, altered conscious level, peripheral temperature, oliguria and metabolic acidosis as discussed above. Due to physiological compensation, hypotension is a late feature of cardiovascular dysfunction.

At this stage of the assessment all patients should have, if not already established:

- Intravenous access – via two large bore 12 or 14G cannulae in the antecubital fossae and blood sent for FBC, urea and electrolytes, clotting and, if indicated from the history, a group and save.
- Urinary catheterization.
- Arterial blood-gas sampling (Figure 6).

Depending on the assessment so far it may also be necessary to insert a central venous line at this stage. From the above assessment it should be possible to make a working diagnosis of the underlying cause of the shock. This may subsequently prove to be incorrect but this should not alter the immediate emergency management of the patient. The majority of patients who are clinically shocked will require aggressive fluid

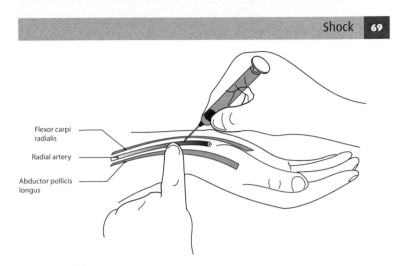

Figure 6 Arterial gas sampling

resuscitation. The actual fluid requirement may vary considerably, however, between types of shock and individual patients, but all patients should receive an initial fluid challenge, usually 250–500 ml of colloid as a stat dose over 30 minutes, during which time effect on the blood pressure or CVP, if any, should be noted.

■ In general, response to a fluid challenge in the different types of shock can be seen below

Hypovolaemic: dependent on volume lost but fluid challenge produces a transient increase in BP(CVP) which will only be sustained once the lost volume is replaced.

Cardiogenic: initial blood pressure (or CVP) may be normal, low or high. If the underlying cause is myocardial infarction, fluid challenge may be tolerated badly and lead to a sustained rise in pressure and pulmonary oedema.

Distributive: due to peripheral vascular dilation, BP (or CVP) may remain persistently low despite large volume resuscitation. In this setting very unwell patients may require vasopressor agents or inotropes such as noradrenaline to cause vasoconstriction and maintain blood pressure before hypovolaemia has been completely corrected.

Obstructive: initial BP (or CVP) especially in tamponade or tension pneumothorax may be high, and there may be little detectable response to fluid challenge. In both of these cases it is essential to treat the underlying cause with insertion of an intercostal drain or by performing pericardiocentesis.

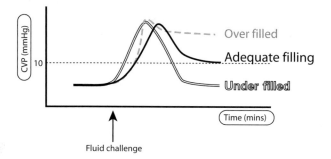

Figure 7 Graph demonstrating under filled, adequately filled and over filled CVP responses to a fluid challenge

Fluid management

ANDREW HARTLE AND MICHELE HENDRICKS

■ Introduction

It is essential to understand how fluids are distributed in the human body: see Figure 8.

Euvolaemia is important because:

It achieves an adequate cardiac output and circulating volume.
It ensures good organ perfusion.
It allows normal cell homeostasis to occur.

With hypovolaemia, the following are evident:

Hypotension
Vital organ hypoperfusion
Metabolic acidosis
Oliguria.

To avoid the above, fluids must be given early and the patient's response to fluids must be monitored.

■ Daily fluid requirements

Adults (of approximately 70 kg) require approximately 3000 ml of fluid/24 hr, which equates to 20–30 ml/kg/24 hr.

Children require fluid (per hour) according to their weight, based on the 4–2–1 rule:

A 25 kg child requires 4 ml/kg for the first 10 kg, 2 ml/kg for the second 10 kg and 1 ml/kg for the remaining weight, adding up to 65 ml/hr.

Hospital Surgery: Foundations in Surgical Practice, ed. Omer Aziz, Sanjay Purkayastha and Paraskevas Paraskeva. Published by Cambridge University Press. © Cambridge University Press 2009.

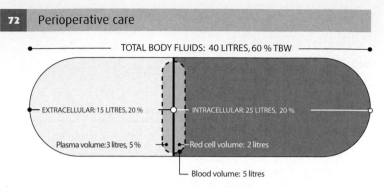

Figure 8 Diagram of fluid distribution in the normal human body

■ Fluid requirements in hypovolaemia

Depending on the cause, adults may require as much as 2000 ml of crystalloid (e.g. normal saline) or colloid (Gelofusine (succinylated gelatin), blood) for resuscitation. Colloids remain in the intravascular compartment longer, and may be preferred in trauma and haemorrhage. Children need 20 ml/kg crystalloid, or 10 ml/kg blood. Third space loss is the sequestration of fluid in a pathological compartment which is not in the ICF or ECF (e.g. in the GI tract during bowel obstruction) and leads to the patient becoming hypovolaemic.

■ Preoperative fluid management

ROUTINE SITUATION

Follow local nil-by-mouth protocols. Electrolyte abnormalities often include hypokalaemia and hyponatraemia.

Give maintenance fluid and electrolytes to:

- Patients receiving bowel preparation
- Patients who have GI upset (vomiting, diarrhoea, fistulae)
- Patients who have experienced prolonged fasting
- Diabetics (give dextrose, insulin and potassium)

- Children
- Those using diuretics.

EMERGENCY SITUATION

These patients have:

- Intravascular volume depletion
- Hypotension
- Tachycardia
- Oliguria.

Give them adequate fluid resuscitation, as well as maintenance fluids and electrolytes (0.9 % sodium chloride + 1 mmol/kg potassium chloride).

■ Postoperative fluid management

Sequestration of fluids perioperatively (i.e. third space losses) may lead to relative hypovolaemia. Replace losses early, e.g. colloid boluses of 500 ml as well as maintenance fluids. Essential monitoring includes temperature, heart rate, blood pressure, respiratory rate, and urine output. Remember to replace potassium, magnesium and phosphates. These can all be given via a central intravenous line.

Ideal monitoring includes central venous pressure measurement and hourly urine output. This allows better assessment of the patient's response to fluid management.

■ Special circumstances

1. **Cardiac and renal disease:** fluids are essential, but response must be monitored by CVP measurement. Check renal function 1–2 times daily.

2. **Burns:** these patients have spectacular fluid loss and sequestration. Fluid resuscitation must be aggressive. ATLS guidelines suggest 2–4 ml Ringer's Lactate/kg/% burn/24 hours (see chapter on burns). Aim for urine output of 30–50 ml/hr in adults, and 1 ml/kg/hr in children.

3. **Sepsis:** these patients are pyrexial, tachycardic, tachypnoeic and often have a focus of infection. They need aggressive fluid resuscitation in order to maintain a good cardiac output, and vital organ perfusion. Give colloid boluses (250–500 ml) as well as electrolytes such as potassium.

■ Daily fluid requirements

An average 70 kg adult also requires 3 l of water intake per day, and with this approximately 60–70 mmol of potassium and 140 mmol of sodium.

■ Types of fluids available on the ward, and their constituents

1. **Crystalloids**: substances which form true solutions and pass freely through semi-permeable membranes:
   - 1 l normal saline (0.9 % sodium chloride): 1 l water, 154 mmol Na, 154 mmol Cl = 0 J energy.
   - 1 l 5 % dextrose: 1 l water, 50 g dextrose = 837 kJ energy.
   - 1 l dextrose saline (0.18 % sodium chloride, 4 % dextrose): 1 l water, 30 mmol Na, 30 mmol Cl, 40 g dextrose = 668 kJ energy.
   - 1 l Hartmann's solution: 1 l water, 131 mmol Na, 111 mmol Cl, 5 mmol K, 29 mmol HCO_3, 2 mmol Ca = 0 J energy.
2. **Colloids:** substances which do not form true solutions and do not pass through semi-permeable membranes. There are many different types of colloid, and all stay in the intravascular compartment for varying lengths of time, depending on molecular size; e.g. Gelofusine, Haemaccel (polygeline), hetastarch, albumin, blood.

- 1 l Gelofusine: 154 mmol Na, 125 mmol Cl, 0.4 mmol K, 0.4 mmol Ca.
- 1 l Haemaccel: 145 mmol Na, 145 mmol Cl, 5.1 mmol K, 6.25 mmol Ca.

Typical prescription of the normal daily requirement of fluid (for a nil-by-mouth patient): 1 l 0.9 % sodium chloride + 20 mmol potassium chloride (KCl) over 8 hours; 1 l 5 % dextrose + 20 mmol KCl over 8 hours; 1 l 5 % dextrose + 20 mmol KCl over 8 hours. **Plus replacement of any additional losses e.g. if vomiting, diarrhoea, high stomal output etc.** The most important aspect of assessment for fluid therapy is clinical evaluation, e.g. looking for dry mucous membranes, tachycardia, low urine output, low CVP, hypotension etc.

Electrolyte management

ANDREW HARTLE AND MICHELE HENDRICKS

■ Why are electrolytes important?

- They maintain cell homeostasis and cell volume, see Figure 9.
- They cause gradients between the inside and the outside of the cell, allowing ions to move into or out of the cells.
- These movements cause physiological effects such as action-potential propagation, protein kinase phosphorylation and protein synthesis.
- These physiological effects give rise to physical changes such as muscle relaxation or contraction, inotropy and bradycardia.

Average adult daily requirements:

Sodium: 2 mmol/kg
Potassium: 1 mmol/kg
Calcium: 0.1–0.2 mmol/kg
Magnesium: 0.1–0.2 mmol/kg
Chloride: 1.5 mmol/kg
Phosphate: 0.2–0.5 mmol/kg.

■ Potassium (K): normal range 3.5–5.0 mmol/l

- Most abundant intracellular cation (+ve).
- Essential for maintenance of the cell membrane potential and for generation of action potentials.
- Depletion often seen pre- and postoperatively.

Hospital Surgery: Foundations in Surgical Practice, ed. Omer Aziz, Sanjay Purkayastha and Paraskevas Paraskeva. Published by Cambridge University Press. © Cambridge University Press 2009.

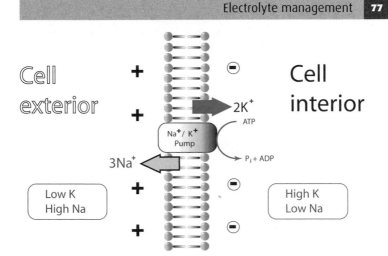

Figure 9 Schematic of Na-K cell-membrane ion-channel pump involved in regulation of cell homeostasis and volume

Hypokalaemia: seen with diuretic use, insulin and catecholamine use, excessive GI tract losses, alkalosis, hyperaldosteronism.

Effects: muscle weakness, arrhythmias (S-T depression, lengthens Q-T and P-R intervals, T wave inversion), metabolic alkalosis, impaired renal concentrating ability.

Treatment of hypokalaemia: oral supplements up to 200 mmol/day, or intravenous potassium chloride 40 mmol in 1 l, infused over a minimum of 1 hour. Monitor ECG if infusing potassium rapidly. Monitor electrolyte levels in perioperative situation, as derangements are very common, and need correcting.

Hyperkalaemia: seen with renal failure, adrenocortical insufficiency, drugs (ACE inhibitors, potassium-sparing diuretics), trauma, crush syndrome, acidosis, rapid blood transfusion.

Effects of hyperkalaemia: nausea, vomiting, muscle weakness, cardiac depression (peaked T waves, wide QRS), arrhythmias including VF and cardiac arrest.

Treatment of hyperkalaemia: Insulin (Actrapid) 15 units in 50 ml of 50 % dextrose (this drives K into the cell).

Calcium gluconate 10 % (10 ml) acts as an antagonist of K.

Polystyrene sulphonate resins 15 g, 8 hourly. Consider dialysis or haemofiltration.

■ Sodium (Na): normal range 135–145 mmol/l

- ■ Main ECF cation, accounts for a large percentage of the osmotic action of plasma, thus determines ECF (plasma) volume.
- ■ Plays central function in excitable cells.

Hyponatraemia: caused by water excess (increased intake (polydypsia), intravenous administration of sodium-deficient fluids, TURP syndrome, hepatic and cardiac failure, nephrotic syndrome), or reduced concentration of Na (SIADH, drugs with anti-diuretic effect e.g. oxytocin).

Features of hyponatraemia: hypovolaemia, dehydration. If Na < 120 mmol/l, may see convulsions and coma (as water enters cells).

Treatment of hyponatraemia: treat underlying cause, restrict water, iv saline to correct plasma levels slowly (by 5–10 mmol/l every day). Too rapid correction can lead to subdural haemorrhage, central pontine myelinosis and cardiac failure.

Hypernatraemia: caused by excess Na (Cushing's syndrome, hyperaldosteronism, iatrogenic), water loss (renal loss, insensible loss), GI tract loss (vomiting, diarrhoea).

Features of hypernatraemia: dehydration, thirst, confusion, coma.

Treatment of hypernatraemia: oral or iv water. Too rapid an infusion can cause cerebral oedema. Aim to reduce plasma Na slowly (by 5–10 mmol/l every day).

■ Calcium (Ca): normal range 2.2–2.6 mmol/l

Mostly found in bone; ionized plasma Ca acts as a second messenger, involved in various cellular responses to stimuli.

Involved in:

- Neuromuscular transmission
- Muscle contraction
- Cell division
- Coagulation
- Cardiac inotropy.

Clinical uses:

To treat hypocalcaemia.
As an inotropic agent in cardiac surgery.

Hypercalcaemia: caused by hyperparathyroidism, malignancy, high bone turnover states e.g. Paget's disease, vitamin D metabolic disorders, hyperthyroidism, renal failure, lithium use. Treatment with fluid rehydration, loop diuretics e.g. frusemide (care with K and Mg depletion and bisphosphonates).

Hypocalcaemia: caused by hypoparathyroidism, e.g. post thyroid/parathyroid surgery, pancreatitis, chronic renal failure, lack of vitamin D. Can cause perioral tingling, tetany, Chvostek's and Trousseau's sign, arrhythmias, seizures and laryngeal spasm. Treat cause and give calcium as iv infusion +/− orally.

■ Magnesium (Mg): normal range 0.75–1.0 mmol/l

Acts as a cell membrane stabilizer. Required for protein synthesis, including ATP.

Uses:

- As a bronchodilator in severe asthma – given as 2 g intravenous infusion over 20 minutes.
- As a membrane stabilizer and vasodilator in pre-eclampsia – given as stat dose of 4 g, then 1 g/hr.
- As an anti-arrhythmic, especially where hypokalaemia is present – give 8 mmol intravenously over 15 minutes.
- As a nutritional supplement in critically-ill patients.
- Remember to check Mg levels, as toxic effects are seen above 4–5 mmol/l. Reflexes disappear at this level, so monitor them regularly.

Pain control

MATT JARRETT AND MIKE PLATT

■ Introduction

What is pain? 'An unpleasant sensory or emotional experience, associated with actual or potential tissue damage or expressed in terms of such damage' (definition from: The International Association for the Study of Pain, 1996).

Acute pain is defined as pain lasting less than 3 months, chronic pain lasting more than 3 months.

■ Steps to good pain control

Pain assessment:

- Site
- Character
- Time course
- Radiation
- Aggravating factors
- Relieving factors
- Associated factors (nausea, sweating etc.)
- Affective (emotional) setting.

Pain treatment is optimized by following the basic principles: analgesia according to individual need, by mouth, by the clock, and by the pain ladder.

The need for regular assessment of pain scores cannot be overemphasized. (For special considerations see below.) Management of co-morbidity, such as sleep disturbance is important.

Hospital Surgery: Foundations in Surgical Practice, ed. Omer Aziz, Sanjay Purkayastha and Paraskevas Paraskeva. Published by Cambridge University Press. © Cambridge University Press 2009.

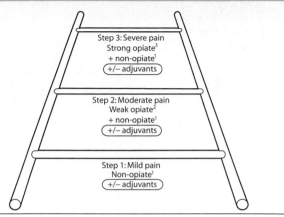

An adjuvant is any drug or technique used to enhance analgesia at any step on the ladder. They include anxiolytics, anti-convulsants, local anaesthetics, neuroleptics, steroids and anti-emetics.

1: Non-opiates include paracetamol, aspirin and non-steroidal anti-inflammatory drugs (NSAID)

2: Mild opiates include codeine, dihydrocodeine and tramadol

3: Strong opiates include diamorphine, fentanyl, morphine and oxycodone.

NB: Patients can move both up and down the analgesic ladder.
Include regular anti-emetics and laxatives as Steps 2 and 3.

Figure 10 Analgesic ladder

■ Analgesic pain ladder (after WHO 1986–90)

Introduced by the World Health Organization as an easy, cheap and effective method of controlling cancer pain. It is effective in approximately 90 % of patients. It has been subsequently modified and extended to include non-cancer patients.

Surgical patients differ from cancer patents in that whatever their background level of pain, which may be negligible (e.g. talipes) or severe (e.g. peritonitis), their postoperative pain is often significantly worse than preoperatively. This gives no time for use of the analgesic ladder (see Figure 10), consequently analgesia is often pre-emptively prescribed at Step 3.

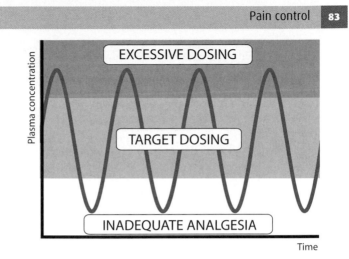

Figure 11 Inadequate analgesia: infrequent, excessive doses of opiate

Unlike cancer pain, post surgical pain usually wanes over a matter of days. As such, it is important to regularly review analgesic requirements and reverse down the analgesic ladder, to prevent opiate narcosis.

■ Modes of administration

Regular vs. on request (PRN: *pro re nata*) prescribing. To achieve a steady state with the plasma drug concentration in the therapeutic range, pharmacokinetics dictates a balance between dose size, frequency and drug clearance. Regular dosing ensures maintenance of therapeutic plasma levels (see Figures 11 and 12).

Remember the old maxim 'PRN = *Pain Relief*? *None*.' PRN dosing should be reserved for patients with minimal discomfort or to top up plasma levels in addition to a regular regime. Ward practicalities mean patients on PRN regimes rarely receive adequate analgesia when it is required.

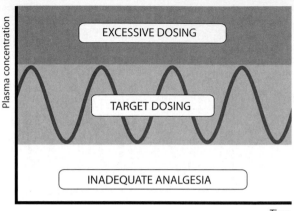

Figure 12 Adequate analgesia: correct dose size and schedule

■ Polypharmacy

Analgesics targeted against various forms of nociception have a synergistic effect, i.e. $(1 + 1$ may $= 3)$: this may be avoided by the prescription of a simple analgesic, plus an anti-inflammatory, plus an opiate to affect different parts of the nociceptive pathway, and achieve analgesia at lower doses and with fewer side-effects than with fewer drugs at higher doses (see Figure 10).

■ Routes of administration

1. Enteral – oral/non-oral: sublingual, intranasal, rectal.
2. Parenteral: topical, transcutaneous, subcutaneous, intramuscular, intravenous, neural blockades (perineural, epidural, intrathecal).

ENTERAL

Oral (po): easily administered, tolerated and preferred by the majority of patients. Beware impaired swallow/absorption. Drugs may be liquid or tablet/capsule, immediate or modified release. Non-oral analgesics avoid first pass metabolism, and sublingual or intranasal opiates act rapidly. Rectal (pr) administration avoids problems of gastric stasis and ileus.

PARENTERAL

Topical (top.)

Local anaesthetic creams used extensively in paediatric and needle-phobic patients prior to venepuncture. Need to be put on for approximately 30 minutes to work effectively. NSAID preparations exist, but are not routinely used in the inpatient environment.

Transcutaneous

Opiate patches provide an effective and simple method of analgesia in special situations such as chronic pain and palliative care.

Overdose range: sedation, respiratory depression and nausea predominate.

Subcutaneous (sc)

Similar kinetics to intramuscular injection, but less painful. Used in palliative care with continuous infusions, but can be used in any situation. Placement of a labelled sc cannula avoids repeat needling and is therefore preferable to im injections. Absorption may be delayed if skin perfusion is low.

Intramuscular (im)

Traditionally the parenteral route of choice for staff, if not patients. Nurses in the UK do not have to be iv licensed to administer. Relatively predictable kinetics, rapid absorption (<20 min). **NB:** im diclofenac may cause sterile abscesses – give po or pr if possible.

Intravenous (iv)

Rapid onset (<5 min), easy to titrate to pain. Used extensively perioperatively, especially in the recovery room. Reliable kinetics. Advent of patient controlled analgesia (PCA) pumps have revolutionized surgical analgesia: a computer-controlled, syringe driver giving small fixed doses of iv opiate as demanded by the patient. A lock-out function means that the patient cannot overdose, and the psychological benefit of giving the patient control over their pain is enormous. PCAs allow rapid response to changes in pain levels, and allow pre-emptive analgesia, e.g. prior to coughing or physiotherapy. Problems can occur after sleep, when plasma opiate levels drop and the patient experiences a delay in regaining pain control. Beware patients titrating to nausea rather than pain: prescribe regular anti-emetics in conjunction.

Neural blockade

Perineural blocks: usually performed perioperatively by anaesthetists (e.g. brachial plexus block, sciatic nerve block), these can be useful in the emergency setting. Intercostal nerve blocks for fractured ribs, or femoral nerve block for fractured femur are particularly useful.

Neuraxial analgesia/anaesthesia: epidural or intrathecal blocks. Currently almost entirely the preserve of anaesthetists, they allow profound analgesia from the thorax down, enabling abdominal, pelvic and lower-limb surgery with a light general anaesthetic or minimal or even no sedation. Postoperative analgesia is often total, and is regarded as the gold standard. Also used in other fields such as palliative care.

Epidural drugs (usually a dilute local anaesthetic plus an opiate) are administered outside the dural sac, diffusing across the sac and cerebrospinal fluid (CSF) to block pain transmission over a region of the spinal cord, but often leaving lower regions intact. It is particularly suited to indwelling catheter techniques. Intrathecal blocks involve the injection of drugs directly into the CSF. Smaller doses can be used, and the block is often a dense sensorimotor one. Indwelling catheters can be inserted. The potential for a serious adverse event with neuraxial block-ade is relatively high, and care of these patients is a specialized area.

■ Special considerations

Most NHS Hospital Trusts in the UK have a Consultant led acute pain team: if in doubt, discuss the patient with the team.

■ Pain scoring

Pain is entirely subjective. To convey this to the clinician, various scoring methods are used, most commonly as a fraction: 0 out of 10 for no pain, to 10 out of 10 for the worst pain imaginable. A descriptive scale of mild/moderate/severe is equally valid. Scores should be checked regularly, noted and acted upon. Anything maintained over 3–4 (>mild) is unacceptable. Children and adults with reduced capacity are more difficult to assess, however the Oucher facial scale is commonly used. It consists of photos or line drawings of children's faces expressing increasing degrees of pain. These are presented and explained in suitable terms. The patient then points to the most appropriate picture. Effective analgesia is when a score of <3 is achieved.

■ Patient considerations

1. Reduced compliance: postoperatively, mental competency is often reduced, especially in the elderly or chronically ill. This may make them unable to take drugs orally, unable to ask for PRN analgesia and unable to operate PCAs. Adapt your prescribing accordingly, and ensure both regular medical and nursing assessment of patient pain.

2. Gastric emptying: this is reduced by pain, abdominal surgery (ileus) and opiates. Subsequent distension reduces drug absorption and causes both nausea and vomiting.

■ Prescribing in opiate-addicted patients

This is often a problem area, due largely to the perceived differences between the aims of the team and patient. In the acute situation, the majority of addicts are not looking for a recreational 'hit' in hospital, and are only concerned with avoiding withdrawal and pain. Addicts in treatment are often on stable doses of opiate, and the equipotent dose may be given by iv or infusion to prevent withdrawal, with a modified PCA regime being given as well. Untreated addicts are unlikely to know how much opiate they require to avoid withdrawal, and prescribing in these cases is best done under expert guidance. A single prescriber may help limit communication difficulties.

■ Affective component of pain

Pain is a multifactorial experience, and rated pain will depend on the context and meaning of the pain. Pain scores for a laparotomy will differ wildly between a patient who has undergone an 'open and shut' for inoperable cancer, compared to a laparotomy for a curative procedure. Analgesic requirements will be considerably higher in the former patient, and it is important to adapt accordingly. Early involvement of specialist support is essential (e.g. palliative care).

■ Drug considerations

1. **Anticoagulation:** it is vital that epidural and spinal blocks are performed in patients with relatively intact coagulation systems. Similarly, epidural or spinal catheters should only be removed from non-anticoagulated patients. The risk is of precipitating an epidural haematoma. This is a neurosurgical emergency, and will require an immediate laminectomy to prevent permanent neurological damage. Consequently, heparin should be prescribed in the evening, outside of the risk period.

2. **Epidurals:** Catheters should be removed from patients 2 hours before the prescribed heparin, to allow clotting to occur. Ideally, the epidural should be stopped in the morning, and only when the patient is requiring <6 ml/hour of low dose epidural solution (LDE: 0.1 % bupivacaine and 2 µg/ml fentanyl) with minimal motor block. As long as the pain can be controlled by other means (po or PCA) over the next 4–6 hours, the epidural is suitable for removal 2 hours prior to the next dose of heparin. If in doubt, ask the pain team.

3. **Epidurals, spinal blocks and lower limb compartment syndrome**: this is a perennial area of conflict between orthopaedic surgeons and anaesthetists, the argument being that neuraxial blockade will mask the pain associated with the development of the syndrome. A search of the literature shows that the connection is controversial. Communication between surgeon and anaesthetist remains the best course.

4. **Non-steroidal anti-inflammatories:** this group of drugs is very useful, but needs careful prescribing. The recent Vioxx(rofecoxib)/COX 2 controversy has further muddied the waters. COX 1 inhibitors, regardless of route, will cause gastric erosion and compromise renal blood flow, precipitating renal failure in vulnerable groups. Avoid in extremes of age, and limit administration to short (3–5 day) courses with food. Consider a proton pump inhibitor or H_2 antagonist. COX 2 inhibitors largely avoid gastric side-effects in the short term, but renal effects are identical to COX 1 inhibitors and cardiovascular events are suggested. (A more detailed report can be found in: BMJ **330**, 2005, 1366–69.)

5. **Opiates and epidurals:** do not prescribe an opiate if the patient has an opiate-containing epidural running, or respiratory depression will occur. Ask the pain team.

6. **Opiates and renal function:** diamorphine and codeine are pro-drugs, being converted to morphine after administration. Morphine (the active drug) is metabolized in the liver to pharmacologically active metabolites, which are then excreted renally. Renal failure causes a build up of active metabolites, which cause opiate toxicity.

Consequently, fentanyl and oxycodone (hepatic excretion) are preferred in renal failure. Help should be sought from the pain team.

■ Other useful facts for complete pain management

Pain acts as a physiological antagonist to opiate-induced respiratory depression and sedation. Acute reduction in pain will reduce this antagonist effect, thereby causing sedation and possibly respiratory depression. If pain is suddenly reduced (e.g. following local anaesthetic), reduce the opiate prescription.

All opiates constipate, as does bed rest. Co-prescribe laxatives.

All opiates nauseate. Co-prescribe anti-emetics.

Warfarinized patients and elective surgery: these will need early admission for conversion to iv heparin at an appropriate APTR prior to surgery.

Nutrition

DAVID WALKER AND HUW J. W. THOMAS

An appreciation of the nutritional status of the patient is an important part of inpatient management. A number of factors may be involved, including poor intake (anorexia associated with illness, chronic illness, neglect), malabsorption (pancreatitis, inflammatory bowel disease, following bowel resections), and increased requirements (malignancies, acute illness). A malnourished patient has a significantly impaired immune system, delayed wound healing and reduced strength that manifests itself as decreased ventilatory function.

Modern surgical management of surgical patients puts increasing importance on adequate nutrition. The current areas of intense discussion are when and how nutrition should be administrated, and how it changes outcome. From the point of view of the junior doctor, it is important to involve the dietician early on, and ideally this should be done preoperatively.

■ Nutritional requirements

As with fluid requirements, the nutritional status and the requirements of the patient will change according to their state of health. The aim in the surgical patient is to prevent a depletion of protein stores due to increased catabolism that leads to a negative nitrogen balance. The average carbohydrate stores are depleted in 24 hours, whereas protein and fat stores are depleted over the next month. Younger patients require a higher number of calories per kg than older ones. However in some patients, e.g. those with severe burns and trauma,

Hospital Surgery: Foundations in Surgical Practice, ed. Omer Aziz, Sanjay Purkayastha and Paraskevas Paraskeva. Published by Cambridge University Press. © Cambridge University Press 2009.

the calorie requirements may increase by 100 % above basal resting requirements.

ADULT DAILY CALORIE REQUIREMENT = 30 kcal/kg/day,
ADULT DAILY PROTEIN REQUIREMENT = 1 g protein/kg/day.

Since 6.25 g of protein provide 1 g of nitrogen, the average nitrogen requirement is approximately 12 g/day.

■ Subjective global assessment of nutritional status

This incorporates the following points:

1. **Weight history** (loss of >10 % body weight suggests significant malnutrition)
2. **Dietary intake**
3. **Gastrointestinal symptoms** (including diarrhoea, vomiting and poor appetite)
4. **Functional status** (bed bound vs. active)
5. **Disease state:** active disease will increase metabolic demands on the body
6. **Physical assessment:** loss of subcutaneous fat (triceps, chest), muscle wasting (quadriceps, deltoids), ankle oedema, sacral oedema and ascites.
7. **Body mass index** = weight/height^2.

■ Biochemical assessment of nutritional status

Albumin is an important indicator in the absence of other pathology that may cause hypoalbuminaemia (liver disease, nephropathy). Albumin does however have a 21-day half-life, making it unreliable in the short term. Albumin < 30 mg/dl suggests malnutrition. **Lymphocyte count** may be low. Other more rapid turnover proteins that may be used to evaluate nutritional status include **transferrin**, **thyroid binding pre-albumin** and **retinol-binding protein**.

■ Anthropometric measurements

Skin-fold thickness (e.g. triceps, iliac crest), arm circumference, and grip strength.

Taking these variables into account, the patient can be classified as **well-nourished**, **moderately malnourished** or **severely malnourished**. Patients who are nutritionally depleted or at risk of nutritional depletion should be considered for supplemental feeding regimes. The decision to start nutritional support and the planning of the route of feeding should be as part of a multidisciplinary decision always involving the dietician, nurses, the patient and if appropriate the speech and language therapist.

■ Enteral feeding

If the patient can swallow and has a functional gastrointestinal tract, oral nutritional support is preferable as it results in fewer complications. Also early enteral nutrition has been advocated to preserve intestinal structure and the role of the intestine in immune function (the absence of enteral feeding has been related to villous and cellular atrophy).

ENTERAL FEEDING ROUTES

If the patient cannot swallow he or she will need to be fed through a fine-bore *nasogastric, nasoduodenal,* or *nasojejunal tube* (surgical). If long-term feeding is required in a patient who is not going to be able to swallow they should be considered for a *gastrostomy*. Gastrostomies can be performed endoscopically (percutaneous endoscopic gastrostomy – PEG) or radiologically (radiologically inserted gastrostomy – RIG).

ENTERAL NUTRITION SUPPORT

This can be in the form of food supplements, liquidized food, or palatable enteral diet. If this is not sufficient then an elemental diet can be given through a fine-bore nasogastric tube that is placed directly into the stomach or small bowel. These types of feeds can provide approx 8000 kJ of energy with about 70 g of protein in 2–3 litres (e.g. Osmolite). Types of enteral nutrition include:

1. Polymeric – near normal
   These contain intact proteins, starches and long-chain fatty acids; they are useful in patients who have a functioning stomach and normal digestive capacity.
2. Disease specific
   These are feeds that are tailored to meet the requirements of specific diseases, e.g. feeds for patients with liver disease are deficient in branched amino acids, which can exacerbate encephalopathy.
3. Elemental
   These are chemically-defined feeds that contain simple amino acids, oligo and monosaccharides. These require minimal digestion. They are useful in patients with intestinal fistulae, but are far from palatable.

INDICATIONS FOR ENTERAL NUTRITION

In practice each patient needs to be considered individually and the decision to begin enteral feeding requires the advice of dieticians, speech and language therapy (SALT) nurses and even relatives if there are difficult issues such as a poor prognosis to be addressed. Indications include:

1. Long-term feeding
2. Dysphagia, e.g. stricture, stroke
3. Chronic disease, e.g. neoplasia
4. Malnutrition

5. Sepsis
6. Burns
7. Major surgery
8. Coma/ICU.

COMPLICATIONS

1. Malposition or blockage of the tube
2. Aspiration pneumonia
3. Feeding intolerance
4. Diarrhoea
5. Vomiting
6. Metabolic imbalance (hyperglycaemia)
7. Electrolyte imbalance (hyperosmotic non-ketotic coma).

■ Total parenteral nutrition (TPN)

TPN is used if the patient does not have a functioning gastrointestinal tract. If TPN is unlikely to be needed for more than two weeks then feed can be given via a large peripheral cannulae. However, if long term feeding is required a central vein (central venous line or a Hickman line) will need to be used.

INDICATIONS FOR TPN

1. Unable to swallow, e.g. oesophageal tumour
2. Burns, where upper GI tract is severely burnt
3. Prolonged obstruction, high output fistula
4. Prolonged ileus
5. Short bowel syndrome
6. Severe Crohn's disease
7. Severe sepsis
8. Severe malnutrition
9. Severe pancreatitis.

TPN COMPOSITION

While the exact composition of TPN should be guided by dietician guidelines most formulations contain a varying amount of carbohydrate, amino acids, lipid emulsions, vitamins, trace elements (Zn, Cu, Cr, Mn, Se) and electrolytes.

PATIENT MONITORING WITH TPN

This includes qds vital signs measurement and BM testing, strict fluid balance, weight measurement every two days. The frequency of biochemical tests is as follows:

1. Daily: FBC, U&E, BM
2. Weekly: LFTs, Ca, PO_4, albumin, trace elements
3. Fortnightly: vitamin B_{12}, Zn, Mg, Se, Cu, Fe, transferrin

■ TPN complications

These can be thought of as complications of the feed itself, and those related to the insertion and presence of a central line:

1. **Line insertion** – pneumothorax, haemorrhage, cardiac tamponade
2. **Line *in situ*** – vein thrombosis, infection, sepsis
3. **Feed (metabolic) complications** – hyper/hypoglycaemia, abnormal LFT, electrolyte imbalance, mineral overload, vitamin and mineral deficiencies.

Meticulous attention should be paid to ensuring an aseptic technique during line handling as infections are common and can be fatal.

REFEEDING SYNDROME

Once the need for enteral/parenteral nutrition has been established, a baseline biochemical assessment must take place before feeding is commenced, and monitoring should continue during the period of nutritional support in order to reduce the risk of 'refeeding syndrome'. This is a serious metabolic consequence of malnourished patients who undergo refeeding. It can result in severe and rapid reduction in potassium, calcium, phosphate and magnesium, leading to cardiac, renal and gastrointestinal abnormalities. Patients who are at risk of refeeding syndrome include chronic alcoholics, patients without nutrition for >7 days and oncology patients receiving chemotherapy. In these patients thiamine 200 mg bd should be prescribed prior to feeding.

Routes and methods of enteral/parenteral feeding

Route	Indications	Possible contraindications
Nasogastric (NG)	– Unsafe swallow – Those patients requiring extra nutrition to supplemental oral intake – For short term use (<21 days)	– Obstruction of oropharynx or oesophagus preventing passage of tube – gastric outlet obstruction – delayed gastric emptying
Gastrostomy – percutaneous endoscopic gastrostomy (PEG)	– Patients requiring nutritional support for >21 days, e.g. trauma patients, head injury, risk of lung aspiration	– Oesophageal/gastric obstruction – Gastric outlet obstruction – Large ascites – Unable to pass endoscope
Gastrostomy – radiologically guided (RIG)	– Unable to pass endoscope to inert PEG	– Oesophageal/gastric obstruction – Gastric outlet obstruction – Large ascites
Nasojejunal feeding tube	– Patients at risk of gastric aspiration – Acute pancreatitis – Intractable vomiting	– Inability to pass NJ tube due to oesophageal/gastric obstruction
Needle catheter jejunostomy	– Upper GI surgery (e.g. Gastrectomy) where patients likely to require nutritional support – Long-term feeding into the jejunum	– Non-functioning gut post surgery
Intravenous (TPN)	– Mechanical obstruction – Non-functioning gut	– Poor venous access

Potential problems of enteral feeding

Problem	Action
Blocked NG, NJ or PEG tube	– Flush the tube with 10 ml warm water (use 20 ml syringe) – Now try 10 ml fizzy fluid e.g. soda water. Leave for at least 30 min – Now try 10 ml pineapple juice – If all unsuccessful consider tube replacement (Note: a common cause of a blocked tube is putting crushed tablets down it. Always use liquid preparations if possible)
Vomiting, gastric distension	– Stop feed. Start slowly and gradually build up rate. – Consider prokinetics, e.g. domperidone, erythromycin
Diarrhoea	– Review medication – Send stool sample for *Clostridium difficile* – Consider loperamide if no infection – Review infusion rate and feed content

Antibiotic prescribing in surgery

SANJAY PURKAYASTHA

This encompasses both prophylactic and treatment regimes for elective and acute cases. Local policies may vary and communication between the surgical and microbiology team is essential.

■ Important principles to remember

1. Are you prescribing for prophylaxis or treatment?
2. What is the duration of therapy planned?
3. Is the infection being treated bacterial?
4. Have the necessary specimens been taken prior to starting antibiotics?
5. Is empirical treatment necessary?
6. Can oral antibiotics be used, or will parenteral therapy be needed?
7. How will the effectiveness of the antibiotic therapy be monitored?
8. Are you sure that the patient does not have antibiotic allergies?
9. Is surgical treatment needed with antibiotic therapy? for example incision and drainage.

How to choose the right antibiotic: think of patient factors and likely causative organism. *Patient factors:* how unwell is the patient; co-morbidities e.g. diabetes, renal impairment, immunocompromised, hepatic impairment etc.) *Likely causative organisms:* see the table for common surgical infections in surgical patients and antibiotics to use.

Hospital Surgery: Foundations in Surgical Practice, ed. Omer Aziz, Sanjay Purkayastha and Paraskevas Paraskeva. Published by Cambridge University Press. © Cambridge University Press 2009.

Surgical infection	Common organisms	Therapy
Peritonitis	Gram negatives and anaerobes	Cephalosporin + metronidazole
Biliary tract infection	Gram negatives and anaerobes	Cephalosporin + metronidazole or ciprofloxacin
Urinary tract	Gram negatives and anaerobes	Trimethoprim or cephalosporin or co-amoxyclav* or ciprofloxacin
Osteomyelitis/septic arthritis	Gram positives	Flucloxacillin* or clindamycin or vancomycin*
Cellulitis	Gram positives	Benzylpenicillin* + flucloxacillin*
Hospital-acquired pneumonia	Gram positive or gram negative	1st line: co-amoxiclav 2nd line: cefuroxime If poor response after 48 hours: ciproflaxicin

* Care with potential penicillin allergy

Usual intravenous doses of the common treatment antibiotics given to surgical patients: cefuroxime 1.5 g tds; metronidazole 500 mg tds; co-amoxiclav 1.2 g tds; ciprofloxacin 400 mg bd; benzylpenicillin 1.2 g qds; flucloxacillin 1 g qds.

Guide for length of antibiotic courses:

Cellulitis: 7–10 days

Gram negative sepsis without focus: 10 days

Lower urinary tract infection: 3–5 days; upper urinary tract infection: 7–10 days

Pneumonia: 10 days; infective exacerbation of COPD: 7 days.

■ When should intravenous prescriptions be converted to oral?

It is best to use the oral route whenever possible and the following drugs are all very well absorbed enterally and have good cellular penetration: ciprofloxacin, clarithromycin, clindamycin, metronidazole and rifampicin. Therefore there is no advantage to prescribing these parenterally unless gut absorption is affected, e.g. bowel obstruction. The majority of the drugs listed above are considerably more expensive in their intravenous forms. However if intravenous antibiotics are prescribed, after 72 hours consider changing to oral regimes if all of the following criteria are met:

Oral fluids are tolerated; there are no potential problems with gut absorption; high tissue concentrations of antibiotics are not needed (e.g. endocarditis, osteomyelitis, *Staphylococcus aureus* bacteraemia, etc.); pyrexia has been <30 °C for >48 hours; WCC and other inflammatory markers are returning to normal; there is no unexplained tachycardia; the patient is not immunocompromised.

Which antibiotics to use when switching from intravenous to oral	
Intravenous	Oral
Ciprofloxacin, gentamicin	Ciproflaxacin
Cefuroxime (for peritoneal infections)	Cefalexin
Cefuroxime (for pneumonia)	Co-amoxiclav or moxifloxacin

■ Prophylactic antibiotics in surgery

Prevention of gas gangrene for contaminated limb amputations: benzylpenicillin 300–600 mg qds for five days or, if penicillin allergic, 500 mg metronidazole tds for five days.

Prevention of infection during gastrointestinal procedures: intravenous single dose of cephalosporin + metronidozole, co-amoxiclav ± gentamicin.

Prevention of infection in orthopaedic surgery: especially for joint replacement surgery, single dose of intravenous cefuroxime or flucloxacillin. If penicillin allergic then use vancomycin.

Prevention of infection in urological procedures: transrectal prostate biopsy: single dose of intravenous cefuroxime and metronidazole; TURP: single dose of oral ciprofloxacin or intravenous gentamicin or cefuroxime.

■ Prevention of endocarditis in patients with prosthetic heart valves

For patients undergoing gastrointestinal procedures and genito-urinary procedures: amoxicillin 1 g intravenously and gentamicin

120 mg intravenously on induction and then oral amoxicillin 500 mg six hours later (NB if urine is infected, prophylaxis should cover infective organism).

Urinary catheterization: antibiotic cover needed if UTI suspected – use single dose of intravenous prophylaxis that will cover urinary infections, e.g. cefuroxime, gentamicin.

■ Patients with orthopaedic implants

Patients that have prosthetic joints do not need any special prophylactic measures if they are having any of the procedures described above.

■ Special infections in surgery

All of the following should be treated in conjunction following communication with the microbiology team in the local NHS Trust.

1. **MRSA:** treat with vancomycin. Initial dosage depends on renal function, so this and creatinine clearance must be checked first:

   Creatinine clearance (ml/min)

   $= [A \times (140 - age) \times weight\ in\ kg]/serum\ creatinine\ in\ \mu mol/l,$

   where $A = 1.23$ for men and 1.04 for women. The above formula may change for obese patients, for whom it is advisable to contact the ward pharmacist.

   Vancomycin is administered as a slow intravenous infusion for MRSA sepsis, combined with 0.9 % sodium chloride or 5 % dextrose. Maximum concentrations are 5 mg/ml (500 mg/100 ml or 1 g/250 ml). Vancomycin level must be monitored using trough levels which should be taken immediately prior to the next dose. Trough levels should be 5–10 mg/l. Levels should be monitored every three days if renal function is normal or daily if this is abnormal. Renal function should be monitored three times a week at least. Teicoplanin is another option.

2. **Clostridium difficile colitis:** although this usually responds well to treatment with oral metronidazole or vancomycin, approximately 15 to 20 % of patients will experience re-appearance of diarrhoea and other symptoms weeks or even months after initial therapy has been discontinued. The usual therapy for relapse is to repeat the 10 to 14 day course of either metronidazole or vancomycin and this is successful in most patients.

Critical care: the critically-ill patient, decision making and judgement

PARASKEVAS PARASKEVA AND RICHARD LEONARD

■ Objectives

1. Identify signs of impending critical illness
2. Understanding and managing critical illness early on ICU
3. Appreciate limitations of intensive care.

Advice on critically ill patients must be provided at a senior level. Trainees should **never** take it upon themselves to manage the sickest patients in the hospital without asking their consultant for support. Events proceed much more quickly in ICU than elsewhere.

Intensive Care is an expensive and limited resource, and should only be offered to those who need it and will benefit from it. It is often said that it is not reasonable to refuse admission to ICU simply on the grounds of advanced age, and that old people have been shown to respond to intensive care just as well as younger ones with similar disorders. While this is true, death cannot be postponed indefinitely, and the humane and reasonable use of Intensive Care over the age of 80 requires particular care in patient selection. Regardless of age, when the appropriateness of ICU admission is in question, an assessing intensivist needs the following information:

- Current diagnosis
- Its prognosis
- Co-morbidities
- Functional status.

The last of these is often the decisive factor, and the personal history, such as exercise tolerance, whether patients can get out of the home and

Hospital Surgery: Foundations in Surgical Practice, ed. Omer Aziz, Sanjay Purkayastha and Paraskevas Paraskeva. Published by Cambridge University Press. © Cambridge University Press 2009.

how, whether they manage to shop and do their own housework, and so on.

Clearly such judgements regarding the possible withholding of life-sustaining treatment can be difficult; they must be made at a senior level, wherever possible involving the patient. If the patient is not competent, the role of the next of kin is to represent the likely wishes of the patient regarding treatment. However, it is inhumane and morally irresponsible to leave such decisions to the relatives alone. The recent fashion for seeking written agreement from the next of kin before making an order not to attempt resuscitation often leaves families feeling that they bear ultimate responsibility for their relative's death. However in tune this may be with current ideological imperatives, such an outcome is a gross dereliction of care. Discussions should be couched in terms of 'working together to decide what the patient would want us to do', not of 'asking consent to withdraw or withhold treatment'. Dealing explicitly with death can be painful and difficult, but should not be avoided until it is too late; patients and their families are sometimes surprisingly grateful for the chance to discuss these issues openly. On the other hand, intensivists often receive requests for manifestly inappropriate admission to ICU, justified by the words 'The family wants everything done.' Such requests represent failures of communication during the decision-making process outlined above. The result is that the intensivist takes on a responsibility for communication which should lie with the referring specialist. Sadly, this phenomenon seems likely to become more common.

It has been shown that some patients are admitted to ICU too late in the course of their disease. Earlier treatment might improve outcome and perhaps even avoid ICU admission altogether. For this to happen, it is necessary to detect deterioration early and then provide staff capable of intervening effectively. The concept of a medical emergency team, called in response to defined physiological criteria, has been suggested as a solution. While this is theoretically attractive, outcome benefits have yet to be demonstrated. It is possible that such systems are simply unable to detect deterioration soon enough to affect the course of the disease.

Successful management of the critically-ill patient requires that two processes occur simultaneously:

1. Resuscitation from the pathophysiological derangement
2. Diagnosis and specific treatment of the underlying disease.

Either of these alone is doomed to failure. For example, appropriate surgical management of faecal peritonitis is futile without resuscitation from the profound septic shock that may accompany it. On the other hand, a ruptured abdominal aortic aneurysm requires rapid surgery, not merely adequate volume replacement. Unfortunately, the resuscitative skills of anaesthetists are not always accompanied by a clear understanding of the need for specific diagnosis and treatment, while physicians and surgeons are often deficient at identifying and correcting severely abnormal physiology.

The rest of these chapters on critical care will concentrate on the physiology of critical illness and how to correct it. The focus will be primarily on the pre-ICU management rather than on the technical details of mechanical life support. While each vital system is considered in turn, in reality they must be dealt with simultaneously. In order to provide useful practical guidance, safe threshold limits are given for physiological values. Naturally there will be some patients for whom the limits chosen are too permissive or too stringent. However, trainees who ignore these limits without seeking senior advice are asking for trouble, and will find it sooner rather than later.

■ Key points

1. Intensive Care requires careful coordination among many specialties and disciplines.
2. Do not advise on critically-ill patients without seeking senior support.

3. Respond quickly to requests for assistance in ICU.
4. Intensive Care is a valuable and limited resource and is not simply a final common pathway to the morgue or a means of reassuring patients' relatives.
5. When referring to Intensive Care, be ready with the following information:
   - Current problem and reason for referral
   - Prognosis of present condition
   - Co-morbidities
   - Functional status.
6. Critically-ill patients need simultaneous resuscitation, diagnosis and specific treatment.
7. Communication with the patient, relatives, nursing, and other medical staff is crucial to managing these patients optimally.

Critical care: cardiovascular physiology and support

PARASKEVAS PARASKEVA AND RICHARD LEONARD

■ Cardiovascular pathophysiology

The function of the circulation is to transport oxygen and nutrients to the tissues and to remove metabolic waste products. For this to happen, there must be:

- Enough **oxygen in the blood**
- Enough **blood flowing (cardiac output)**
- Enough **blood pressure** to let tissues regulate their own perfusion.

The **oxygen content** of the blood is determined by haemoglobin concentration and saturation.

■ Blood pressure

This is determined by the equation $BP = CO \times TPR$.

(BP = blood pressure, CO = cardiac output, TPR = total peripheral resistance.)

Thus hypotension can be due either to low cardiac output or to inappropriate vasodilation. Treatment usually requires correction of the abnormal variable.

■ Cardiac output

Cardiac output is determined by the following:

1. **Rate:** too high a heart rate prevents adequate filling of the ventricle and reduces preload and cardiac output. Bradycardia reduces cardiac output as ejection simply does not happen often enough.

Hospital Surgery: Foundations in Surgical Practice, ed. Omer Aziz, Sanjay Purkayastha and Paraskevas Paraskeva. Published by Cambridge University Press. © Cambridge University Press 2009.

2. **Rhythm:** loss of atrial contraction in junctional rhythms or atrial fibrillation also reduces preload and hence cardiac output by up to 30 %.

3. **Preload:** Starling's law states that the force of contraction of a cardiac muscle fibre is proportional to its initial length. The fibre length is determined by the ventricular volume. However volumes are difficult to measure clinically, and the simplest substitute is the central venous pressure (CVP). The relationship between pressure and volume is not linear and is described by the ventricular compliance, which varies both between individuals and within each individual over time. Because of this and the shape of the ventricular compliance curve, it is often not possible to determine the true preload or volume status from a single measurement of the central venous pressure. We get far more information about volume status from the CVP by observing, first, the trend over time and, second, the response to a **fluid challenge** (see figure 7 in the chapter on Shock).

   Give 250 ml colloid over 10 minutes. The response indicates the volume status:

   - CVP rises by more than 7 mmHg   hypervolaemic
   - CVP settles to within 3 mmHg of original value   euvolaemic
   - CVP rises by less than 3 mmHg   hypovolaemic.

4. **Contractility** is defined as the intrinsic ability of the myocardium to contract, independent of loading conditions. It is impossible to measure directly even under laboratory conditions, and must be inferred clinically from the CVP, blood pressure and assessments or measurements of the cardiac output. If preload is adequate and blood pressure remains low, with evidence of a low cardiac output, contractility is usually impaired.

5. **Afterload:** cardiac output is inversely related to the afterload, which may be defined either as the aortic input impedance or as the systolic ventricular wall tension. Afterload is reduced by the following manoeuvres:

   - Vasodilation (including re-warming of hypothermic patients)
   - Positive intra-thoracic pressure

■ Intra-aortic balloon counter pulsation.

Manipulation of afterload in cardiogenic shock is complex and difficult, and is outside the scope of this introduction.

It is not often necessary to measure cardiac output in clinical situations. There has recently been much debate about a possible association between the use of pulmonary artery catheters to measure cardiac output and an apparent increase in mortality. The quality of both evidence and debate is low. However, partly in response to this controversy, less invasive methods of monitoring cardiac output are gaining in popularity. For some reason the British seem excessively interested in such devices, to the exclusion of proper understanding of the diseases being treated.

Inadequate tissue perfusion produces the signs of *shock* listed below (See chapter on Shock). As can be seen the disorder involves several systems. Patients with these signs are critically ill and are liable to rapid decompensation. They need urgent resuscitation.

Signs of inadequate tissue perfusion:

1. Hypotension (BP < 90 mmHg)
2. Tachypnoea
3. Oliguria
4. Abnormal mentation
5. Slow capillary refill (not in early sepsis).

■ Hypotension

In the non-pregnant adult, a systolic blood pressure of less than 90 mmHg represents dangerous hypotension and requires immediate action. While there may be patients for whom a slightly lower BP is acceptable (for instance the rule does not necessarily apply under anaesthesia), inexperienced trainees should not take such a decision alone. Conversely, if a patient has a systolic BP of 100 mmHg, but shows all the other signs of inadequate tissue perfusion, they should be treated with the same urgency as a shocked hypotensive patient.

MANAGEMENT OF HYPOTENSION

Check for airway, breathing and circulation

Check the BP yourself

Give high flow oxygen

Check for signs of shock

Establish large bore venous access (14G or 16G) and draw blood for:

Investigations: FBP, coagulation studies, U&E, amylase, cardiac enzymes, arterial blood gases, chest X-ray/ECG

Quickly examine for signs of pulmonary oedema. If a hypotensive patient has pulmonary oedema, he or she is desperately ill and needs expert assistance from the ICU immediately. If there is no pulmonary oedema it is safe to give fluid

Give 500 ml of any fluid except 5% dextrose, and repeat as necessary

Take a history, examine the patient, **make a diagnosis and give specific treatment**.

If there is no response after between 1000 and 2000 ml fluid, insert a central venous catheter and titrate filling using serial fluid challenges as described above.

If hypotension persists despite adequate filling, vasoactive drugs are needed.

Inotropes (adrenaline) if cardiac output is low or uncertain.

Vasoconstrictors (noradrenaline) if cardiac output is high.

It is sometimes necessary to measure cardiac output directly in order to make this distinction.

■ Goals of resuscitation

- Mean BP > 70 mmHg
- Resolving tachycardia
- Improved peripheral perfusion
- Urine output improved above at least 0.5 and preferably 1 ml/kg/hour
- Resolving acidosis and falling lactate.

■ Key summary points

1. Systolic BP < 90 mmHg requires urgent treatment.
2. Hypotension is due to either reduced cardiac output or pathological vasodilation.
3. In the absence of clinically obvious pulmonary oedema, it is safe to give fluid.
4. The response of the CVP to a fluid challenge indicates volume status.
5. Cardiac output is determined by contractility, rate and rhythm, afterload, and preload.

Critical care: respiratory pathophysiology and support

SERENE SHASHAA AND RICHARD LEONARD

The function of the respiratory system is to transport oxygen to the blood and remove carbon dioxide from it. Success requires an adequate volume of gas to ventilate the alveoli and close matching of the degree of ventilation and perfusion of each lung unit. Failure results in hypoxaemia, hypercarbia or both.

Hypercarbia is caused by a reduction in alveolar minute ventilation, due to:

- *Decreased minute ventilation* (respiratory rate or tidal volume) such as in drug overdose and neuromuscular disorders
- *Increased dead space ventilation* (e.g. rapid shallow breathing, COPD)
- *Increased physiological dead space ventilation*
- *Increased CO_2 production* (e.g. sepsis, fever, seizure).

All of these can be corrected or compensated by an increase in the respiratory rate.

Hypoxaemia may be caused by:

Hypoventilation: if the rate at which fresh inspiratory gas is presented to the alveoli falls but oxygen consumption remains the same, the partial pressure of oxygen within the alveoli falls. The oxygen tension within the pulmonary capillary and systemic arteries (PaO_2) is reduced. Postoperative surgical patients are vulnerable to hypoxaemia due to *pain* from upper abdominal incisions and *opioid* analgesia causing respiratory suppression. Hypoxaemia from hypoventilation can be corrected by:

Hospital Surgery: Foundations in Surgical Practice, ed. Omer Aziz, Sanjay Purkayastha and Paraskevas Paraskeva. Published by Cambridge University Press. © Cambridge University Press 2009.

- *Increasing the respiratory rate*, either pharmacologically or mechanically
- *Increasing the inspired FiO$_2$* (oxygen fraction).

Shunting: *true anatomical shunting* cannot be corrected by an increased FiO$_2$, because by definition no gas exchange occurs. *Physiological shunting* caused by imperfect V/Q matching can be partially corrected by increasing the FiO$_2$. Postoperative surgical patients are vulnerable to shunting due to *basal atelectasis, ARDS, pulmonary oedema,* and *chest infection*. Techniques available to reduce shunt involve raising the mean airway pressure in order to recruit collapsed lung units. Management includes:

- *Oxygen*
- *Continuous positive airway pressure* (CPAP)
- *Mechanical ventilation* (invasive or non-invasive).

[Note: *chronic obstructive pulmonary disease (COPD) patients* – as with all patients, hypoxaemia is a far more dangerous and rapidly lethal state than hypercarbia. Although hypoxic COPD patients do experience an increase in arterial carbon dioxide tension (due to a suppression of their respiratory drive) when given oxygen, it is extremely important to give them oxygen to treat the hypoxia. The increase in arterial carbon dioxide tension (P$_a$CO$_2$) rarely causes problems so long as oxygen therapy is controlled to ensure safe but not excessive oxygen saturations (say 90–92 %). If hypercarbia does occur, and is causing problems, the treatment is to ventilate the patient, not to add hypoxaemia to their difficulties.]

Other causes include:

- *Ventilation/perfusion mismatch* (e.g. pulmonary embolus)
- *Diffusion impairment* (e.g. interstitial lung disease)
- *Low cardiac output*
- *Anaemia.*

Types of ventilation can be divided into:

- *Invasive:* requires an artificial airway, e.g. endotracheal intubation.

- *Non-invasive:* via nasal or full-face mask. Includes CPAP and BiPAP (see below). The need for emergent intubation is an absolute contraindication to non-invasive ventilation.

■ 1. Oxygen therapy

This can be delivered through the following devices:

- *Nasal prongs* delivering 2–4 l/min O_2
- *Hudson masks* delivering up to 15 l/min O_2.

[Note: nasal prongs and Hudson masks deliver a known flow of oxygen, but the FiO_2 is determined by amount of air entrained by the patient during inspiration. This in turn is determined by the peak inspiratory flow rate, which of course varies.]

- *Venturi masks* delivering 24–60 % O_2.

[Note: Venturi devices use *Bernoulli's principle* in order to deliver a high enough flow of known FiO_2 to exceed the patient's peak inspiratory flow rate, thus avoiding entrainment of further air.]

In surgical patients, oxygen therapy is always prescribed in the early postoperative period to treat hypoxaemia from the causes mentioned. These patients are known to continue to experience episodic nocturnal hypoxaemia for at least three days after surgery, which is also a period that coincides with a high risk for perioperative myocardial infarction. Anaesthetists commonly prescribe oxygen for three days after surgery in patients who are at particular risk of this dangerous complication and it is important for surgical teams to ensure that this takes place.

■ 2. Continuous positive airway pressure (CPAP)

This represents the next level of respiratory support from oxygen supplementation. A tight-fitting mask connected to either a large reservoir or high gas flow permits an FiO_2 of up to 1.0, while at the same time a positive pressure is applied continuously to the patient's upper airway. This positive pressure recruits alveoli which are collapsed due to lung disease, and results in:

- *Reduced shunting* and therefore increased PaO_2
- *Increased lung volume* and therefore (usually) improved pulmonary compliance and reduced work of breathing.

CPAP is not usually recommended in patients with hypoxaemic respiratory failure, unless in the setting of CHF exacerbation. In this case the patient should be closely monitored in an ICU setting for clinical improvement. If in 2–3 hours the patient is not better, one should pursue immediate intubation. In a patient with severe pneumonia or ARDS, consider intubation early.

[Note: CPAP usually has little effect on $PaCO_2$, despite the reduced work of breathing.]

■ 3. Bi-level positive airway pressure (BiPAP)

BiPAP provides two levels of pressure (one for inhalation and a lower pressure for exhalation). In the setting of a COPD exacerbation, BiPAP can be used to improve both P_aO_2 and P_aCO_2. The patient should be watched closely and have regular blood gases done. They should also receive their steroids and nebulizer treatments. Failure to improve after several hours suggests the need to intubate.

[Note: *contraindications to NIPPV (non-invasive positive pressure ventilation) include:* (1) Cardiac or respiratory arrest. (2) Non-respiratory organ failure. (3) Severe encephalopathy (GCS < 10). (4) Severe upper gastrointestinal bleeding. (5) Haemodynamic instability or unstable cardiac arrhythmia. (6) Facial or neurological surgery, trauma, or deformity. (7) Upper airway obstruction. (8) Inability to cooperate/protect airway. (9) Inability to clear secretions, and (10) High risk for aspiration.]

■ 4. Mechanical ventilation

This commonly involves endotracheal tube intubation (and later a tracheostomy for prolonged ventilation)

AIMS

Improve oxygenation
Improve ventilation (hypercapnoeic respiratory failure)
Protect the airway (e.g. stroke, drug overdose)
Provide pulmonary toilet (e.g. excessive secretions).

INDICATIONS

Respiratory failure refractory to less-invasive treatments
Elective postopcrative ventilation
Physiological control (e.g. raised intra-cranial pressure).

The decision to ventilate a patient with respiratory failure is complex, taking into account:

- Respiratory distress
- Respiratory drive
- Conscious level
- Natural history of underlying disease
- Arterial blood gas results.

Elective postoperative ventilation is often used in anticipation of respiratory failure following:

- Major surgery (e.g. cardiac surgery, thoraco-abdominal aneurysm repair)
- Hypothermia
- Massive transfusion
- Haemodynamic instability

- Staged procedure (e.g. following penetrating abdominal trauma or faecal peritonitis).

[Note: elective intubations are much less risky than emergent ones. As a result the decision to intubate is an important one with delays likely to result in devastating consequences for the patient.]

COMPLICATIONS OF MECHANICAL VENTILATION

Complications of artificial airway

- Trauma of insertion
- Tracheal stenosis.

Complications of positive pressure ventilation

- Pneumothorax
- Pneumomediastinum
- Ventilator-associated lung injury
- Decreased cardiac output
- Fluid retention.

Complications of artificial ventilation

- Ventilator-associated pneumonia
- Oxygen toxicity
- Sedation-related ileus
- Stress ulcers
- Myopathy
- Psychosis.

MODES OF VENTILATION

These can be confusing, and classifications of them are usually unhelpful. Essentially, it is important to understand that other than the basic goal of delivering tidal volumes of respiratory gas to the lungs a certain number of times a minute, the different modes are aimed at:

- Facilitating the patient's spontaneous respiratory efforts
- Improving oxygenation in refractory hypoxaemic patients by increasing FiO_2 and/or positive-end-expiratory pressure (PEEP)
- Reducing hypercarbia by increasing tidal volume or respiratory rate
- Limiting dangerously high airway pressures.

■ Identifying respiratory distress

Signs of respiratory distress are one of the earliest indicators of impending critical illness, as well as the major determining factor of the need for mechanical ventilation. They are:

- Tachypnoea
- Tachycardia
- Agitation, confusion or coma
- Use of accessory muscles of respiration
- Difficulty speaking
- Rapid shallow breathing
- Cardiovascular instability
- Refractory hypoxaemia (e.g. $SpO_2 < 90\%$ despite 100% oxygen).

A patient with any of the following is potentially seriously ill and requires **immediate** treatment:

- Respiratory rate > 30 or < 8
- Unable to speak half a sentence
- Agitation or coma
- Refractory hypoxaemia (e.g. $SpO_2 < 90\%$ despite 100% oxygen).

Unless such patients improve rapidly they are likely to require intubation and ventilation in the near future. In the setting of respiratory distress, agitation or coma are particularly worrying, as they make it very difficult to manage the patient without securing the airway.

[Note: $SpO_2 < 90\%$ in a patient not known to have COPD requires immediate correction, as further desaturation is likely to be rapid. Additionally, a satisfactory SpO_2 reading does not rule out severe respiratory problems, as oxygen therapy can often maintain normal saturations until shortly before respiratory arrest occurs. The respiratory rate is a crucial component of monitoring the potentially unstable patient.]

■ Common postoperative pulmonary complications

Atelectasis: very common; may cause significant hypoxaemia. Prevent it by using incentive spirometry, deep breathing and adequate pain control.

Infection: including bronchitis and pneumonia.

Prolonged mechanical ventilation and respiratory failure.

Exacerbation of underlying lung disease.

Bronchospasm: may be secondary to medications (e.g. morphine) or exacerbation of an underlying pulmonary condition (COPD, asthma). Treat by removing any possible instigators, administer inhaled β2 agonists. Systemic steroids may be needed.

Pleural effusions: managed with observation in patients with otherwise uncomplicated course, especially if the effusion layers are <10 mm on the decubitus film. A sub-phrenic abscess should be considered when a pleural effusion develops ≥10 days after abdominal surgery and is associated with signs and symptoms of systemic infection.

Pulmonary oedema: may be cardiogenic, non-cardiogenic or a combination of both. Treat with oxygen, diuresis, and mechanical ventilation if indicated.

ANISHA TANNA AND RICHARD LEONARD

■ Renal dysfunction

Renal failure is a frequent problem in surgical wards and in the ICU. By far the commonest cause is acute tubular necrosis (ATN) resulting from inadequate renal perfusion, which in turn is usually due to a combination of:

- Hypovolaemia
- Hypotension
- Sepsis
- Nephrotoxic drugs
- Pre-existing renal disease.

In the case of sepsis, renal failure may occur as part of the syndrome of multiple organ dysfunction, when it carries a grim prognosis. However if the patient survives the acute illness, renal function usually recovers.

■ Oliguria

The initial manifestation of renal dysfunction is oliguria. **Urine output of less than 0.5 ml/kg/hr must be corrected.** If any underlying renal hypoperfusion can be corrected at an early stage, it may be possible to prevent the development of acute tubular necrosis. Management of oliguria should therefore be to:

- Correct hypovolaemia, if necessary using CVP guidance as described above.
- Correct hypotension and low cardiac output, using vasopressors or inotropes.

Hospital Surgery: Foundations in Surgical Practice, ed. Omer Aziz, Sanjay Purkayastha and Paraskevas Paraskeva. Published by Cambridge University Press.
© Cambridge University Press 2009.

In previously hypertensive patients it may be necessary to raise the blood pressure to levels close to their normal pressure (which may be higher than the usual target mean arterial pressure in ICU of around 70 mmHg). Only then can the kidneys autoregulate their blood flow, allowing renal perfusion to occur.

Use of other protective strategies is not founded on evidence of clinical benefit. In particular, low-dose '*renal' dopamine* has recently been shown to be ineffective in the critically ill. The use of *frusemide* to promote a diuresis is common, and though it appears not to affect the course of the disease, it does at least have the theoretical benefit of reducing renal oxygen consumption and protecting the struggling kidney against ischaemia. However, **it is essential to correct hypovolaemia first. One of the commonest errors in surgical management is the use of frusemide to treat oliguria caused by hypovolaemia. Do not commit it.**

In a surgical patient, the other common causes of oliguria are:

■ Urinary obstruction, of which the commonest cause by far is a blocked catheter.
■ Sodium and water retention due to the neuroendocrine stress response to surgical trauma.

If oliguria persists despite the above measures, established renal failure is likely. A high urinary sodium (>20 mmol/l) or a low urinary osmolality (280–320 mOsm/l) in the absence of recent diuretic use are suggestive of renal failure. **The advice of an intensivist or nephrologist is necessary**. During this time:

■ Maintain euvolaemia, which will usually involve fluid restriction to 20 ml/hr plus the previous hour's output. Avoidance of fluid overload is much more important in patients who are not ventilated.
■ Monitor closely for hyperkalaemia and metabolic acidosis.
■ Measure serum creatinine and urea twice daily.

Renal replacement therapy in the form of haemofiltration or haemodialysis is indicated for:

- Hyperkalaemia
- Acidosis
- Fluid overload
- Inexorably rising creatinine.

Once dialysis is inevitable there is nothing to be gained from procrastination, and it should be instituted without delay.

Surgical juniors are usually called to see patients with the following common renal problems: reduced urine output, raised creatinine and hyperkalaemia.

For all renal conditions in surgical patients, including the three above, it is important to remember the types of renal failure:

1. Pre-renal: hypotension/dehydration, sepis, iatrogenic under filling.
2. Renal: toxins, e.g. NSAIDs, ACE inhibitors, antibiotics (especially gentamicin).
3. Post-renal: urinary tract outflow obstruction – prostatic disease, blocked catheter, clot retention etc.

How to assess patients with failure; evaluate the following:

1. Fluid balance: skin turgor, JVP/CVP, pulse, BP, check for pericardial rub or other signs of pericarditis or pericardial effusion (will need dialysis).
2. Cognitive state – declines with uraemia.
3. Urine output.
4. Drug chart for potential causes and to change doses of renally handled medications still needed e.g. renal dose antibiotic prescription.
5. Previous blood results/imaging and renal investigations, especially baseline creatinine.

■ Management

1. *Patient*: move to area of close monitoring; ensure rehydration if under filled; if postoperative bleeding then give blood and call senior

surgeon involved for assessment to go back to theatre; urinary catheter and careful fluid balance recording; if overloaded consider frusemide bolus/infusion; regular assessment; consider early central access (CVP line).

2. *Electrolytes*: hyperkalaemia: ECG and cardiac monitor. Consider 10 ml 10 % calcium gluconate as soon as possible for cardioprotection and then 10–15 U of actrapid insulin in 50 ml of 50 % dextrose with regular blood glucose monitoring. Acidosis: if bicarbonate is less than 20 and patient is clinically dehydrated consider physiological strength sodium bicarbonate (1.26 %, 500 ml to 1000 ml over 6–12 hours, depending on volume and cardiac status) and call renal team as soon as possible.

3. *Medication*: stop renotoxic drugs e.g. NSAIDs and ACE inhibitors. Alter (reduce) doses of renally handled drugs.

4. *Investigations:*
   a. Urine (MC&S and electrolytes and osmolality)
   b. Bloods (FBC, U&E, clotting, renal screen if appropriate)
   c. CXR – check for volume overload
   d. Renal USS – exclude obstruction.

Regular assessment and reassessment is vital. If there is no improvement in the urine output, or if the creatinine continues to rise, or hyperkalaemia persists despite treatment, contact senior member of renal team or ICU as soon as possible.

■ Indications for dialysis

- Persistent acidosis
- Persistent hyperkalaemia
- Symptomatic uraemia
- Persistent oliguria/anuria (where simple causes are excluded)
- Persistent fluid overload.

■ Key points

1. Urine output of <0.5 ml/kg/hr represents oliguria and must be corrected.
2. Do not treat hypovolaemia with frusemide.
3. Low dose 'renal' dopamine is ineffective.
4. Careful clinical examination and regular assessment and reassessment along with the use of appropriate investigations will ultimately work to avoid ATN.

Critical care: other considerations

PARASKEVAS PARASKEVA AND RICHARD LEONARD

■ Acute neurological problems

Surgical trainees will encounter many patients with an acutely depressed conscious level resulting from:

- Trauma
- Drugs
- Acute intracranial event (e.g. infarction, haemorrhage)
- Encephalopathy of critical illness.

There are two important points to make:

- Never forget to check the blood sugar level.
- Any patient with a Glasgow coma score (GCS) < 8 or who fails to localize to pain requires intubation and ventilation, as well as investigation and specific treatment.

There is a tendency to try and avoid intubating such patients pending investigation. Unless the patient should not have active management of an intra-cranial disaster under any circumstances (in which case investigation is pointless), this is a mistake. **A patient with a GCS < 8 needs to be intubated.** If a CT scan shows an unrecoverable situation, then treatment can be withdrawn at that point as described in the introduction.

■ Nutrition

Nutritional support is needed when the patient is unlikely to resume normal oral intake within 7–10 days of it ceasing. If nutritional support is inevitable it should be started as soon as the patient is stabilized.

Hospital Surgery: Foundations in Surgical Practice, ed. Omer Aziz, Sanjay Purkayastha and Paraskevas Paraskeva. Published by Cambridge University Press. © Cambridge University Press 2009.

The timing of commencement of feeding is often a bone of contention between surgeons and intensivists. A mutually acceptable compromise can usually be worked out.

PREFERRED ROUTES FOR FEEDING

The ideal route of nutrition is the subject of much dogma and little evidence. There is no doubt that enteral feeding is cheaper and easier, and therefore preferable. The evidence for a protective effect on the intestinal mucosa is much weaker than commonly realized, and the complications of enteral feeding are generally under-reported in the literature. In particular, enteral feeding has been definitely established as an independent risk factor for ventilator-associated pneumonia. Thus it is a reasonable position to consider parenteral feeding in patients whose ability to tolerate enteral feeding within seven days is in serious doubt. In the meantime strenuous efforts should be made to establish enteral feeding. When nasogastric feeding is not tolerated despite the use of prokinetic agents, a nasojejunal tube is often successful. This route is now commonly used in patients with pancreatitis. Traditionally, such patients were fed parenterally, but jejunal feeding is now known to be safe and perhaps associated with better outcomes.

COMPOSITION OF FEED

The optimal content of feeding solutions is also uncertain. Carbohydrates, essential lipids, protein, vitamins and trace elements are needed, and it is clear that there is an upper limit to the amount of both energy and protein which the body can use. Excessive feeding is at least as dangerous as under feeding. There is a vogue for the use of regimes which contain immunologically active nutrients such as arginine, glutamine, RNA and omega-3 fatty acids. These feeds are expensive and the methodology of some of the studies evaluating them is poor.

■ General considerations

Much of Intensive Care medicine consists not of the melodrama surrounding admission and resuscitation but rather of the mundane, unexciting but nonetheless vital process of nursing patients back to health. This aspect requires meticulous attention to detail, and is as important as the initial resuscitation. Four areas deserve mention:

- **Nosocomial infection** with resistant organisms is an enormous problem in ICU. *Infection control measures must be adhered to*; surgeons who think themselves above such concerns are putting all their patients at risk and will incur the anger and contempt of ICU staff. The following minimum measures must **always** be applied:
  - Wash hands before and after touching any patient.
  - Wear gloves and plastic apron when examining a patient, and wash hands afterwards.
  - Use full sterile technique as for a surgical procedure when inserting a central venous catheter, whether in ICU or on the wards. This reduces catheter-related bacteraemia rates 6-fold, and it is indefensible not to do so.
- **Thromboembolism prophylaxis:** this is needed for most patients. Subcutaneous heparin is appropriate for the majority. Compressive stockings may be useful.
- **Stress ulcer prophylaxis** is also necessary at least until enteral feeding is established. Proton pump inhibitors (PPIs) are the drug of choice for this. If the patient has no history of or special risk factors for peptic ulceration then feeding alone is adequate protection.
- **The patient's family** is in an extremely stressful situation. Frequent communication and support can alleviate this to some extent. Good communication early on can make subsequent management of difficult decisions much easier. While this can sometimes be burdensome to ICU staff, it is also one of the most rewarding aspects of the specialty.

■ Key points

1. Patients with a GCS < 8 who merit active treatment must be intubated.
2. Always check a blood sugar level in an unconscious patient.
3. Enteral feeding should usually be started once the patient is stabilized.
4. Infection control measures must be adhered to.
5. Time spent talking to patients' families is time well spent.

Postoperative complications

DAVID JAMES AND OMER AZIZ

A careful appreciation and understanding of postoperative complications that a patient may face during their recovery period is required by clinical staff in order to respond early and reduce associated morbidity.

■ Classification

This can be done:

1. **Temporally:** *immediate* (<24 hours); *early* (<30 days); *late* (>30 days).
2. **By type of complication:** complications of anaesthesia; general complications of surgery; complications specific to type of surgery.

■ Common presentations

Postoperative pyrexia: *Day 0–2:* atelectasis, response to trauma (beware of aspiration pneumonia). *Day 3–5:* UTI, wound infection, cannula site infection, catheter-related sepsis. *Day 5–10:* wound infection, anastomotic leak, intra-abdominal abscess, DVT/PE (beware of acute acalculous cholecystitis in ICU/HDU (high dependency unit) patients). *Weeks/months:* prosthesis/implant-related infections.

Postoperative pain: best to avoid this with adequate planning of a patient's analgesic requirement. Pain can significantly affect recovery by: impaired respiratory function (reduced breathing, coughing and secretion clearance), reduced mobility (increases DVT/pressure sore risk), increased cardiac output (myocardial oxygen demand), impaired bowel function, urinary retention and anxiety. For analgesic recommendations see the Pain Control Chapter. *Calf pain* – beware of DVT (see Haematological Considerations Chapters).

Hospital Surgery: Foundations in Surgical Practice, ed. Omer Aziz, Sanjay Purkayastha and Paraskevas Paraskeva. Published by Cambridge University Press. © Cambridge University Press 2009.

Poor urine output: *oliguria* is defined as a urine output of ≤ 30 ml/hr. *Anuria* means no urine production at all. Most common causes include a blocked urinary catheter, poor fluid replacement (dehydration), or acute renal failure following direct renal injury due to drugs, prolonged hypoperfusion during surgery, transfusion or trauma. Each of these should be ruled out with bladder washout, fluid challenge, and serum urea, creatinine and electrolyte measurement, respectively.

Shortness of breath: important causes include fluid overload (and LVF), pneumonia, PE, unrecognized COPD, pneumothorax (particularly following CVP line, thoracic surgery and thoracic drain insertion). Early intervention by sitting patient up, oxygen therapy, and prompt examination (chest auscultation) with appropriate investigation (ABG, CXR).

Tachycardia $+/-$ **hypotension:** beware of postoperative haemorrhage, sites of trauma, or unrelated haemorrhage, and look for sites of bleeding (including po/pr/pu). Also consider cardiogenic causes (MI, arrhythmia), PE, pain, anaphylaxis secondary to drugs (See Shock Chapter). Adequate iv access and resuscitation is mandatory.

Chest pain: beware of angina and MI. Prompt examination and investigation with ECG is the least that should be done. If suspicious of cardiac disease, sublingual GTN may be both diagnostic and therapeutic and serum troponin can be performed (not usually raised within first eight hours). Seek early cardiology advice. Gastritis and PUD may also present in which case use alginates such as Gaviscon and a PPI (lansoprazole).

Confusion: patient may be agitated, disorientated, aggressive, have lowered level of consciousness or perceptual abnormalities. Common causes include hypoxia, drug-related (opiates), infections, urinary retention, renal failure, hepatic disease, CVA, endocrine cause.

Nausea and vomiting: beware of mechanical obstruction (adhesional), paralytic postoperative ileus (commonly within the first three days), opiate-induced ileus and drug reaction. Early examination with avoidance of oral intake, NGT, iv resuscitation and anti-emetic treatment (with cyclizine 50 mg tds iv/im or metoclopramide 10 mg iv/im tds) may be used to manage this.

Wound complications: *wound dehiscence* following laparotomy may be due to inadequate closure, poor healing, or wound infection. An early warning sign is a serosanguinous (pink) discharge from the wound followed by separation at days 7–10. This is a serious complication associated with significant mortality (up to 30 %). *Infections* begin as erythema and cellulitis around the wound, eventually resulting in purulent discharge associated with fever. Deep wound infections may require exploration under either LA or GA. Early bacterial swabbing and culture, adequate cleaning and drainage, and antibiotic treatment are all important.

Postoperative bleeding: this may be classified as: *primary haemorrhage* that starts during or very shortly after surgery, directly from operative site, usually due to inadequate haemostasis or rise in blood pressure postoperatively. If continuous and not reducing it requires re-operation and haemostasis. Resuscitate patient and use blood products if necessary. *Secondary haemorrhage* occurs after 7–14 days, usually due to infection. Resuscitate and arrange for blood products as above.

Classification of general complications of surgery	
Immediate	Haemorrhage Allergic reaction Primary haemorrhage
Early	Secondary haemorrhage Atelectasis Anastomotic breakdown Wound dehiscence/infection UTI Chest infection DVT/PE
Late	Chronic infection (prosthesis) Disease recurrence (cancer) Scar (keloid/hypertrophic) Psychological

Examples of complications specific to types of surgery

Bowel resection	Anastomotic leak Intra-abdominal abscess Incisional hernia Disease recurrence (cancer)
Laparoscopy (pneumoperitoneum)	Visceral damage Air embolism Hypercapnoea/acidosis Arrhythmias/vagal reaction Atelectasis
Laparoscopic cholecystectomy	Bile duct injury/stricture/leak Cystic artery haemorrhage
Thyroidectomy	Haematoma Tracheal compression Nerve injury (recurrent laryngeal)

Surgical drains

TIM BROWN AND OMER AZIZ

■ Definition

A material (such as tubing, sheet, gauze, or sponge) inserted into a wound or cavity to facilitate discharge of fluid, gas or purulent material from that cavity. An ideal drain is easily managed by both staff and patient, easily removed, inexpensive, safe (preventing introduction of infection and damage to surrounding structures), and allows adequate cavity drainage.

Tubular drains are traditionally sized using the 'French' scale. 1 Fr = 0.33 mm.

■ Classification

1. OPEN VS. CLOSED

Open drains allow effluent to drain directly into overlying dressings or collecting appliances, i.e. 'open' to the environment. These are typically low pressure systems that rely on pressure gradients, capillary action or gravity to allow flow of material. Some open drains work by preventing wound closure and allowing fluid to exude around the drain (e.g. corrugated drain). *Advantages:* low pressure, therefore unlikely to cause surrounding tissue damage. No collecting system attached, allowing greater patient mobility. *Disadvantage:* they are open to air with the potential to introduce infection to the cavity being drained. *Examples:* 'wick drain' used for drainage of abscess cavities, 'corrugated drain' used for contaminated wounds and superficial cavities (see Figures 13, 14).

Hospital Surgery: Foundations in Surgical Practice, ed. Omer Aziz, Sanjay Purkayastha and Paraskevas Paraskeva. Published by Cambridge University Press. © Cambridge University Press 2009.

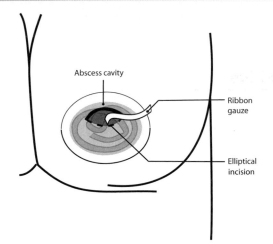

Abscess cavity

Ribbon gauze

Elliptical incision

Figure 13 Wick drain

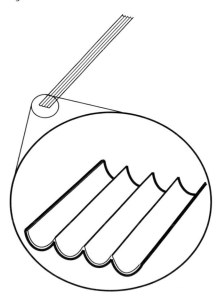

Figure 14 Corrugated drain

Closed drainage systems typically consist of a drainage tube, a connecting tube and a closed collection container, i.e. they are 'closed' to the external environment. They can be low or high pressure depending on whether the system is attached to a vacuum device. *Advantages:* closed systems tend towards lower infection rates than open systems. The collecting device can prevent caustic skin damage. They are cleaner, therefore potentially safer to ward staff. There is increased accuracy when measuring output. *Disadvantages:* usually more traumatic to insert and remove, closed system failure can lead to development of 'open' drainage system. *Examples* include 'Robinson's drain' used for prophylactic drainage of the abdominal cavity following surgery, 'radiologically guided' drains, 'T-tubes' draining the biliary tree, 'nasogastric tubes' and 'urinary catheter' draining the stomach (Figure 16) and bladder, respectively (Figure 15).

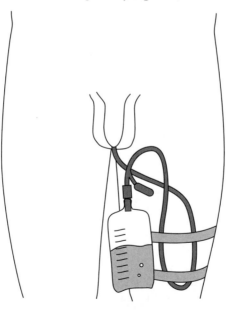

Figure 15 Urinary catheter

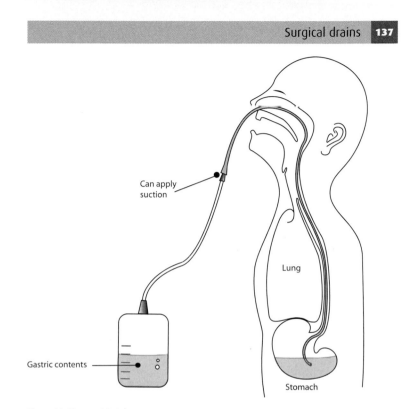

Can apply suction

Lung

Gastric contents

Stomach

Figure 16 Nasogastric tube

2. UNDERWATER SEAL DRAINAGE

This type of drainage system is used following chest drain insertion, with the drainage fluid or air passing through an underwater seal prior to entering the drain (Figure 17). This seal prevents the re-entry of air into the pleural space, preventing pneumothorax. Chest drain insertion and management is further described elsewhere in this book.

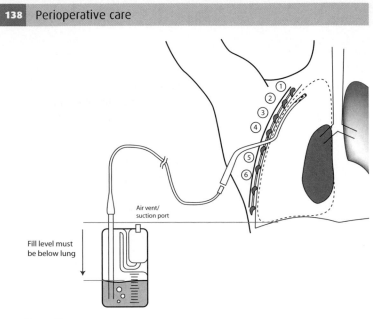

Figure 17

3. ACTIVE (SUCTION) VS. PASSIVE (GRAVITY)

Suction drainage systems are 'closed' systems that are connected to a vacuum device. This may be a vacuum drainage bag or a wall vacuum device. *Advantages:* negative cavity pressure prevents fluid accumulation within the cavity (e.g. haematoma or seroma formation). External pressure gradient theoretically prevents bacterial migration into the drainage cavity. Continuous suction can prevent build up of material that may precipitate and cause the drainage tube to become blocked. *Disadvantages:* the drain may erode into the cavity causing further complications. For example suction drains are not used in the abdominal cavity. Examples of suction drains include 'Redivac drains' used following breast and hernia surgery, and 'vacuum dressings' used for closure of large fascial defects in plastic surgery.

4. 'SUMP' SUCTION VS. 'CLOSED' SUCTION

The sump is the collection of fluid within a cavity that requires drainage. A sump drain has an inner and outer tube. The outer tube has air vents just proximal to the tip that encourage air flow into the emptying sump. The inner tube is connected to a wall suction device and drains the 'sump' and circulating air via a vacuum effect. The purpose of air flow into the sump cavity is to maintain a positive sump pressure. This will theoretically prevent cavity walls from collapsing onto the drainage tube as well as attempting to prevent solid tissue from blocking the drainage tube. *Advantages*: prevention of mechanical damage to surrounding tissue; other advantages of suction drainage. *Disadvantages*: 'open' drainage system, therefore has risk of introducing infection into the cavity. This risk can be minimized by the addition of a microbial filter device. The drain is connected to a wall-mounted vacuum device, thereby reducing patient mobility.

When are drains required?

To drain a collection of fluid or gas that may potentiate infection.
To remove dead space and promote wound healing.
To allow access to a body cavity (e.g. intrathecal drug administration).
To monitor leakage (e.g. volume of ascites after ascitic tap).
To relieve pressure within a closed system.
To allow injection of contrast into a system (T-tube cholangiogram).

Note: drainage is not a substitute for haemostasis.

■ When are they removed?

The simple answer is 'as soon as possible'. Time is proportional to complications and so when the drain has ceased to perform its job, it should be removed. Timing of drain removal is a very contentious issue and varies from surgeon to surgeon. If in any doubt, consult a senior member of the team before removing a drain. Once removed, it almost always cannot be easily re-inserted.

■ Drain management

When called about drain problems, a systematic approach is adopted. Remember to approach and think about the patient first and the drains second!

1. **Blocked drain**: when the output slows suddenly or stops, or if fluid starts to bypass the drain, there is a suspicion that the drain may be blocked. *Solution*: rule out mechanical blockage (e.g. kinked tube, tight suture). Ensure connectors are intact. Check for foreign material in the drain lumen. This may require aspiration, flushing or changing the apparatus. (NB only flush a drain under aseptic conditions and only after seeking senior advice.)

2. **Broken drain tubing, drain retraction, loosening or falling out.** *Solution*: re-secure the drain to the skin using an appropriate method. If the drain has fallen out, it is important to ensure that there are no drain fragments left within the cavity. Inspect the drain to ensure it is in its entirety. If in doubt, perform a radiograph looking for radio-opaque fragments. This problem may require exploration and/or re-insertion in theatre. Never attempt to re-insert a drain that has previously fallen out. This will be a dirty procedure and risks introducing micro-organisms into the patient.

3. **Loss of suction (vacuum drains):** this may be due to failure of the equipment, erosion into, or leak from, an air-containing cavity (e.g. bowel) or having a drainage hole migrating away from the skin. *Solution*: look very carefully at the drain system. Ensure that all connectors, seal caps and tubes are in their entirety and applied properly. Ensure that there are no drainage holes appearing through the wound. If an air leak is found in the drain apparatus, this should be replaced or occluded with adhesive tape. If no cause is found then investigation for a leaking viscus should be employed. Notify senior team member.

Abdominal stoma care

ELAINE CRONIN

■ Stoma classifications

There are three basic types of **eliminating** stomas:

Ileostomy: opening into the ileum (small intestine)
Colostomy: opening into the colon (large bowel)
Urostomy: opening into the urinary tract.

A fourth, but less common, eliminating stoma is that of a jejunostomy – an opening into the jejunum.

■ Different stoma types

1. Ileostomy: constructed mainly from terminal ileum. Usually sited in the right iliac fossa (RIF). Output is variable (loose/watery) but mostly a thick porridge consistency. Daily output is approximately 600–800 ml. An ileostomy is spouted, protruding 6–25 mm from the abdominal wall surface (Figure 18). A drainable bag is required. The bag is emptied 3–7 times in 24 hours. A low-fibre diet is recommended.
2. Colostomy: constructed from ascending, transverse, descending or sigmoid colon. Usually situated in the left iliac fossa. Output is thicker/more formed/contains less fluid. A colostomy is flush with the abdominal wall surface (Figure 18). A closed bag is required. The bag is changed 1–3 times in 24 hours. A high fibre, high fluid intake is usually recommended.
3. Urostomy/ileal conduit: constructed from 10–15 cm of ileum (implantation of the ureters into ileum). Usually situated in the RIF.

Hospital Surgery: Foundations in Surgical Practice, ed. Omer Aziz, Sanjay Purkayastha and Paraskevas Paraskeva. Published by Cambridge University Press. © Cambridge University Press 2009.

With a fluid intake of 2–2.5 litres a day, 1.5–2 litre output is expected. A Urostomy is spouted (6–25 mm). The mucosal lining produces mucus on a daily basis. A bag with a tap outlet is required. The bag is emptied 3–7 times in 24 hours. (Night drainage system is also used.) A high fluid intake is advised (to reduce the risk of infection).

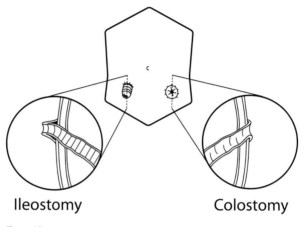

Ileostomy   **Colostomy**

Figure 18

■ End and loop stomas

End: a single segment of bowel (the afferent or proximal limb from the digestive tract) is exteriorized, i.e. following a Hartmann's procedure, abdominoperineal excision of rectum (APER) or panproctocolectomy.

Loop: two openings that sit side by side (the afferent or proximal limb from the digestive tract and the efferent/distal limb which opens into redundant intestine (ileum or colon) are exteriorized, e.g. covering loop ileostomy following anterior resection (an example of a *defunctioning stoma*), loop colostomy following procedures for the treatment of colo-vesical fistula, carcinoma of the rectum and perianal Crohn's disease).

■ Mucus fistula

The efferent/proximal limb that opens into redundant bowel is exterior-ized as a mucus fistula (mucus producing). It is usually situated at the bottom of the midline incision (e.g. following a sub-total colectomy) but can be found along the transverse or descending colon. Mucus is passed at irregular intervals (anteriorly and posteriorly) and a gauze/lint dress-ing or a small stoma bag (cap) is required.

■ How to site a stoma

The patient should be asked to lie semi-recumbent, sit forward and stand during which time the following anatomical features should be identified and avoided (see Figure 19).

- Umbilicus
- Bony prominences of the hip, rib cage and symphysis pubis
- The natural waistline
- Previous scars (dense scar tissue)
- Deep skin creases and fatty folds
- The groin flexure (on either side)
- Pendulous breasts.

The location of the abdominal incision (usually midline) must be taken into account so that the stoma is not placed in too close proximity to the wound. The patient's general physique should also be considered, i.e. BMI, any abdominal distension or pre-existing skin conditions (e.g. psoriasis).

NB: always site higher in those patients with abdominal distension since its position will fall postoperatively following bowel decompres-sion and a reduction of intra-luminal oedema. The optimal stoma site should (where possible) be visible and accessible to the patient either on standing or sitting and movement (i.e. bending, sitting) should not adversely affect the site.

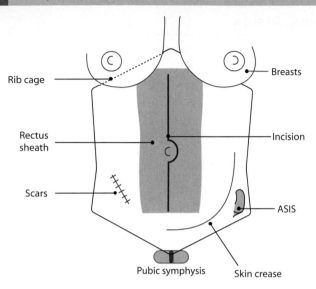

Rib cage

Breasts

Rectus sheath

Incision

Scars

ASIS

Pubic symphysis

Skin crease

Figure 19 Anatomical features to identify during stoma siting

■ Stoma sites

The ileostomy (RIF) and colostomy (LIF) are positioned one-third to half way between the umbilicus and the anterior superior aspect of the iliac crest. A transverse colostomy is positioned 5–8 cm below the lower rib cage (right or left) and either central to the umbilicus or to one side depending on disease type/location (i.e. tumour). The urostomy is positioned as for an ileostomy. Jejunostomies are usually constructed under emergency conditions and are therefore not sited preoperatively.

■ Stoma complications (immediate/early/late)

Necrosis: the blood supply to the stoma is compromised. The stoma will appear dusky initially and black when the mucosa becomes truly necrotic. Necrosis can occur during surgery or within 72 hours post-operatively. Surgical revision may be required.

Retraction: the stoma is pulled back below skin level (as a result of tension or inadequate bowel mobilization), making management and containment of faecal fluid difficult.

Muco-cutaneous separation: separation occurs between the bowel mucosa and the skin (can be partial or full – 360 degrees) creating a noticeable gap/defect. Faeces can irritate exposed nerve endings in this gap causing pain and discomfort. Occlusion therapy (i.e. Aquacel, cohesive) or Orabase paste are required for healing.

Stitch fistula: effluent seeps from the lumen of the bowel through a peristomal stitch site that has not closed/healed, pouring straight onto the abdominal surface.

Prolapse: the stoma (one or two limbs) falls out onto the exterior of the abdomen. The stoma becomes bulky and oedematous and the bowel is at risk of superficial necrosis or friction ulcers.

Herniation: an abnormal bulge develops around the stoma distorting the shape of the abdomen. The base of the stoma enlarges and stoma function often becomes erratic.

Stenosis: the lumen (opening) of the stoma becomes narrowed. Scar tissue continues to develop around the mucosal junction and evacuation becomes difficult. Laxatives (if a colostomy) are required to keep the output soft.

■ Product types

The diameter of the stoma should be measured so that the flange from the stoma bag fits snugly and does not leak (Figure 20).

1 Piece: the base (flange) and bag (closed, drainable or tap) are welded together as one inseparable unit. When the bag needs changing (as for a colostomy patient) the whole appliance is renewed. The adhesive needs renewal every 24 hours.

2 Piece: the base (flange) and bag (closed, drainable or tap) come as two separate units. One is joined to the other by way of a coupling mechanism. The flange can stay in place 3–4 days prior to renewal (it has a thicker adhesive). The patient changes the base 2–3 times a week, renewing the bag as often as required or as preferred.

Convex Product: used in the management of complex stomas (i.e. retracted, stenosed) where product adhesion and further stomal spouting is desired.

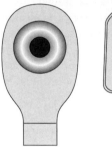

One piece   Two piece

Figure 20 Stoma bags

Trauma: adult trauma

ABOSEDE AJAYI AND PATRICIA WARD

■ An approach to managing the multiply-injured patient

The incidence of trauma (both blunt and penetrating) is rising in the UK. Associated with significant morbidity and mortality, trauma is the commonest cause of death in the first four decades of life and mostly affects people in their third decade. Males are more likely to be injured than females. Death from trauma follows a *tri-modal distribution* where 50 % of deaths occur at the time of trauma followed by another peak at an hour *(golden hour)* followed by a subsequent peak weeks or months later.

Trauma is frequently associated with multi-system injury. Such injuries may be difficult to identify and can be life threatening. The 'Primary survey' provides a simple and effective method for identifying and treating life-threatening injuries in the multiply-injured patient by treating the greatest threat to life first.

Assessment, investigation and treatment of the trauma patient are performed simultaneously. It may not be possible to take an accurate history until life-threatening problems have been addressed. Key information about mechanism of injury should be collected from paramedics who attended the scene. Several members of a 'trauma team' have specific roles using the same principles of trauma management under the guidance of an experienced Team Leader.

There are potential pitfalls with respect to the management of patients at the extremes of age, and pregnant women – this is because of altered physiology (senescent or iatrogenic).

Hospital Surgery: Foundations in Surgical Practice, ed. Omer Aziz, Sanjay Purkayastha and Paraskevas Paraskeva. Published by Cambridge University Press. © Cambridge University Press 2009.

■ Underlying principles

Systematic approach: ABCDEs.

Initial assessment and regular reassessment.

Correct life-threatening abnormalities before moving on to the next part of assessment.

Always assess the effect of any intervention or treatment.

Initial interventions should be considered to be 'holding measures' until definitive treatment can be initiated, which often involves operative intervention.

Recognize the need and ask for senior surgical opinion early.

Use and communicate effectively with all members of the trauma team.

If there is any deterioration in the patient's condition go back to the beginning of the system and reassess the patient.

■ Primary survey

AIRWAY WITH CERVICAL SPINE CONTROL

- Maintain inline spinal immobilization; either manually or with cervical collar, blocks and tape.
- Is the patient able to talk? If not, is there stridor, or paradoxical chest and abdominal movement?
- If the airway is compromised try jaw thrust/chin lift but **not** head tilt, and consider oropharyngeal or nasopharyngeal airway.
- If endotracheal intubation is required, inline C-spine immobilization **must** be maintained throughout.
- Give oxygen in high concentration (using mask with reservoir bag).

BREATHING

- Count the respiratory rate and attach oxygen saturation monitor.
- Look for signs of chest trauma: bruising, deformity, penetrating wounds, crepitus, and paradoxical movements.

- Look for signs of respiratory distress.
- Examine the chest comparing expansion, palpation, percussion and auscultation on both sides of the chest.
- Think of and treat tension pneumothorax (immediate needle decompression) and haemothorax (early chest drain).

CIRCULATION WITH HAEMORRHAGE CONTROL

- Assess patient's colour, skin temperature.
- Assess pulse rate, character, volume and blood pressure.
- 2 × large intravenous access and bloods for FBC, U&E, clotting, and crossmatch.
- Give warmed fluids and watch for a response.
- Examine the abdomen and limbs for sites of haemorrhage.
- Treat obvious haemorrhage with direct pressure and elevation.
- Splint obvious fractures. Splint pelvis (reduces blood loss).

DISABILITY (BRIEF NEUROLOGICAL ASSESSMENT)

- Use the Glasgow coma score (GCS) to assess consciousness.
- Pupils – size, reaction to light.

EXPOSURE/ENVIRONMENT/EVENTS

- Expose the patient fully to enable assessment of injuries.
- Do not allow the patient to become hypothermic, therefore make use of blankets and heating apparatus.
- Review the events of the trauma with the patient and any witnesses available.

INVESTIGATIONS IN THE PRIMARY SURVEY

- Arterial blood gas
- Exhaled CO_2 (end tidal pCO_2)

- ECG
- Urinary catheter
- NG tube
- **X-rays: AP chest X-ray, AP pelvis X-ray, lateral C-spine X-ray**
- Consider diagnostic peritoneal lavage (DPL) on abdominal USS (see Abdominal Trauma Chapters).

LOG ROLL

The timing of this is variable depending on the clinical status of the patient. The pelvis should be examined and fractures stabilized prior to the log roll.

The log roll requires a minimum of five people. The first coordinates the procedure and takes control of the head and neck of the patient by maintaining continuous inline cervical spine immobilization. Three assistants are responsible for rolling the trunk and legs. The fifth examines the neck, back and sacrum and performs a digital rectal examination. Other personnel can assist in the removal of clothing or equipment and in the application of any required dressings.

■ Secondary survey

This involves a brief history as indicated by the AMPLE below. This is then followed by a top-to-toe examination including otoscopy, rhinoscopy, digital rectal examination and insertion of a urinary catheter. The adage 'fingers and tubes in every orifice' is a useful reminder.

AMPLE history:

Allergies
Medication (i.e. drug history)
Past medical history
Last meal
Events.

Specific information regarding the mechanism of injury, some assessment of forces involved, time to extrication and time from the incident to arrival in hospital should be sought from the ambulance personnel. These can serve to predict patterns of injury as well as to serve as prognostic indicators.

PHYSICAL EXAMINATION

1. *Head and maxillofacial* – inspect and palpate for injuries (lacerations, contusions, fractures), pupils, GCS score, eyes (injury, acuity, contact lenses), gross cranial nerve function, ears and nose (CSF leak), mouth (injuries, loose teeth).
2. *C-spine and neck* – inspect for injury and tracheal deviation. Palpate (maintaining inline neck traction) for tenderness, swelling, deformity, subcutaneous emphysema, symmetrical pulses. Auscultate for carotid bruits. Lateral C-spine X-ray.
3. *Chest* – inspect and palpate thoracic cage for blunt/penetrating injury, use of accessory muscles, fractures (ribs, sternum and clavicle), and subcutaneous emphysema. Percuss for resonance. Auscultate for heart and breath sounds.
4. *Abdomen* – inspect anterior and posterior surface for blunt or penetrating injury, palpate for tenderness, guarding, rebound tenderness. Percuss to elicit peritonism. Auscultate for bowel sounds. Pelvic X-ray. DPL/USS if warranted. Consider abdominal CT if patient is stable.
5. *Perineum (rectum/vagina)* – look for contusions, haematomas, lacerations, rectal examination (bleeding, tone, bowel wall integrity, bony fragments, prostate position), vaginal examination (bleeding, lacerations).
6. *Musculoskeletal* – inspect and palpate upper and lower limbs for lacerations, contusions, fractures, bleeding, deformity and pain. Evaluate joints. Palpate peripheral pulses. Evaluate X-rays for fractures. Look for thoracic, lumbar and sacral spine injury (log roll). If in doubt X-ray to exclude fracture.

7. *Neurological* – GCS, upper and lower limb sensory and motor function (gross), look for localizing signs.

Careful documentation of findings and procedures is paramount and should be performed by a dedicated member of the trauma team.

RADIOLOGY

The use of radiological investigations and their timing can be difficult. Plain radiographs of the C-spine, chest and pelvis are imperative together with imaging of suspected long-bone fractures.

Ultrasound scan is helpful in assessing intra-abdominal injury. However, although sensitive, it is not very specific and is operator-dependent. It is generally accepted that the presence of free fluid on abdominal ultrasound acts as an indication for laparotomy. It is important to note that the absence of any positive finding on ultrasound does not exclude major intra-abdominal pathology.

Computed tomography should only be considered in the haemodynamically normal patient. The decision to undertake a transfer of a patient from the emergency department (to CT scanning or theatre) should always be made in consultation with senior doctors.

OTHER INVESTIGATIONS

Diagnostic peritoneal lavage is not commonly undertaken as it is less specific than ultrasound and computed tomography which have now largely superseded it. There are rare occasions when it may be appropriate to undertake diagnostic peritoneal lavage, but the procedure must always be performed by an appropriate operator.

■ Transfer

This needs to be safe, efficient and necessary, to a place where an appropriate level of care can be provided. This may be to the operating theatre or to an intensive care unit. An appropriate escort must accompany the patient. There needs to be a safe handover of the patient in terms of the history, initial findings, treatment and response thus far. It is often not possible to complete the secondary survey prior to transfer; it is therefore important that documentation of the injuries found, and their treatment up to that point are clear – including any items of the primary and secondary survey that have not been completed.

■ Potential pitfalls

There are certain groups of patients who may present potential difficulties in management due to altered physiological states.

Children: see *Paediatric Trauma* chapter.

Elderly: among this group there is a reduction in physiological reserve and therefore a decreased ability to deal with the physical challenges of trauma. Many will be on drugs (often numerous), which can impair the ability to produce an appropriate response to trauma; e.g. β blocker use will prevent an appropriate tachycardia in the hypovolaemic patient.

Pregnancy: in this context, although there are two patients, it is maternal health that is the first priority. The obstetric team and paediatricians should always be involved in the care of these patients. It is important to remember that the gravid uterus will cause compression of the IVC if the patient is supine. Therefore a wedge should be placed under the right hip to displace the uterus off the IVC, otherwise, manual manoeuvres can be employed. Pregnancy involves a relatively hypervolaemic state and therefore, haemorrhage may not be associated with any signs.

This chapter is an overview of these principles and offers an approach to managing the multiply-injured trauma patient. Participation on an *Advanced Trauma Life Support course* is recommended for trainees in relevant specialties.

Trauma: paediatric trauma

PRIYA BHANGOO

Trauma is the leading cause of death in childhood, with a higher incidence in boys, with road traffic accidents and falls accounting for 80 % of injuries. The initial assessment follows the same principles as in adults, the first priority being Airway, Breathing and then Circulation, but there are additional considerations at every step of the assessment.

Additional points to consider when preparing for the arrival of a paediatric trauma patient:

- Delegating team member roles: this is particularly important with children as not only are the trauma team present but the pediatricians, paediatric intensive care unit (PICU) staff and paediatric anaesthetists may all be present. Swift and clear team leadership is required to run an efficient trauma team, with relevant specialists called upon when required.

- Unlike adult trauma victims, childhood trauma also involves the parents. Early on the parent(s) needs to be cared for by a single delegated member of staff who can provide ongoing support to the family and also take a considered history during the resuscitation. Parents may often request to be present during the resuscitation; such requests need to be respected and given due care and consideration but reassessed repeatedly during the ongoing resuscitation. To calm children during a trauma, it may be helpful for a familiar voice and face (a single member of the family/friend) to be present at the head end of the child.

- Since children are usually under adult supervision, witnesses/parents often accompany the child to hospital. A clear history needs to be taken with due care and consideration documenting clearly not only

Hospital Surgery: Foundations in Surgical Practice, ed. Omer Aziz, Sanjay Purkayastha and Paraskevas Paraskeva. Published by Cambridge University Press. © Cambridge University Press 2009.

the event history, but also who is providing the history. This allows not only an appreciation of potential injuries but may also raise concerns regarding the possibility of non-accidental injury.

- Vital parameters vary with age. In all resuscitation rooms there should be easy access to normal values for respiratory rate, pulse rate and blood pressure. Become familiar with these before the child arrives as active resuscitation is dependent on these as well as a child's weight.

- Weight can be estimated from age or from head-to-toe length. The Broselow tape provides details of normal parameters for height as well as extensively detailing doses of medication and size of equipment required during a paediatric resuscitation. Easily memorizable formulae also provide similar guidance, e.g. Weight $= (age + 4) \times 2$.

- Children compensate for illness and injury more effectively than adults. They have a greater reserve to mask shock, whatever the aetiology. By careful repeated assessments, along with a high index of suspicion, the aim is to prevent the sudden deterioration from compensated shock to catastrophic decompensation.

■ Primary survey

Treat life-threatening conditions as they are encountered during the initial survey.

A useful mnemonic for possible aetiology:

A irway obstruction
T ension pneumothorax
O pen pneumothorax
M assive haemothorax
F lail chest
C ardiac tamponade.

■ 1. Airway with cervical-spine control

- **Oxygen** – high flow, 10–15 l/min through a face mask and reservoir bag. If, after further assessment, breathing is inadequate, bag and mask ventilation will be required.

- As with adult trauma. Collars are sized according to the size of the child's neck. A collar alone is insufficient, either sandbags or tape are required or in a smaller child manual immobilization is often better tolerated. If a child is uncooperative, senior judgement is required as to whether more harm than good is being done by forceful immobilization. It may be appropriate to immobilize the child, if there is a high index of suspicion, once the child is intubated and ventilated.

- The optimal airway position in a child is different from that of an adult. The neutral position is advocated as opposed to 'sniffing the morning air' in adults. This can be achieved either manually or with a small support placed under and at the level of the shoulders, thus reducing overextension at the neck. Jaw thrust and chin lift is done as for adults.

- Once optimal positioning is achieved the patency of the airway can be assessed.

- **Look** for effort of breathing/cyanosis, **listen** for breath sounds and voice, **feel** for breath.

- Airway adjuncts can be used to improve airway patency if tolerated:
  Oropharyngeal airways (Guedel) are sized from the level of the incisors to the angle of the jaw and are placed with the concave side nearest the roof of the mouth.

  Nasopharyngeal airways are often better tolerated, the estimated size is one that is the same as the patient's little finger. **Do not insert np airways when head injury is suspected**.

- Definitive airway if indicated – a secure tube placed within the trachea. This is done by an experienced member of the trauma team after discussion with the team leader:
  Endotracheal airway size: newborn size 3.0
  From age of 1 year: internal diameter size (mm) = (age/4) + 4
  Length (cms) = (age/2) + 12.

ANATOMICAL DIFFERENCES IN CHILDREN

Infants less than six months are obligate nasal breathers.
Relatively larger head and tongue.

Larynx is higher and epiglottis is proportionally bigger and horseshoe shaped.

Cricoid is narrowest part of the larynx which limits the size of the endo-tracheal tube (ETT). In adulthood, the narrowest part is at the cords, hence the use of uncuffed ETT in children to reduce ulceration and sub-glottic swelling.

C-spine: interspinous ligaments are more flexible, facet joints are flat, children have larger head compared to neck – all these result in greater flexibility and movement of the head on the neck. Spinal cord injuries without any evidence of a fracture are more common compared to adults. Bear this in mind when addressing potential C-spine injuries (SCIWORA – spinal cord injury without radiological abnormality).

■ 2. Breathing

- Assess respiratory effort as with adults, noting the normal rate corrected for age.
- **Look, feel, auscultate**.
- Check midline tracheal position – if deviated with evidence of pneumothorax (pushes trachea away) then immediate needle decompression required. A large bore cannula is inserted into the affected side, second intercostal space in the mid-clavicular line. This is then to be followed with insertion of a chest drain.
- Identify any life-threatening conditions and treat immediately.

T   ension pneumothorax
O   pen pneumothorax
M   assive haemothorax
F   lail chest.

ANATOMICAL DIFFERENCES IN CHILDREN

Relatively smaller upper and lower airways. Resistance to flow is inversely proportional to the fourth power of the radius (so halving the radius will result in a 16-fold increase in resistance); so small obstructions have significant effects on air entry.

Infants' ribs lie more horizontally, contributing less to chest expansion. They rely mainly on diaphragmatic breathing.

The majority of chest trauma in children is due to blunt injury, principally caused by road traffic accidents.

Children have a more pliable chest wall, this increases the frequency of pulmonary contusions without overlying rib fractures. When rib fractures do occur they indicate severe force.

Chest injuries are managed as with adults. Chest drains in adults are 28–32F size; in children the largest drain that fits between the rib spaces is used.

■ 3. Circulation with haemorrhage control

- Assess as with adults, noting the normal values corrected for age.
- In infants and children it is easier to assess the pulse at the brachial and femoral/carotid artery, respectively.
- Normal capillary refill is taken at the sternum for five seconds and should return within two seconds.
- Cool peripheries.
- Blood pressure: according to age. As a rough guide systolic BP $= 80 + (2 \times Age)$; diastolic 2/3 of this value.
- Intravenous access is gained as in adults but intraosseous (io) is considered in young children (<6 years of age) if iv access is poor (after two attempts) in an unwell child. The most common site is over the relatively subcutaneous area 1–2 finger breadths below the tibial tuberosity (venous cut down is another alternative although more time-consuming and requiring more skill).
- Request FBC, blood request (O negative, type specific and full crossmatch dependent on urgency) and bedside glucose test as a minimum.
- Fluid boluses: 10 ml/kg followed in quick succession by another 10 ml/kg.

  Circulation is then reassessed. If required, this is then repeated. Again reassess. When starting the third bolus, blood should be considered (10 ml/kg) **and urgent surgical opinion is needed.**

- Look for source of blood loss and aim to control it. Think of the body in compartments as you carry out your primary assessment; blood can be lost into any of these and may not be recognized unless actively looked for.

Thoracic cavity, abdominal cavity, pelvic cavity, long bones, and don't forget to look on the floor!

ANATOMICAL DIFFERENCES IN CHILDREN

A child's circulating volume per kg of body weight (70–80 ml/kg) is greater than an adult, but the actual total volume is small.

Heart rate contributes significantly to their ability to compensate; BP fall is a much later sign of shock relative to adults.

Pain relief is particularly important after gaining iv access. Children become much more cooperative when they are comfortable; as they get older their compliance improves with their comprehension.

■ 4. Disability (brief neurological assessment)

- Hypotension and hypovolaemia must be corrected to prevent secondary injury to the brain.
- Assess neurological status using the modified paediatric Glasgow coma score which changes the verbal component in those under the age of four years. A much simpler method is using the AVPU scale in which responding to pain only is equivalent to 8/15 GCS.
- Check papillary responses, fontanelle, lateralizing signs.

A – Alert; V – Verbal; P – Pain; U – Unresponsive.

■ Glasgow coma scale: document best score

- If each side is different document this clearly.
- Clearly specify score in each of eyes (E), verbal (V), and motor (M) response.

Glasgow Coma Scale		
Eye opening		Score
Spontaneously		4
To speech		3
To pain		2
Nil		1
Best motor response		Score
Obeys command		6
Localized stimulus (above level of clavicle)		5
Withdraws		4
Abnormal flexion		3
Extensor response		2
Nil		1
Verbal response >4 yrs	<4 yrs	Score
Orientated	Appropriate words, smiles, follows	5
Confused	Cries but consolable	4
Inappropriate words	Persistently irritable	3
Incomprehensible words	Restless and agitated	2
Nil	None	1
Reprinted with permission from Elsevier © 1974		

ANATOMICAL DIFFERENCES IN CHILDREN

Although uncommon, and unlike adults, children may become hypotensive after a head injury. Fontanelles and mobile cranial sutures are more tolerant of expanding intra-cranial lesions. Patients with bulging fontanelles, in the absence of coma, should be treated as having a more severe injury.

■ 5. Exposure

- Keep children warm from early on in resuscitation with warm/heated blankets.
- Manage as with adults.

ANATOMICAL DIFFERENCES IN CHILDREN

Ratio of a child's body surface area to blood volume is highest at birth, diminishing as child grows. Children subsequently become hypothermic more quickly than adults.

■ Investigations in the primary survey

Invasive procedures are avoided unless necessary and this is dependent upon clinical indication:

- Blood glucose
- X-rays – chest, pelvis, C-spine: AP and lateral (+ peg view if >8 years)
- Urinary catheter – NG tube used to catheterize
- ECG
- Remaining investigations as with adults.

Log roll – number of people required is dependent on size of child. Take this opportunity to examine not only the spine but also the back of the head and limbs, clearly documenting the presence or absence of injuries. Rectal examination although performed in adults is rarely indicated in children.

■ 6. Secondary survey and AMPLE history

See adult trauma section.

■ 7. Further investigations, transfer and definitive care

See adult section.

■ 8. Non-accidental injury

This should be suspected if:

- There is delay in seeking medical help
- Vague, or inconsistencies in re-calling events, either from the same or different people

- Repeated presentations in different emergency departments
- Inappropriate parental behaviour and interaction with the child
- Discrepancy between injuries and history
- Concerning injuries and patterns: bites, burns in unusual sites, perianal or genital injuries
- Injuries of different ages
- Injuries inconsistent with the child's developmental age.

Paediatric trauma victims are not only challenging due to the anatomical and physiological differences, but also psychologically. A de-briefing session should be offered to all staff after the resuscitation to discuss management issues as well as coping with potentially traumatizing experiences.

This chapter is based on the principles advocated on Advanced Trauma Life Support and Advanced Paediatric Life Support courses.

Trauma: trauma scoring systems

ABOSEDE AJAYI AND PATRICIA WARD

Trauma scoring refers to the use of physiological and anatomical parameters as prognostic indicators in trauma. *Physiological scoring systems* incude the Glasgow coma scale (GCS), Revised trauma score, and Trauma and injury severity score (TRISS). *Anatomical scoring systems* include the Abbreviated injury score (AIS) and Injury severity score (ISS). While no single system is accepted as the gold standard some important examples are given below:

■ Glasgow coma score

(Note that a score of <8 indicates need for definitive airway such as endotracheal tube.)

Feature	Scale responses	Score notation
Eye opening	Spontaneous	4
	To speech	3
	To pain	2
	None	1
Verbal response	Orientated	5
	Confused conversation	4
	Words (inappropriate)	3
	Sounds (incomprehensible)	2
	None	1
Best motor response	Obey commands	6
	Localize pain	5
	Flexion – normal	4
	– abnormal	3
	Extend	2
	None	1
Total coma 'score'		3/15–15/15

Hospital Surgery: Foundations in Surgical Practice, ed. Omer Aziz, Sanjay Purkayastha and Paraskevas Paraskeva. Published by Cambridge University Press. © Cambridge University Press 2009.

■ Revised trauma score

One commonly used system is the revised trauma score, which can be used as a triage tool, and has been shown to have high inter-rater reliability. As with most scoring systems it is based on physiological parameters as at the time of presentation. A composite of scores, given for respiratory rate, systolic blood pressure and Glasgow coma score, is calculated. It is heavily weighted towards the Glasgow coma score to compensate for major head injury in the absence of multi-system injury or major physiological changes. The probability of survival rises with trauma score. Various threshold values have been suggested to demand treatment of patients at a fully equipped trauma centre.

Revised trauma score		
Component	Finding	Score
A Respiratory rate (breaths/min)	10–29	4
	>29	3
	6–9	2
	1–5	1
	0	0
B Systolic BP (mmHg)	>89	4
	76–89	3
	50–75	2
	1–49	1
	0	0
C GCS score conversion	13–15	4
	9–12	3
	6–8	2
	4–5	1
	<4	0
Revised trauma score (A + B + C)		

■ Paediatric trauma score

There are important physiological and anatomical differences between adults and children which make trauma scoring difficult. These relate to body surface area, different size and shape of the airway and different

Assessment component	Score		
	+2	+1	−1
Weight	>20 kg	10–20 kg	<10 kg
Airway	Normal	Oral or nasal airway	Intubated/surgical airway
Systolic BP	>90 mmHg; good peripheral pulses and perfusion	50–90 mmHg; carotid/femoral pulses palpable	<50 mmHg; weak or absent pulses
Consciousness	Awake	Obtunded	Coma/unresponsive
Fracture	None seen/suspected	Single, closed	Open or multiple
Cutaneous	None visible	Contusion, abrasion, laceration <7 cm not through fascia	Tissue loss, any gun shot wound/stab wound, through fascia
Totals			

Paediatric trauma score

Reprinted with permission from Elsevier © 1987

ranges of physiological parameters such as heart rate, respiratory rate and blood pressure.

The respiratory rate observed may or may not represent respiratory compromise e.g. in the crying or frightened child. Assessment of the Glasgow coma score requires knowledge of the normal behaviour of a child of any given age, and in the pre-verbal child it is even more difficult to determine. The paediatric trauma score represents the sum of the severity of grade of each category and has been demonstrated to predict potential for death and severe disability.

■ Injury severity score (ISS)

This is an anatomical scoring system that provides an overall score for patients with multiple injuries. An *Abbreviated injury scale (AIS) score* is assigned to each injury, allocated to one of six body regions (head, face, chest, abdomen, extremities and pelvis, external). Only the highest AIS score in each body region is used. The three most severely injured body regions have their score squared and added together to produce the ISS score. The ISS takes some time to formulate so is not a useful triage tool, but it has important uses as a prognostic indicator as it correlates with morbidity, hospital stay and mortality. Ranging from 0–75, a score of <15 points, for example, indicates a better prognosis than one of >56 points.

Trauma: traumatic brain injury

ANDREAS DEMETRIADES AND JOAN GRIEVE

■ Introduction

Head injury can be defined as any alteration in mental or physical functioning related to a blow to the head. The most affected are young adults and societal cost is significant (emotional and financial), estimated at $25 billion per annum in the USA alone, excluding inpatient costs.

■ Classification

- Neurological impairment: **mild** (GCS 14–15), **moderate** (GCS 9–13) or **severe** (GCS 3–8). See Trauma Scoring Systems Chapter for GCS.
- Anatomical: **focal** (extradural, subdural and intra-cerebral haematoma) vs. **diffuse** (concussion, multiple contusions, diffuse axonal injury (DAI), hypoxic injury).
- Mechanism: **blunt** vs. **penetrating**.

■ Incidence

180–220 cases per 100 000 population (US), approximately 600 000 each year. Of these 10 % are fatal, 75 % are minor, the remainder equally divided between moderate and severe. Males are affected more than females (2:1) and it is commoner in the under 35s.

■ Aetiology

Road accidents are the commonest cause. Also falls, occupational injuries, sports and leisure accidents. Violence and penetrating trauma increases in cities with a population >100 000.

Hospital Surgery: Foundations in Surgical Practice, ed. Omer Aziz, Sanjay Purkayastha and Paraskevas Paraskeva. Published by Cambridge University Press. © Cambridge University Press 2009.

■ Pathophysiology concepts

Monro-Kelly doctrine: total intra-cranial volume (1500 ml) is *fixed* due to the inelastic nature of the skull and is composed of brain (85–90%), blood (10%), and CSF (<3%). Cerebral oedema, haemorrhage, focal haematoma and hydrocephalus increase these components. An increase in one of these compartments will require a compensatory decrease in the others in order to maintain intracranial pressure (ICP). Normal ICP = 10–15 mmHg. At the point where the compensatory mechanisms are exhausted, ICP exponentially rises (see Figure 21).

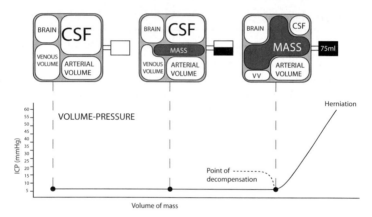

Figure 21

Compliance: the change in volume per change in pressure. Brain compliance is limited and volume changes from oedema or haematoma are not easily tolerated.

Cerebral blood flow (CBF): the critical parameter for brain function and outcome following trauma. CBF can only be measured continuously by invasive means. It is, however, dependent on cerebral perfusion pressure.

Cerebral perfusion pressure (CPP) = mean arterial pressure (MAP) – ICP.

Autoregulation: CBF is maintained in the normal brain when MAP is 50–150 mmHg. Below 50 mmHg there is a risk of ischaemia and above 150 mmHg a risk of high ICP caused by pressure-passive flow. In traumatic brain injury (TBI) autoregulation is often impaired when CBF becomes directly dependent on CPP.

■ History

A complete history may be impossible and collateral history (family, witnesses and paramedics) is therefore crucial. Consider non-accidental injury in children and discuss with appropriate authorities (subdural haematomas of different ages, bilateral or multiple skull fractures, retinal haemorrhages and contusions). Consider mechanism of injury: could there be associated injuries? (e.g. cervical spine). Establish degree of retrograde and antegrade amnesia. Past medical history should include investigation of the cause of traumatic brain injury (e.g. arrhythmia, epilepsy), establishing co-existing disease (diabetes, coagulopathy) and alcohol intake – **never** assume that decreased GCS is due to alcohol and always look for a head injury. Allergies and tetanus status are important.

■ Symptoms

Headache, nausea, vomiting, focal neurological symptoms (weakness, dysphasia, sensory changes, double vision) may all lead to suspicion of TBI. Ask about symptoms of skull fracture (otorrhoea, rhinorrhoea) and seizures (collateral history).

■ Signs

Vital signs: heart rate, blood pressure, Glasgow coma scale (GCS)
Eyes: pupil size and symmetry (consider third nerve palsy or local orbital trauma), extraocular eye movements, visual fields and acuity, and fundoscopy

Neurological assessment: cranial nerves, limb tone, power, coordination, reflexes and sensation. Gait if appropriate

Signs of skull base fracture: haemotympanum, haemorrhage from ear, rhinorrhoea or otorrhoea (CSF will give a halo sign on blotting paper), anosmia, subconjunctival haemorrhage, *Battle's sign* (mastoid bruising from petrous temporal bone fracture) (see Figure 22) and *racoon eyes* (bilateral periorbital bruising (see Figure 23)).

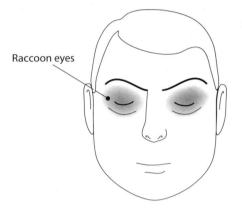

Figure 22

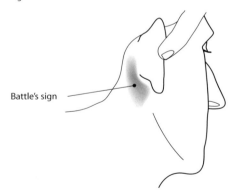

Figure 23

■ Investigation

Blood tests: FBC, U&E, LFTs, G&S, glucose, blood alcohol level.

Urine toxicology screen.

Skull X-ray has been largely replaced by CT but may still have a role in penetrating injury to assess foreign body presence.

CT scan is the mainstay of TBI assessment. It is rapid, reliable and easily interpretable but patients must be fully assessed and stable prior to transfer.

■ NICE guidelines in England and Wales for brain CT with head injury (www.nice.org.uk)

- GCS < 13 at any point after the injury.
- GCS of 13 or 14 two hours after injury.
- Suspected open or depressed skull fracture.
- Any sign of basal skull fracture.
- Post-traumatic seizure.
- Focal neurological deficit.
- Retrograde amnesia (events before injury) over 30 minutes.
- Vomiting more than once.
- Amnesia or LOC with any of age > 65, coagulopathy or warfarinization.
- Dangerous mechanism of injury.

■ CT scan interpretation

Although the CT scan should always be seen and reported by a radiologist, below are a few things to look out for when commenting on the scan.

1. Examine bone windows for fractures.
2. Assess tissue windows for intra-axial haematoma (intra-cerebral, subarachnoid or intraventricular haemorrhage); extra-axial

haematoma (extra- or subdural); contusion with or without a contre-coup injury. Note that an acute subdural haematoma (freshly clotted blood) is more opaque on CT than a chronic subdural which is more liquid.

3. Check for intracranial air (pneumocephalus); hydrocephalus (temporal horn dilatation is often the earliest indicator); mass effect and midline shift; oedema and obliteration of the basal cisterns.

■ Other imaging

MRI has a limited role in acute trauma evaluation, however its greater anatomical accuracy is useful in the subacute stage to assess for small *contusions* and *diffuse axonal injury*, neuronal injury in the subcortical gray matter or brainstem due to rotational or acceleration/deceleration forces, which is often the cause of persistently low GCS with no significant injury visible on CT.

Types of brain haematoma (Figures 24–27)

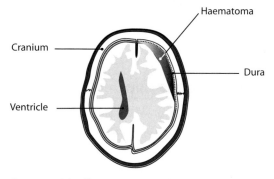

Figure 24 Subdural haematoma

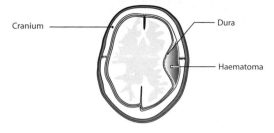

Figure 25 Extradural haematoma

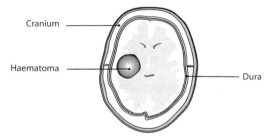

Figure 26 Intracerebral haematoma

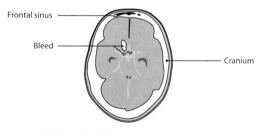

Figure 27 Subarachnoid haematoma

■ Management

MINOR HEAD INJURY

Admit for observations until the picture is any concern.

Indications for admission:

- Seizure
- Focal deficit
- ↓GCS
- Skull fracture
- Severe headache and vomiting
- Bleeding diathesis
- Difficulty in assessment e.g. alcohol, age, epilepsy, language barrier
- Social circumstances.

Regular neurological observations are essential.

If deterioration occurs:

- Resuscitate
- Discuss with a senior and/or neurosurgery
- Consider an urgent CT scan.

Discharge after 12–24 hours if the patient has GCS 15 and is asymptomatic with no focal neurological deficit. Otherwise consider CT scan. Ensure a responsible adult will be present for 24 hours following discharge. Give advice card warning of post-concussion symptoms. Ensure adequate analgesia.

MODERATE HEAD INJURY

ABCDE of ATLS protocol

All require CT scan

All require admission and observation

80 % will improve – manage as minor head injury

10–20 % will deteriorate – manage as severe head injury.

SEVERE HEAD INJURY

ABCDE of ATLS protocol.

Give oxygen and maintain full spinal precautions unless spinal injury excluded – always assume there is an associated neck injury.

Check breathing and provide assistance as necessary. Comatose patients will require intubation and ventilation to protect airway and maintain oxygenation.

Aim at pCO_2 of 4–4.5 kPa. Hypocapnia causes vasoconstriction. If patients are over-aggressively hyperventilated, the brain is made further hypoxic, compounding the primary injury.

Correct hypovolaemia.

Treat any cause of major continuing blood loss.

Urgent CT and discuss with neurosurgery.

Check BM and correct hypoglycaemia.

Give tetanus cover and iv antibiotics (cefuroxime 1.5 g) for compound skull fractures (check local policy).

Avoid nasogastric tube in skull base or facial fractures (use orogastric instead).

Clean and close scalp lacerations but not at the expense of CT or transfer to neurosurgery.

Treat seizures with iv diazepam 5–10 mg and load with phenytoin (15 mg/kg iv slowly with ECG and BP monitoring then 3–4 mg/kg as a single dose per day).

■ Further management

1. **Look closely for signs of raised ICP/herniation:** *Cushing's triad:* hypertension, bradycardia and reduced LOC suggest increased ICP. *Signs of raised ICP with a risk of imminent herniation* include a fixed and dilated pupil ipsilateral to pathology with contralateral (occasionally ipsilateral Kernohan's notch) hemiparesis (not always assessable). *In either case discuss immediately with neurosurgeon.*

2. **Consider the need for osmotic diuresis with mannitol:** (0.5 g/kg bolus or 200 ml of 20 % in adults). Note this is only a temporizing manoeuvre but may buy time to allow for neurosurgical transfer.

3. **Avoid causes of secondary brain injury:** hypoxia, hypotension, hyperthermia and infection.

4. **In intensive care units where intracranial pressure monitoring is used, CPP can be accurately controlled.** Aim at ICP < 25 and CPP > 65 mmHg. Maintain a head-up body tilt of 20–30 degrees.

■ Prognosis

Risk of *intracranial haematoma* after traumatic brain injury is as follows:

- GCS 15 with no skull fracture 1:6000
- GCS < 15 with no skull fracture 1:120
- GCS 15 with skull fracture 1:30
- GCS < 15 with skull fracture 1:4.

Up to 50 % may have late-onset epilepsy (>7 days from injury) after penetrating trauma. With *CSF fistula* 80 % of acute rhinorrhoea resolves within a week; *meningitis risk* with CSF leak is 10–15 %, but prophylactic antibiotics have not been proven to reduce this. *Post-concussion symptoms* (headache, dizziness, poor concentration, depression, lethargy) are common after head injury and may persist for months. Symptoms are exacerbated by alcohol, and decreased functional status will affect return to work, predisposing to stress and anxiety. 100 % of severe and approximately 65 % of moderate head injuries will not return to pre-morbid functional level due to permanent disability.

■ Head injury advice (on discharge)

Rest quietly and avoid alcohol for 48 hours.
A responsible adult should remain with you for the next 24 hours.

You should return to the hospital immediately if you:

1. Vomit more than twice
2. Become dizzy or develop a severe or persistent headache not relieved by normal painkillers (e.g. paracetamol)
3. Become restless or drowsy
4. Have a convulsion or fit or twitching of face, arms, legs etc.
5. Develop any sign of weakness anywhere in the body.
6. Have double vision or blurred vision.

Common symptoms (these may persist for some days) include:

1. Mild headache
2. Tiredness
3. Poor concentration
4. Mild memory loss.

Trauma: thoracic trauma

GEORGE KRASOPOULOS AND THANOS ATHANASIOU

Incidence: 10 % of all trauma cases. 25 % of trauma deaths in the United Kingdom.

Prognosis: less than 15 % of the victims with thoracic injuries require surgery and 80 % are managed conservatively with or without a chest drain. Overall mortality of 10 %.

Classification: injuries can be described broadly as due to *blunt trauma* and those due to *penetrating injuries* (gunshot or stab wounds).

Pathophysiology: blunt injuries may be more difficult to diagnose, often require additional imaging, and are mainly managed with simple interventions like intubation, ventilation and chest-tube insertion. In contrast, penetrating injuries are more likely to require emergency surgery. Patients with penetrating trauma generally deteriorate more rapidly and recover more quickly than patients with blunt injury.

Clinical features: major thoracic trauma can occur without chest wall damage, and the presence of other injuries may delay diagnosis, so high index of suspicion is paramount. The examination and diagnosis should be guided by mechanism and suspicion of injury rather than a direct manifestation.

Initial management and investigation: this follows the basic tenets of resuscitation of all critically injured patients as per ATLS guidelines. The primary goal is to provide oxygen to vital organs. Airway control (A), adequate breathing and ventilation (B), circulation and volume replacement (C) are the top priorities. The patient should be monitored with pulse oximetry and a cardiac monitor (ECG) to ensure adequate ventilation and look for common arrhythmias such as premature ventricular contractions and pulseless electrical activity (PEA). The first-line

Hospital Surgery: Foundations in Surgical Practice, ed. Omer Aziz, Sanjay Purkayastha and Paraskevas Paraskeva. Published by Cambridge University Press. © Cambridge University Press 2009.

approach to managing the clinical entities of thoracic trauma is given below. The cardiothoracic team should be involved early on.

■ Primary survey of life-threatening injuries

TENSION PNEUMOTHORAX

Thoracic injury resulting in a 'one-way valve' air leak through either the chest wall or from the lung itself; allows air to enter (but not leave) the thoracic cavity. This completely collapses the affected lung, displacing both mediastinum and trachea away from the affected side.

Clinical features: chest pain, shortness of breath, respiratory distress. Examination reveals tachycardia, hypotension, tracheal deviation away from the affected side, neck vein distension, absent breath sounds on affected side, and hyperresonance on percussion. *Tension pneumothorax is an emergency clinical diagnosis that should be acted on prior to CXR.*

Management: patient should be placed on high-flow oxygen and large-bore needle decompression (14G or 16G cannula) of the affected side in the second intercostal space anterior axillary line immediately performed. Follow with iv access and fluid resuscitation. Definitive treatment involves placement of a chest drain in the fifth intercostal space anterior axillary line on the affected side.

FLAIL CHEST

Occurs with two or more consecutive rib fractures in two or more places, resulting in an unstable thoracic wall segment. Subsequent paradoxical motion of this segment in relation to thoracic wall, and reduced chest expansion due to pain. If untreated results in respiratory failure and hypoxia. Associated with contusion of underlying lung and a haemo-pneumothorax.

Management: respiratory support (high-flow oxygen, positive-pressure ventilation or intubation) and analgesia. Gain iv access and fluid resuscitate but do not fluid overload as this is likely to precipitate pulmonary oedema. Arterial blood gas monitoring (arterial line insertion) and HDU admission mandatory. Normal chest wall stability restored within 5–10 days. Physiotherapy. Surgical repair rarely indicated.

OPEN PNEUMOTHORAX OR '*SUCKING CHEST WOUND*'

Results from a large chest wall defect through which air enters the thoracic cavity (if the opening is greater than the diameter of the trachea, air enters preferentially through this wound).

Management: high-flow oxygen, iv access, resuscitate. Close defect with a sterile occlusive dressing taped on three sides, acting as a valve allowing air to escape from the pleural space on expiration (see Figure 28), and insert a chest drain. Definitive closure is required.

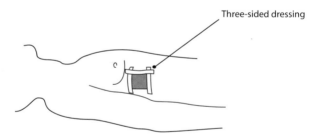

Three-sided dressing

Figure 28

MASSIVE HAEMOTHORAX

An accumulation of more than 1500 ml (or 1/3 blood volume) of blood within the thoracic cavity.

Clinical features: severe hypovolaemia with shock, flat neck veins (unreliable as tension pneumothorax may distend the neck veins), absent breath sounds or dullness to percussion.

Management: high-flow oxygen, large-bore iv access and volume replacement with colloid and crystalloid, and type specific blood.

Urgent blood crossmatch, FBC, U&E, clotting. Chest drain insertion on the affected side. Over 1500 ml blood drainage usually requires a thoracotomy so cardiothoracic team should be contacted immediately if this is suspected. Autotransfusion may also be set up to restore volume. Other indications for thoracotomy include continuing blood loss (200 ml/hr for 2–4 hours), requirement for repeated transfusion, persistent hypovolaemic shock, and penetrating chest-wall injuries (especially those between nipples anteriorly and scapulae posteriorly). *Thoracotomy should only be performed by a surgeon qualified to deal with and control the site of haemorrhage.*

CARDIAC TAMPONADE

The collection of blood within the pericardium (a fibrous sac surrounding the heart), resulting in inadequate cardiac filling and low cardiac output.

Clinical features: *Beck's triad* of raised JVP (raised CVP), hypotension and muffled heart sounds. Exaggerated *pulsus paradoxus* (systolic BP drops more than 10 mmHg during inspiration) and *Kussmaul sign* (paradoxical rise in CVP on inspiration) may be noted but are soft signs. Prompt echocardiogram (as part of a FAST scan) may be useful provided patient is stable. In PEA with the absence of hypovolaemia and tension pneumothorax, cardiac tamponade should be excluded.

Management: *pericardiocentesis* (see Pericardiocentesis Chapter) is diagnostic and therapeutic. Positive pericardiocentesis from trauma requires further surgical management by cardiothoracic team, either to fully drain blood with a pericardial window, or to perform emergency thoracotomy/sternotomy and pericardiotomy to inspect the heart. Note that the presence of clotted blood will result in ineffective pericardiocentesis and require emergency drainage by a qualified surgeon.

EMERGENCY THORACOTOMY

Indicated mainly for penetrating injuries with vital signs on presentation (survival 25 %). Any penetrating injury traversing the mediastinum is an indication for thoracotomy. It is not indicated for the vast majority of blunt injuries (mortality >98 %). The preferable incision is the 'clam-shell' as it can give you access to both pleural spaces and to the mediastinum. The possibility of survival is enhanced if it is performed by a cardiothoracic surgeon and in the operating theatre.

Indications:

- Cardiac arrest with penetrating injury
- Any penetrating injury traversing the mediastinum
- Massive haemorrhage (>1.5 l or >0.3 l/hr)
- Cardiac tamponade
- Large open wounds
- Major thoracic vascular injuries
- Major tracheobronchial injuries
- Oesophageal perforation.

■ Secondary survey of life-threatening injuries

During the secondary survey there is an opportunity to examine the patient in depth, look at the CXR, ABG, pulse oximetry and ECG. In thoracic trauma the clinician should have a high index of suspicion for the following injuries:

SIMPLE PNEUMOTHORAX (Figure 29)

Air enters the space between visceral and parietal pleura (either from the lung via a laceration or through the thoracic wall) resulting in collapse of the affected lung.

Clinical features: patient may be short of breath and hypoxic. Absent breath sounds, subcutaneous emphysema, and hyper-resonance on percussion of affected side.

Management: CXR confirms diagnosis. Chest drain should be inserted. A patient with a pneumothorax should not be intubated and ventilated or given positive pressure ventilation (PPV) until a chest drain is inserted to avoid turning this into a tension pneumothorax.

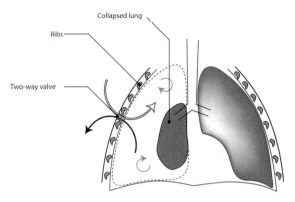

Figure 29 Simple pneumothorax

HAEMOTHORAX

Blood enters the interpleural space from a bleeding intercostal vessel, internal mammary artery, or lung laceration most commonly.

Management: if seen on CXR, insert a chest drain and monitor output (as for Massive haemothorax).

RIB FRACTURES

A common injury usually occurring in the space between the fourth to tenth ribs. *If lower ribs are involved*: think about the possibility of an associated abdominal (hepatic or splenic) injury. *If upper ribs are involved*: think about the possibility of a major neurovascular injury, haemo/pneumothorax, or abdominal injury.

Management: pain control (see Figure 10 Analgesic ladder), and identification of complicated injuries. The presence of lung injury or haemothorax requires chest drain insertion. Early physiotherapy is imperative.

PULMONARY CONTUSION

May develop over time as contusion matures following injury, and present with progressive respiratory failure.

Management: pulse oximetry, serial ABG, ECG monitoring, high-flow oxygen and appropriate ventilatory support (including intubation and ventilation if severe hypoxia), HDU/ICU admission, repeat CXR.

TRACHEOBRONCHIAL TREE INJURY

Injuries to the trachea, larynx and major bronchi carry a significant mortality, and are often overlooked in blunt trauma.

Clinical features: haemoptysis, subcutaneous emphysema, tension pneumothorax, mediastinal shift.

CARDIAC INJURIES

Can occur with blunt or penetrating injuries of the thorax and include:

Penetrating injuries

1. **Simple lacerations of the chambers:** resuscitate the patient and call for urgent cardiothoracic assistance. Clam-shell or median sternotomy is indicated to inspect all sides of the heart and major vessels. Septal or valvular injuries can be repaired later unless haemodynamically important.
2. **Simple lacerations of the coronary arteries:** resuscitate the patient and call for cardiothoracic assistance. Surgery involves ligation for distal arterial involvement, and cardiopulmonary bypass and repair if proximal artery is involved.

Blunt injuries

They are the cause of myocardial contusion in 90 % of the cases. Patients may complain of chest discomfort, and present with arrhythmias (premature ventricular contractions, sinus tachycardia, AF, RBBB, S-T segment changes), right ventricular failure (raised CVP) and hypotension. Patients should be on a monitor for at least 24 hr.

TRAUMATIC AORTIC DISRUPTION

Specific symptoms and signs are absent, high index of suspicion in deceleration injuries. CXR may raise suspicion showing:

1. Widened mediastinum
2. Fractures of scapula, first or second ribs
3. Obliterated aortic knuckle
4. Left haemothorax
5. Presence of apical pleural cap
6. Right tracheal/oesophageal deviation
7. Obliterated space between pulmonary artery and aorta
8. Depressed left main bronchus.

Management: resuscitate the patient. If suspected contact cardio-thoracic team early. Further investigation includes aortography and helical contrast-enhanced CT. Surgery or stenting is indicated if there is massive blood loss, tamponade or an expanding haematoma. This decision should be made by a cardiothoracic surgeon.

DIAPHRAGMATIC INJURIES

These are present in 25 % of penetrating injuries of the thorax. Blunt injuries of the thorax and/or abdomen can cause diaphragmatic injuries. In these cases the left side is more commonly affected (90 %) although bilateral injuries can be present. They are often associated with lower-rib fractures. The stomach is the most frequent herniating organ.

Clinical features: include respiratory distress, bowel sounds in the chest, hypovolaemia (80 % chance of gastric volvulus in three years if untreated).

Management: resuscitate and refer to cardiothoracic team early.

OESOPHAGEAL INJURIES

Can be due to penetrating and blunt trauma. Diagnosis requires a high level of suspicion especially in gunshot or stab-wound transversing the mediastinum. Spontaneous oesophageal rupture (*Boerhaave's syndrome*) is usually precipitated by severe vomiting, resulting in a sudden onset of severe thoracic or epigastric pain. Diagnosis is often delayed as the clinical picture mimics other emergency conditions, such as myocardial infarction, acute gastritis and acute pancreatitis.

Clinical features: presence of pleural effusion without rib fractures, chest pain, subcutaneous and/or mediastinal emphysema, pneumo/haemothorax, presence of gastric contents in the chest tube.

Management: resuscitate the patient, nil by mouth, analgesia, chest drain insertion, prompt referral to cardiac team. CT scan may help confirm diagnosis, Gastrografin (diatrizoate meglumine and diatrizoate sodium) swallow may be used, and early oesophagoscopy is useful to confirm diagnosis (50–90 %).

STERNAL FRACTURES

Usually linear and in middle third. Have high index of suspicion for underlying major vascular injuries.

Management: adequate analgesia, identify underlying injuries with imaging (CT). Ultimately may require open reduction and fixation as part of another treatment or to improve cosmesis.

SCAPULA FRACTURES

May occur with significant force of impact injuries. The brachial plexus is usually injured.

Management: shoulder immobilization, early physiotherapy and surgical intervention are indicated if complicated shoulder problems are present.

CLAVICULAR FRACTURES

May be extremely displaced and should raise index of suspicion of high velocity blunt thoracic injury.

Trauma: abdominal trauma

ROS JACKLIN AND PARASKEVAS PARASKEVA

Abdominal trauma is an important cause of morbidity and mortality among all age groups. Identification of the site of trauma requires an appreciation of the fact that the external surface of the abdominal cavity is superiorly covered by the lower thorax (the diaphragm may rise up to the fourth intercostal space with full expiration), inferiorly extends down to the pelvis, laterally includes the flanks, and posteriorly is covered by the back (Figure 30). Internally the cavity is divided into:

Peritoneal space: contains diaphragm, liver, spleen, stomach, small bowel, parts of ascending and descending colon, transverse colon, sigmoid colon, and female reproductive organs.

Retroperitoneal space: contains abdominal aorta, inferior vena cava, duodenum, pancreas, kidneys, ureters, parts of ascending and descending colon.

Pelvis: contains rectum, bladder, iliac vessels and female reproductive organs.

■ Types of injury

Blunt abdominal trauma: *compression forces* such as direct blows or compression against a fixed object (seatbelt) commonly cause tears and subcapsular haematomas in solid visceral organs. Hollow organs (bowel) may experience a transient increase in intraluminal pressure resulting in rupture. *Deceleration forces* result in shearing between fixed and free segments of tissue, tearing supporting tissues at their junction.

Hospital Surgery: Foundations in Surgical Practice, ed. Omer Aziz, Sanjay Purkayastha and Paraskevas Paraskeva. Published by Cambridge University Press. © Cambridge University Press 2009.

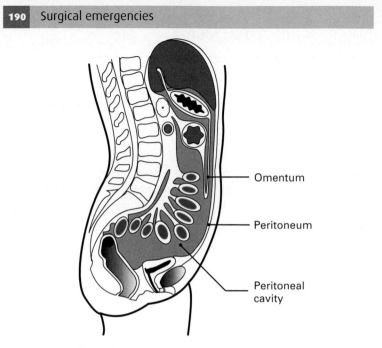

Omentum

Peritoneum

Peritoneal
cavity

Figure 30

Classic injuries include mesenteric tear with splanchnic vessel injuries, and hepatic tear along the ligamentum teres. At laparotomy for blunt trauma, common injuries include splenic (40–55 %), hepatic (35–45 %), and retroperitoneal haematoma (15 %).

Penetrating abdominal trauma: a foreign body breaches the abdominal wall and enters the peritoneal cavity. *Stab wounds* may be deceptive in the injuries they cause and a high index of suspicion for occult injuries must be maintained. Commonly affected organs include liver (40 %), small bowel (30 %), diaphragm (20 %) and colon (15 %). *Gunshot wounds (GSWs)* are high-energy transfer injuries with unpredictable missile track. High-velocity rifle wounds may cause temporary cavitation and secondary missiles (e.g. fragments of bone) may inflict additional injuries.

■ Management of abdominal trauma

Initial assessment and management are described in the Trauma: adult trauma Chapter in accordance with ATLS guidelines. An experienced surgeon should be involved early. In hypotensive patients the goal is rapidly to determine if an abdominal injury is present and whether it is the cause of haemorrhage (indicating immediate laparotomy).

HISTORY

Seek information as to the mechanism of injury, such as the height of any fall. In the context of a road traffic accident (RTA) this would include speed of the vehicle, type of collision, use of seatbelts/restraints and deformity to the passenger compartment. After penetrating trauma, establish time of injury, type of weapon, range (GSW) and the amount of external bleeding at the scene.

EXAMINATION

This should be performed systematically (inspection, palpation, percussion, auscultation), remembering to examine the back and lower chest. Look for penetrating injuries, lacerations, and contusions from restraint devices. Assess pelvic stability and perform penile, perineal, rectal and vaginal examinations. Assess the gluteal region, as up to 50 % of penetrating injuries here are associated with significant intra-abdominal component (including rectum).

INVESTIGATIONS

Blood tests: G&S/cross match, FBC, U&E, clotting, amylase, glucose, alcohol levels. *Urinary catheter* to monitor urine output and *urinalysis* for haematuria (exclude urethral injury first looking for meatal blood, pelvic fractures). Urinary pregnancy test +/– urinary drug screen when appropriate. *NG tube* may be beneficial.

X-rays: trauma series (lateral C-spine, chest and pelvis). Erect CXR may reveal free air, diaphragmatic hernia or rib fractures. AXR of questionable benefit but in blunt trauma may show retroperitoneal air or loss of psoas shadow suggesting retroperitoneal haemorrhage. *Diagnostic ultrasound:* focused assessment sonography in trauma (FAST) scan is a rapid, non-invasive means of diagnosing intra-abdominal fluid, which may be performed by trained individuals (See Radiology – Ultrasound Chapter). Limitations include operator dependency and inability to diagnose diaphragmatic, pancreatic and bowel injuries. *Diagnostic peritoneal lavage (DPL)* is a quick invasive procedure for detecting free blood or gastrointestinal contents in the peritoneal cavity (see DPL Chapter). Limitations include invasiveness, low specificity, inability to diagnose retroperitoneal haemorrhage and inability to localize injury. *Computed Tomography (CT)*: only appropriate for patients who are haemodynamically normal with no existing indication for emergency laparotomy. CT provides information on site of injury including pelvic organs and retroperitoneum. Limitations include time taken, failure to diagnose diaphragmatic/pancreatic injuries, and need for patient transport.

Indications for laparotomy following abdominal trauma		
Mode of evaluation	Blunt abdominal trauma	Penetrating abdominal trauma
Clinical findings	Positive DPL/FAST USS in unstable patients	Uncontrolled haemorrhage from GI/GU tract Any GSW traversing peritoneum/retroperitoneum Evisceration of abdominal contents
	Unexplained hypotension and abdominal distension	
	Signs of peritonitis	
X-ray	Free/retroperitoneal air or rupture of hemidiaphragm	—
CT	Ruptured GI tract or intraperitoneal bladder, renal pedicle injury or severe visceral parenchymal injury	

■ Local exploration of stab wounds

If the patient is haemodynamically stable and has no signs of peritonism, the wound may be explored under local anaesthetic; however this is often not definitive and of questionable value. Confirmation of peritoneal cavity breach either with a CT scan or definitively with diagnostic laparoscopy should be carried out.

■ Observation and serial examination

Admission, observation, and serial examination in apparently asymptomatic patients with blunt or penetrating (stab wounds) abdominal trauma may reveal injuries that were initially missed in the resuscitation room.

Burns

BEN ARDEHALI AND GREG WILLIAMS

Incidence: 250 000 people per annum sustain burn injuries in the UK. Of these, 15 000 require admission to a specialist burns unit. There are 300 deaths per annum from burns.

Types: *Flame injuries* (55 %) account for the majority of the burns. *Scald burns* (40 %) are the second most common type. *Electrical* and *chemical* burns are less common (5 %).

■ Pathophysiology

Local response – three zones of burn:

1. *Coagulation zone* – central area composed of non-viable tissue due to coagulation of constituent proteins.
2. *Stasis zone* – initially blood supply is present but over the ensuing 24 hours hypoperfusion and ischaemia can prevail, resulting in irreversible damage. The aim of burn resuscitation is to increase tissue perfusion and prevent this tissue damage. Hypotension, infection and oedema can render this zone non-viable.
3. *Hyperaemia zone* – contains viable tissue; unless associated with severe sepsis and/or prolonged hypoperfusion this zone tends to recover.

Systemic response: large burns > 30 % total body surface area (TBSA) can have a profound systemic effect on major organs through the release of cytokines and other inflammatory mediators.

Hospital Surgery: Foundations in Surgical Practice, ed. Omer Aziz, Sanjay Purkayastha and Paraskevas Paraskeva. Published by Cambridge University Press.
© Cambridge University Press 2009.

1. *Cardiovascular system*: systemic hypotension and end organ hypo-perfusion can occur from (a) fluid loss from the burn wound, (b) sequestration of intravascular fluid and proteins into the interstitial space due to increase in capillary permeability, and (c) decrease in myocardial contractility due to release of cytokines such as tumour necrosis factor α.

2. *Respiratory system*: bronchospasm is caused by circulating inflammatory mediators, and adult respiratory distress syndrome can occur in severe burns.

3. *Metabolic changes*: hypermetabolic response is common and can increase the original rate upto three fold. Early enteral feeding to meet increased energy requirement and maintain gut integrity due to splanchnic hypoperfusion is imperative.

■ Burn wound assessment

Evaluating size of area involved:

1. *Palmar surface method*: patient's palm (including fingers) is approximately 1 % TBSA. Good at estimating small (<15 %) or very large (>85 %) burns.

2. *Wallace's rule of 9's*: good at estimating medium to large burns in adults. Each arm, anterior aspect of each leg, posterior aspect of each leg, and head = 9 % each, anterior/posterior torso = 18 % each.

3. *Lund and Browder charts*: account for variation in body shape (Figure 31) with age and provide an accurate assessment of burns in children.

(Note: erythema should not be included in the burn area.)

Evaluating depth of burn:

1. *Superficial (First degree)*: e.g. sunburn. Mild erythema and confined to epidermis. Capillary refill present. Pain resolves in 72 hours. No blisters or scarring.

2. *Partial thickness (Second degree)*: this is further sub-divided into three categories.

a. Superficial dermal: pale pink, presence of sensation and capillary refill. Blisters are small. Dermal appendages are intact and the wound will heal in less than three weeks with minimal scarring.

b. Mid-dermal: dark pink, sensation intact, capillary refill slow. Large blisters present and usually heals with minimal scarring.

c. Deep-dermal: fixed staining, absence of sensation and capillary refill. No blisters and will heal in more than three weeks with marked scarring.

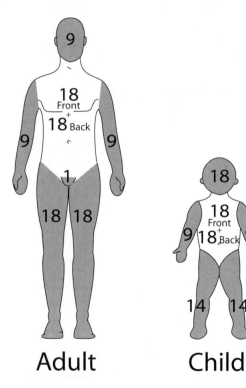

Figure 31

3. *Full thickness (Third degree)*: epidermis and dermis layers are destroyed, no epidermal appendages remain. White/yellow leathery, waxy, charred appearance with thrombosis of vessels. Absence of sensation and capillary refill. No possibility of spontaneous regeneration.

■ Management

Major burns > 15 % TBSA:

History: mechanism (type of burn, duration of exposure, time of injury, type of first aid performed). Any concomitant injury, inhalational risk (enclosed space).

Examination: ABCDE of primary survey as follows:

1. *Airway* – signs suggesting inhalational injury and potential airway compromise include: singed nasal hairs, carbonaceous sputum or carbon particles in the oropharynx, facial burns and history of flame burn in an enclosed space or patient lying unconscious in a fire. A senior anaesthetist should assess the patency of the airway and if in doubt intubate.

2. *Breathing* – inhalational injury can lead to carbon monoxide (CO) poisoning. CO has 250 times the affinity for Hb as oxygen and leads to tissue hypoxia. Blood gas levels of COHb > 25 % warrant intubation of the patient. Treatment with 100 % oxygen displaces CO six times faster than atmospheric oxygen. Smoke inhalation leads to bronchospasm, inflammation and bronchorrhoea. The accumulation of secretion can lead to pneumonia. Nebulizer and non-invasive ventilation can help. Invasive ventilation may be required to allow lung toileting. Circumferential thoracic burn causing mechanical restriction in chest expansion requires escharotomies.

3. *Circulation* – intravenous access with large bore cannula (take blood for urea and electrolytes, full blood count, clotting and group and save). Fluid resuscitation is required for adults with burn > 15 % and children with burns > 10 % (excluding erythema). Fluid formulae are guidelines, and ultimately the monitoring of physiological

parameters is the key to successful resuscitation, e.g. blood pressure, pulse and urine output. Many regimes have been described. We use the Parkland formula based on Hartman's crystalloid fluid.

Parkland formula for total fluid requirement in 24 hours

= 4 ml × kg (body weight) × % burn surface area.

Half of this fluid is given in the first 8 hours (*starting from the time of burn* and not time of admission) and the remaining half is given in the next 16 hours.

Fluid requirements for children: because of their increased surface area, they should receive an additional maintenance infusion of dextrose-saline:

100 ml × kg in 24 hours for the first 10 kg of the child's weight.
50 ml × kg in 24 hours for the next 10 kg of the child's weight.
20 ml × kg in 24 hours for the next 10 kg of the child's weight.

Aim to maintain a urine output of 0.5–1.0 ml/kg/hour in adults and 1.0–1.5 ml/kg/hour in children.

4. *Disability* – Glasgow coma scale (GCS) assessment important, but rule out hypoxia and hypovolaemia as source of confusion.
5. *Exposure* – adequate exposure is essential to correctly estimate the area of burn and assess the depth and temporarily dress the area with cling film. Also look for other concomitant injuries. Minimize heat loss through unnecessary exposure by applying bear hugger to keep patient warm.

(Note: any deep circumferential burn results in limited ability of expansion of tissue oedema. This can lead to tissue ischaemia and necrosis. The burn extremity needs to be elevated and *escharotomy* carried out. This involves making an incision of burned skin to relieve pressure.)

■ Reasons for referral to a burns unit

- Burns covering more than 10 % TBSA in adults and 5 % in children
- Burns involving face, hands or perineum

- Inhalational injury
- Significant electrical or chemical burns
- Suspicion of non-accidental injury
- Burns associated with major trauma
- Extremes of age – under 5 or over 60.

Chemical burns

Usually deeper than they appear; dilution and not neutralization is the rule of management. In cases of hydrofluoric acid burn, however, the wound should be neutralized with 10 % calcium gluconate. Phenol burns need to be washed with polyethylene glycol if available, as phenol is poorly soluble in water.

Electrical burns

Low voltage injuries < 1000 V: can cause local tissue destruction without systemic impact.

High voltage injuries > 1000 V: can cause significant internal destruction through passage of current through tissues. Can be described as a massive crush injury with intact skin. The resultant muscle damage and breakdown can lead to *myoglobinuria* and *acute tubular necrosis*. These patients should be managed by maintaining a high urine output (2 ml/kg/hr) and urine can be alkalinized with sodium bicarbonate to increase the solubility of myoglobin. *Fasciotomies* as opposed to escharotomies may need to be carried out, as deep compartments are involved. *Cardiac damage* is rare but monitoring should be carried out during the first 24 hours along with cardiac enzymes.

Excision and grafting

Deep dermal and full thickness burns need to be excised either tangentially with a hand knife or fascial excision. The resultant defect is then covered with meshed autograft. In cases of inadequate donor site for graft harvest the debrided area can be covered with cadaveric allograft or skin substitutes (Integra, Biobrane) to protect against fluid loss and burn wound infection.

■ Nutritional requirement

In their hypermetabolic state the burn patients have increased daily calorific requirements: adults: (25 kcal × kg) + (40 kcl × % burn), children: 40–60 kcl × kg.

■ Multi-disciplinary approach

Successful outcome in burns patients to pre-injury level of physical, emotional, and psychological well-being relies on a strong multi-disciplinary approach from the onset of the accident. The essential role of fire brigade, paramedics, medics, nurses, pharmacists, nutritionists, physiotherapists, occupational therapists, psychologists and social services cannot be over emphasized.

■ Examples of fluid resuscitation calculations

Case 1: a 48-year-old mechanic weighing 70 kg with a 40 % flame burn was brought to A&E (accident and emergency department) at 5 pm. The accident took place an hour prior to his admission.

- *Question 1.* What is his total fluid requirement in the first 24 hours? *Answer:* 4 ml × 70 kg × 40 % TBSA burn = 11 200 ml in 24 hours.
- *Question 2.* How much should he receive in the first 8 hours? *Answer:* 5600 ml in the first 8 hours and 5600 ml over the next 16 hours.
- *Question 3.* He was given 1000 ml by the paramedic team. What will be his hourly infusion rate in the first 8 hours? *Answer:* subtract what he has already been given from what he should be receiving in the first 8 hours: 5600 − 1000 = 4600 ml. The burn took place at 4 pm and midnight will be his 8 hour point. It is now 5 pm, so over the next 7 hours he should receive: 4600/7 = 657 ml/hour from 5 pm to midnight.

■ *Question 4.* What will be his hourly infusion rate for the next 16 hours?
  Answer: 5600/16 = 350 ml/hour from midnight to 4 pm the next day.

Case 2: calculation of maintenance fluid for a child.

■ *Question 5.* How much maintenance fluid will a 29 kg child require?

  Answer:

100 ml × kg in 24 hours for the first 10 kg of the child's weight = 1000 ml
  in 24 hrs.
50 ml × kg in 24 hours for the next 10 kg of the child's weight = 500 ml in
  24 hrs.
20 ml × kg in 24 hours for the next 10 kg of the child's weight = 180 ml in
  24 hrs.
Total = 1680 ml in 24 hours.
Hourly infusion rate: 1660/24 = 70 ml/hour.

Acute abdomen

HENRY TILLNEY AND ALEXANDER G. HERIOT

■ Definition

Acute abdominal pain of less than one week's duration sufficiently severe to require hospital admission and not previously investigated/treated. Accounts for 1 % of UK hospital admissions, 6 % of A&E referrals and 18 % of surgical admissions.

■ Aetiology

This may be due to thoracic, abdominal or pelvic pathology as shown in the figure.

■ Pathogenesis

Visceral pain is poorly localized and sensed according to the embryological origin of the structure/organ (see figure). *Foregut viscera* (including stomach, duodenum, pancreas, gallbladder and liver) transmit pain to the epigastrium via coeliac plexus. *Midgut viscera* transmit pain to the umbilicus via superior mesenteric plexus. *Hindgut viscera* transmit pain to the hypogastric region via inferior mesenteric plexus. **Parietal pain** is localized pain secondary to direct parietal peritoneal irritation mediated by the somatic nerves (thoraco-lumbar), and may be associated with reflex involuntary abdominal wall rigidity. **Diaphragmatic irritation** (for example secondary to acute cholecystitis) is referred to the shoulder (C3–5 distribution) (Figure 32).

Hospital Surgery: Foundations in Surgical Practice, ed. Omer Aziz, Sanjay Purkayastha and Paraskevas Paraskeva. Published by Cambridge University Press. © Cambridge University Press 2009.

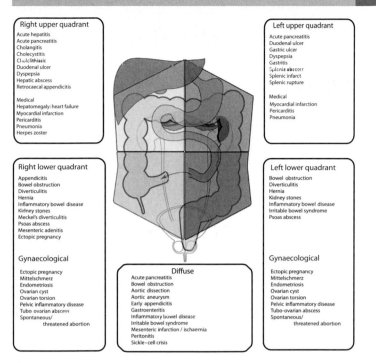

Right upper quadrant

Acute hepatitis
Acute pancreatitis
Cholangitis
Cholecystitis
Cholelithiasis
Duodenal ulcer
Dyspepsia
Hepatic abscess
Retrocaecal appendicitis

Medical
Hepatomegaly: heart failure
Myocardial infarction
Pericarditis
Pneumonia
Herpes zoster

Left upper quadrant

Acute pancreatitis
Duodenal ulcer
Gastric ulcer
Dyspepsia
Gastritis
Splenic abscess
Splenic infarct
Splenic rupture

Medical
Myocardial infarction
Pericarditis
Pneumonia

Right lower quadrant

Appendicitis
Bowel obstruction
Diverticulitis
Hernia
Inflammatory bowel disease
Kidney stones
Meckel's diverticulitis
Psoas abscess
Mesenteric adenitis
Ectopic pregnancy

Gynaecological

Ectopic pregnancy
Mittelschmerz
Endometriosis
Ovarian cyst
Ovarian torsion
Pelvic inflammatory disease
Tubo ovarian abscess
Spontaneous/
            threatened abortion

Left lower quadrant

Bowel obstruction
Diverticulitis
Hernia
Kidney stones
Inflammatory bowel disease
Irritable bowel syndrome
Psoas abscess

Gynaecological

Ectopic pregnancy
Mittelschmerz
Endometriosis
Ovarian cyst
Ovarian torsion
Pelvic inflammatory disease
Tubo-ovarian abscess
Spontaneous/
            threatened abortion

Diffuse

Acute pancreatitis
Bowel obstruction
Aortic dissection
Aortic aneurysm
Early appendicitis
Gastroenteritis
Inflammatory bowel disease
Irritable bowel syndrome
Mesenteric infarction / ischaemia
Peritonitis
Sickle-cell crisis

Figure 32

■ History

Features of the abdominal pain (Figure 33):

- *Location over the abdomen*: localized versus generalized.
- *Character*: sharp, dull, burning, colicky (episodic and of variable intensity, usually secondary to obstruction of hollow muscular viscus with frequency of pain increasing with proximal obstruction).
- *Nature*: constant vs. intermittent. Constant pain is usually secondary to inflammation/necrosis.

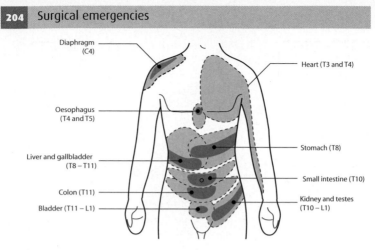

Figure 33

- *Onset/offset*: sudden (signifying acute event such as perforation) versus gradual (progressive inflammatory process such as appendicitis). Change from intermittent to constant pain in a patient with obstructive symptoms is a worrying sign, and is suggestive of infarction or perforation.
- *Intensity*: 1–10 (10 being the worst pain they have ever experienced).
- *Radiation*: renal colic (loin to groin), biliary colic (RUQ to right scapula), and pancreatitis (epigastrium through to the back) are classical examples.
- *Exacerbating/alleviating factors*: for example movement and coughing exacerbates parietal peritonism but has no affect on renal colic, and food alleviates gastric pain but exacerbates biliary colic.
- *Similar previous presentations.*

Associated symptoms such as anorexia, nausea, vomiting, haematemesis, diarrhoea, constipation, rectal bleeding, fever, urinary tract symptoms (dysuria, frequency, nocturia, etc.) and vaginal discharge are important in making the initial differential diagnosis.

Characteristics of vomiting may help, for example, determine the level of intestinal obstruction (food implies above the second part of the duodenum, bilious may be indicative of a lower obstruction, and faeculent is indicative of small bowel obstruction and occurs due to bacterial overgrowth in stagnant small bowel contents).

Bowel habit is an important part of the history. Constipation may indicate obstruction, or ileus (absolute constipation is a worrying feature). Diarrhoea may suggest gastroenteritis, diverticulitis, appendicitis, or partial obstruction. Blood in the stool is a very important clue (see Gastrointestinal Bleeding Chapter). Stool colour and character (pale stools difficult to flush in toilet) may also highlight site of pathology.

Menstrual and sexual history to exclude gynaecological causes and ectopic pregnancy.

Systems review, past medical history and drug history allows not only an appreciation of co-morbidity but may identify a medical cause for the abdominal pain (for example diabetic keto-acidosis or sickle-cell crisis).

■ Examination

General inspection: general appearance (jaundice, dehydration) and level of comfort (lying very still in peritonism versus writhing around unable to get comfortable in colic). Pain with coughing implies parietal peritonism. **Vital signs:** heart rate (tachycardia with pain and shock), respiratory rate (tachypnoea in compensated respiratory acidosis), blood pressure. **Abdominal inspection:** scars, shape (distended), visible peristalsis, hernias. **Palpation/percussion:** site of maximal tenderness and rigidity. *Guarding* is involuntary contraction (rigidity) of underlying musculature. *Rebound tenderness* is pain on removal of examining hand or percussion (due to stretching of the inflamed parietal peritoneum). This is a sensitive guide to underlying inflammation (peritonism). **Auscultation:** absent/scanty/high pitched/obstructive bowel sounds. **Complete the examination by performing** rectal, vaginal, hernial orifices and external genitalia examinations.

■ Investigation and management

Bloods tests: FBC, U&E, LFTs, Amylase, CRP and group and save/crossmatch as indicated. **Urine dip:** infection, haematuria. **Urine β-HCG:**

essential in females of child-bearing age. **Arterial blood gas:** metabolic acidosis (compensated or uncompensated)/lactate (e.g. in bowel ischaemia and pancreatitis). **Erect CXR:** free gas (indicative of visceral perforation), pulmonary pathology. **AXR:** dilated bowel, extraluminal gas (*Rigler's* sign), gallstones, renal stones, calcified pancreas/aorta. **USS, CT and contrast studies** may all be of benefit. Whilst initial management includes patient resuscitation and analgesia while investigations are performed, further management is directed to the underlying condition and described throughout this book.

Acute pancreatitis

DANNY YAKOUB AND GEORGE HANNA

Implies pancreatic inflammation and autodigestion. Acute cases regress and heal while chronic cases persist and progress. It may occur at any age, but most commonly in middle-aged men.

■ Aetiology

Alcoholism and gallstones are the most common causes. It may occur with viral infections e.g. *Coxsackie B* virus, hyperparathyroidism, blunt trauma, iatrogenic injury during surgery or ERCP.

■ Pathophysiology

Aetiological factors might lead to acinar cell injury, leading to release of proteases and lipases which cause local gland and fat digestion. The resulting acute oedematous inflammation may regress or progress to haemorrhagic or necrotizing form. Necrosis of the gland may lead to dysfunction, formation of a pseudocyst, abscess or peritonitis.

■ Presentation

Acute cases: pain (90 %), nausea, vomiting and possibly picture of shock, acidosis and signs of peritonitis as abdominal distension, tenderness, guarding and rigidity. Retroperitoneal haemorrhagic fluid collection may show as pigmentation in the flanks and peri-umbilical region (*Grey Turner* and *Cullen*'s signs). Complications include chronic pancreatitis, biliary obstruction, pseudocyst formation and septicaemia. Chronic

Hospital Surgery: Foundations in Surgical Practice, ed. Omer Aziz, Sanjay Purkayastha and Paraskevas Paraskeva. Published by Cambridge University Press. © Cambridge University Press 2009.

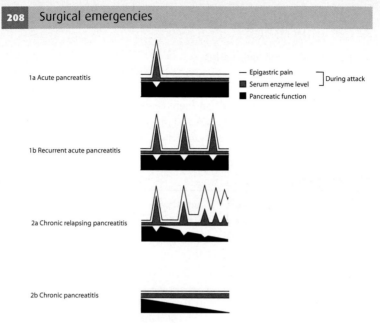

Figure 34 Modified Marseilles definition of types of pancreatitis

pancreatitis may present with relapsing acute attacks or simply by progressive loss of pancreatic function in the form of diabetes and malabsorption. Pancreatitis can be classified according to aetiology, severity or clinical presentation and progression (see Figure 34).

■ Differential diagnosis

Acute cholecystitis, intestinal gangrene, obstruction or perforation, ruptured aortic aneurysm.

■ Assessment of severity and prognosis of acute pancreatitis

Scoring systems include Ranson's, Glasgow and APACHE II scores (see tables). APACHE II (acute physiology and chronic health evaluation) score is the most sensitive and specific and can be used at any time. In addition some biochemical markers have been investigated but none proved robust enough to be used alone e.g. trypsin activated peptide, phospholipase A2, serum trypsinogen 2 and CRP.

■ Investigations

Biochemical tests: increased serum and urinary amylase starts after 12 hours, peaks at 48–72 hr and is back to normal at 5–7 days, sensitivity (75–92 %), specificity (20–60 %). Serum lipase and trypsin are more sensitive (86–100 %) and specific (50–99 %) but are not widely available and disappear rapidly, thus not used routinely. Blood gases are important as they may show signs of acidosis. Others include hyperglycaemia, hypocalcaemia, methemalbuminaemia and hyperlipidaemia. *Plain abdominal X-ray* may show signs of ileus. *CT scan:* invaluable for diagnosis and assessment of severity and complications via a contrast-enhanced CT scoring giving grades A–E according to radiological picture.

■ Management

Acute cases: resuscitation and systems support is the mainstay of treatment, through NG placement, replacement of fluids, electrolytes, blood and plasma with monitoring of vital signs, urine output and central venous pressure. Opiates are used for relief of pain. Premature feeding may cause exacerbation, frequent arterial blood gas monitoring may reveal occult respiratory failure commonly present early, which may need ventilator support and pulmonary artery pressure monitoring. Where sepsis is present, antibiotics should be started early. Frequent re-evaluation of severity and progress is essential to guide further management. *Surgical:* indicated in failed response to medical management or to treat complications such as abscess, haemorrhage or pseudocyst.

Chronic cases: enzyme replacement, adequate nutrition and insulin supplement. For chronic relapsing cases, pain management and rehabilitation of the alcoholic patient. Surgical intervention is indicated in intractable pain not responsive otherwise or for management of a secondary complication.

■ Various scoring systems for assessment of severity and prognosis of acute pancreatitis

Ranson's criteria scoring	
Present on admission	Developing during the first 48 hours
Age > 55 years	Haematocrit fall > 10 %
WBC > 16 × 10^9/l	Urea > 0.9 mmol/l rise
Blood glucose > 10 mmol/l	Uncorrected serum calcium < 2 mmol/l
Serum LDH > 350 IU/l	Arterial pO$_2$ < 60 mmHg (8 kPa)
AST > 120 IU/l	Base deficit > 4 mmol
	Estimated fluid sequestration > 6 l

Ranson score of 0–2: 0.9 % mortality. Score of 3–5: 10 %–20 % mortality. Score of >5 has 50–90 % mortality and is associated with more systemic complications.

Modified Glasgow prognostic criteria		
Parameter	Finding at any time during first 48 hours	Points
Arterial pO$_2$ on room air	< 8 kPa (<60 mmHg)	1
Serum albumin	< 32 g/dl	1
WBC count	> 15 × 10^9/l	1
Serum calcium	< 2 mmol/l	1
Urea	> 16 mmol/L	1
Serum LDH or	> 600 IU/l	1
Serum AST/ALT	>100 IU/l	
Age	> 55 years	1
Blood glucose	> 10 mmol/l	1

*Interpretation: if the score ≥ 3, severe pancreatitis likely while if < 3 it is unlikely. NOTE: a useful acronym is **PANCREAS** (**P**=pO$_2$, **A**=Albumin, **N**=Neutrophils (WBC), **C**=Calcium, **R**=Raised Urea, **E**=Enzymes (LDH/AST/ALT), **A**=Age, **S**=Sugar (Glucose).*

APACHE II Scoring system (Online calculator: www.sfar.org/scores2/apache22.html)

(A) Acute physiology score (each 0–4)	(B) Age points	(C) Chronic health points
1 = Rectal temp (°C)	<44 – 0	Cirrhosis – 2 or 5
2 = Mean arterial pressure (mmHg)	45–54 – 2	Immunosuppression – 2 or 5
3 = Heart rate (bpm)	55–64 – 3	NY Heart Assoc. class IV – 2 or 5
4 = Respiratory rate (bpm)	65–74 – 5	COPD – 2 or 5
5 = Oxygen delivery (ml/min)	>75 – 6	Renal dialysis – 2 or 5
6 = pO_2 (mmHg)		
7 = arterial pH		
8 = Serum sodium (mmol/l)		
9 = Serum potassium (mmol/l)		
10 = Serum creatinine (mg/dl)		
11 = Haematocrit (%)		
12 = White cell count		

Interpretation: A + B + C > 9 suggests severe pancreatitis.

Acute appendicitis

ROS JACKLIN AND PARASKEVAS PARASKEVA

■ Definition

The vermiform appendix is a long diverticulum, rich in lymphoid tissue, extending from the inferior pole of the caecum at the point of convergence of the taenia coli. Appendicitis refers to inflammation of this structure with superimposed infection (Figure 35).

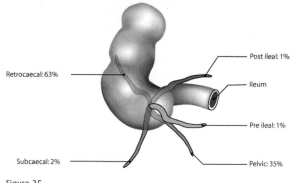

Retrocaecal: 63%

Post ileal: 1%

Ileum

Pre ileal: 1%

Subcaecal: 2%

Pelvic: 35%

Figure 35

■ Incidence

It may occur at any age, but is commonest in the second and third decades, with an overall lifetime risk of 7 %. M > F.

■ Pathophysiology

Luminal obstruction (commonly due to a faecolith) results in an increased luminal pressure, ultimately resulting in an impaired blood

Hospital Surgery: Foundations in Surgical Practice, ed. Omer Aziz, Sanjay Purkayastha and Paraskevas Paraskeva. Published by Cambridge University Press. © Cambridge University Press 2009.

supply to the appendix wall. Infection of the obstructed appendix ultimately results in gangrene and perforation of the wall of the appendix which is either localized (appendix abscess) or leads to generalized peritonitis.

■ Classification

According to the position in which the appendix lies in relation to the caecum: (1) Lies within the peritoneal cavity (exposed to anterior parietal peritoneum), (2) 'Hidden' from parietal peritoneum (pelvic, retroileal or retrocolic positions).

■ History

Progressive history often starting with central abdominal pain eventually localizing to the right iliac fossa. Associated anorexia, nausea, vomiting, and low grade fever. Pain usually has features of peritonism such as worsening on coughing or moving, and is alleviated by lying still. A retrocaecal appendix may present with varying features of abdominal pain depending on the site of peritoneal irritation. Perforation results in diffuse peritonitis with pain throughout the abdomen. Atypical presentations include diarrhoea (irritation of adjacent rectum), urinary frequency (irritation of adjacent bladder), and flank pain (retrocaecal appendix). A urological and gynaecological (menstrual) history should be taken, to exclude urinary tract infection, pregnancy (ectopic or uterine) and ovarian pathology as the cause. Always ask the patient if they have had an appendicectomy before!

■ Examination

Patient may be flushed, dehydrated, tachycardic, have low grade pyrexia and a fetor oris (foul-smelling breath). Patient often bends over when walking holding RIF, or may sit with legs drawn up. Abdominal examination reveals RIF tenderness, with guarding. Classically tenderness from an anterior lying appendix is greatest at '*McBurney's point*' (a point one-third of the distance from the anterior superior iliac spine and umbilicus). Peritonism may be elicited by percussion tenderness or rebound tenderness (the former is kinder to the patient). A palpable mass is indicative of an appendix abscess. Digital rectal examination may reveal tenderness if appendix is located in the pelvis. Vaginal examination should be performed on female patients with vaginal discharge or bleeding. *Rovsing's sign* is demonstrated by palpation in the left iliac fossa reproducing the pain in the right iliac fossa. *Psoas sign* can be elicited by stretching the iliopsoas muscle by extending the thigh. *Obturator sign* is tenderness elicited on passive internal rotation of the flexed hip.

Appendicitis usually evolves over 24–36 hours, and use of a brief period of observation and serial examination are invaluable in making the diagnosis.

■ Investigation

FBC (raised WBC), U&E, CRP (may be raised), G&S, clotting. Urinalysis including β-**HCG** (ectopic pregnancy) and dipstick for UTI, but beware as urine may contain traces of blood, protein and leucocytes in appendicitis. Although mainly a clinical diagnosis radiological investigations may be used in difficult cases. USS may be beneficial in patients with appendix masses, and in women to exclude ovarian pathology. **Note that a negative USS does not exclude appendicitis.** CT has a higher diagnostic accuracy and may visualize an inflamed appendix. Diagnostic laparoscopy is indicated in difficult cases, particularly in women. In patients over the age of 50, alternative diagnoses such as colonic diverticular disease and malignancy should be excluded with a CT scan (see relevant chapters).

■ Management

The patient should be given analgesia and iv fluids while preparations are made for appendicectomy. Antibiotics should be given once a diagnosis and decision to operate has been made by the surgeon, especially if there is a delay in surgery. Appendicectomy may be performed laparoscopically or open. If an apparently normal appendix is removed, the surgeon must exclude a Meckel's diverticulum, acute salpingitis and Crohn's disease. Other sequelae of appendicitis include an *appendix mass* where the appendix becomes walled off by the omentum, typically after a several-day history. These patients should be settled on iv antibiotics and an interval appendicectomy performed after 6 weeks. An *appendix abscess* may be managed with percutaneous drainage under imaging guidance, or drained at appendicectomy. Mortality in unperforated appendicitis is less than 1 %, but approaches 5 % in the very young and the elderly, due in part to delays in diagnosis and a higher rate of perforation. The management of appendicitis is summarized below.

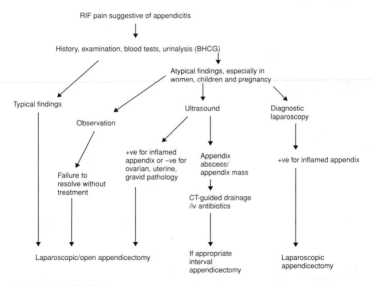

Management algorithm

Acute cholecystitis

ANDRE CHOW AND ARA DARZI

■ Definition

Acute inflammation of the gallbladder. One-third of patients with biliary colic develop acute cholecystitis within two years.

■ Aetiology

90 % of cases associated with obstruction of the cystic duct by a gallstone. Acalculous (absence of gallstones) cholecystitis occurs in 2–5 % of cases and is associated with prolonged fasting, trauma (burns, fractures), severe illness, intensive care admission, parenteral nutrition (TPN) and AIDS.

■ Pathophysiology

Cystic duct obstruction with continued gallbladder secretions leads to an increase in pressure. Concomitant infection by intestinal organisms leads to gallbladder inflammation, diaphragmatic irritation. The stone often slips back into the gallbladder fundus allowing drainage and resolution of inflammation. Continued obstruction of the duct results in collection of mucus (mucocoele) and then pus in the gallbladder forming an empyema (pus-filled gallbladder). Subsequently ischaemia of the gallbladder wall may lead to infarction, necrosis, perforation and ultimately biliary peritonitis.

Acalculous cholecystitis often results from reduced gallbladder contraction due to decreased cholecystokinin release, with viscous bile thought to result in gallbladder obstruction and subsequent bacterial

Hospital Surgery: Foundations in Surgical Practice, ed. Omer Aziz, Sanjay Purkayastha and Paraskevas Paraskeva. Published by Cambridge University Press. © Cambridge University Press 2009.

seeding. Cystic duct compression may also be caused by extrinsic compression (tumour, node, inflammatory mass).

■ Symptoms

Continuous RUQ and epigastric pain (in contrast to the fluctuating pain of biliary colic). Pain may radiate to back or to right scapula (due to peritoneal irritation via T7–9 dermatomes). Note that pain may be very similar to that of acute gastritis or peptic ulcer disease (PUD). Associated nausea, anorexia, fever and vomiting. May have known history of gallstones/biliary colic.

■ Examination

Pyrexia, tachycardia, dehydration and possible tachypnoea with shallow respiration. Jaundice may result due to a common bile duct stone. RUQ palpation reveals localized tenderness with peritonism exacerbated with deep inspiration. *A positive Murphy's sign is produced when the palpating hand is placed in the RUQ and the patient asked to inhale. Descent of the diaphragm pushes the inflamed gallbladder against the examining hand. The resulting pain causes the patient to arrest inspiration, catching their breath.* The inflamed gallbladder is rarely palpable.

■ Differential diagnosis

Peptic ulcer disease (gastritis or perforation), acute pancreatitis, acute appendicitis (with appendix tip in RUQ), right lower lobe pneumonia, pyelonephritis, and myocardial infarction (MI).

■ Investigations

Blood tests: raised WCC and CRP. LFTs often abnormal with ALP more affected than ALT/AST. An elevated serum bilirubin should raise suspicion of CBD stone (choledocholithiasis). Amylase may be mildly elevated. *X-rays*: erect CXR is required to exclude perforated viscus (duodenal ulcer) and right lung lower lobe pathology. AXR is often normal and therefore not indicated, however if performed it is important to look out for a 'sentinel loop' of dilated proximal jejunum (pancreatitis) and air in the biliary tree (gallstone ileus). *Ultrasound* is a good and useful initial investigation (see Hepatobiliary disease: gallstones and biliary colic Chapter). *Endoscopic retrograde cholangio-pancreatography (ERCP)* is indicated in obstructive jaundice to visualize the biliary tree and identify gallstones. *Magnetic resonance cholangio-pancreatography (MRCP)* may be considered if there is no obvious evidence of CBD obstruction on blood tests and ultrasound scan, however clinical suspicion remains.

■ Management

Admit for analgesia, iv fluids, antibiotics (cefuroxime 750 mg–1.5 g/8 hr iv or ciprofloxacin 500 mg bd po + Metronidazole 400 mg/8hr iv) effective against gram negative and coliform organisms. Keep NBM if vomiting. Should signs of obstructive jaundice or cholangitis develop, urgent visualization of biliary tree with MRCP and subsequent drainage is indicated.

Laparoscopic cholecystecomy is the definitive procedure and may be performed within 72 hours of the onset of symptoms, or 4–6 weeks after discharge from hospital. Persistent sepsis with suspicion of gallbladder necrosis/perforation is an indication for emergency surgery. In severe cases of acute cholecystitis or in a moribund patient a cholecystostomy tube may be used to drain the gallbladder.

■ Prognosis

90 % of cases resolve with this conservative management. 10 % require further emergency intervention.

■ Cholangitis

DEFINITION

Obstruction of the biliary tree (such as by a stone in the CBD) results in stasis and subsequent bacterial overgrowth. The biliary tree eventually fills with pus and severe biliary sepsis follows. This life-threatening condition requires early diagnosis and intervention.

CLINICAL FEATURES

Charcot's triad of (1) Fever and rigors, (2) RUQ pain, and (3) Jaundice is seen in 60 % of cases. Worsening of the patient's medical condition may lead to (4) Shock and (5) Altered level of consciousness (*Reynold's pentad*).

INVESTIGATIONS

Elevated WCC together with obstructive jaundice (raised bilirubin and LFTs), with confirmation of biliary tree obstruction and dilatation by urgent USS.

MANAGEMENT

Patient requires intensive resuscitation, antibiotic treatment (consider ciprofloxacin, tazocin, imipenem or meropenem iv) and supportive care in an HDU/ICU setting. Urgent surgical decompression of the biliary tree may be achieved by either ERCP, percutaneous drainage, or intra-operatively with CBD exploration.

■ Choledocholithiasis

DEFINITION

Stones most commonly pass down gallbladder cystic duct into the CBD where they may cause biliary colic, cholangitis, pancreatitis and strictures.

INVESTIGATIONS

An elevated serum bilirubin and LFTs warrant visualization of the biliary tree and determination of evidence of obstructive dilation with first USS and then MRCP.

MANAGEMENT

ERCP and definitive CBD drainage. Failed ERCP is an indication for *percutaneous cholangiography*. Some favour *intraoperative cholangiogram* and *bile duct exploration* at the time of laparoscopic cholecystectomy. *Laparoscopic USS* at the time of laparoscopic cholecystectomy may also be used to locate CBD stones. Note that if surgical opening of the bile duct is required to remove stones, a T-tube is often placed within the CBD through this opening. A T-tube cholangiogram can then be performed at day five, and if no CBD stones/leakage is seen then the tube is clamped. The tube is then removed over a period of 2–3 weeks in the outpatient setting.

Large-bowel obstruction

PIERS A. C. GATENBY AND PAWAN MATHUR

■ Introduction

Incidence: this is a common presentation to the general surgeon on call. It is more common in older patients in line with the three common causes – carcinoma, volvulus, diverticular disease (and the important differential diagnosis of pseudo-obstruction).

Risk factors:

1. Colorectal adenocarcinoma (53 %): age, male sex, previous colonic polyps, familial adenomatous polyposis, hereditary non-polyposis syndromes, long-standing ulcerative colitis.
2. Diverticular disease (12 %): age, poor fluid/fibre diet, previous episodes of diverticulitis.
3. Volvulus (17 %): age, poor colonic motility.

■ Definition and classification

Definition by site: distal to ileocaecal valve.

Causes:

1. Mechanical:
   a. Extraluminal: colonic volvulus (most frequently sigmoid colon, but caecum may fold upwards), metastatic carcinoma (frequently gynaecological/stomach); less frequently: endometriosis, hernia.
   b. Luminal: colorectal carcinoma, diverticular/inflammatory (Crohn's, UC)/ ischaemic stricture.
   c. Intraluminal: foreign body ingestion, intussusception of polyp, faecal impaction; rare: foreign body introduction.

Hospital Surgery: Foundations in Surgical Practice, ed. Omer Aziz, Sanjay Purkayastha and Paraskevas Paraskeva. Published by Cambridge University Press. © Cambridge University Press 2009.

2. Non-mechanical: ileus and pseudo-obstruction (mechanical causes must be excluded).

■ Making the diagnosis and treatment

It is important to differentiate clinically a true (mechanical) obstruction from a failure of bowel motility (pseudo-obstruction), and this may be made on clinical examination and plain X-rays (or CT or contrast scans if doubt still remains).

CT scanning is useful for demonstration of metastatic disease in malignant disease, and in the presence of metastases, relief of the obstruction by endoluminal stent alone may be sufficient surgical treatment of the primary tumour.

■ History

Pain classically colicky in nature (in waves) with individual waves lasting several minutes, felt in the centre of the abdomen; pain becomes constant in strangulation or perforation. Distension progresses as history lengthens.

Vomiting in the presence of an incompetent ileocaecal valve, large bowel ('faeculent') contents will be vomited late in the course.

Constipation will become absolute (no flatus or faeces – also known as obstipation) in complete obstruction after the bowel distal to the obstruction has emptied (often with diarrhoea initially due to increased peristalsis in the early course).

Acute/chronic patients may have chronic features of worsening obstruction (commonly in carcinoma) or previous episodes of acute obstruction (most commonly in volvulus).

Complete/incomplete partially obstructing lesions may give chronic symptoms prior to presentation.

Simple vs. strangulated: simple = mechanical obstruction (most common), strangulated = compromise of vascular supply (especially in sigmoid volvulus).

Closed-loop vs. non-closed-loop: if the bowel is obstructed at two points (e.g. the neck of a hernia or volvulus, or a single obstructing lesion with a competent ileocaecal valve), the segment lying between these will become rapidly distended with vascular compromise and risk of perforation (beware large-bowel obstruction and right iliac fossa tenderness which may indicate that the caecum is at risk of ischaemia/rupture).

Time course: initially in the time course symptoms and signs increase in severity as the intestinal motility and contractile activity increase, followed later by fatigue and dilation of the bowel. Alternatively the increased intraluminal pressure may result in perforation and peritonitis (especially if the blood supply is compromised e.g. in a strangulated hernia, volvulus, sepsis, hypovolaemia). The time course of symptom progression may be several days if the ileocaecal valve is incompetent and the large bowel may decompress proximally into the small intestine. Large quantities of fluid will be sequestered into the third space (outside of the intracellular and intravascular compartments).

Other features: chronic change in bowel habit, weight loss and passage of fresh or altered blood per rectum are common in colorectal carcinoma (but may be present in diverticular disease).

■ Examination

Cardiovascular shock secondary to fluid sequestration, systemic inflammatory response or sepsis.

ABDOMEN

1. Inspection: distension, previous surgical scars, hernia.
2. Palpation: tenderness, peritonism (in the case of perforation), abdominal mass from carcinoma, diverticular segment or distended bowel loop, hernia.
3. Percussion: resonance over gas-filled dilated bowel loops, tender in the case of peritonitis, ascites in previous abdominal malignancy.

4. Auscultation: increase in bowel sound frequency and pitch in earlier stages followed by reduction later in course if there is concomitant small-bowel obstruction. Normal or reduced bowel sounds otherwise.

5. Rectum: after bowel opened may be empty and collapsed, presence of blood indicates possibility of tumour, bowel infarction, diverticular disease or inflammatory bowel disease; rectal tumour may be palpable. A capacious rectum is suggestive of pseudo-obstruction.

MANAGEMENT ALGORITHM

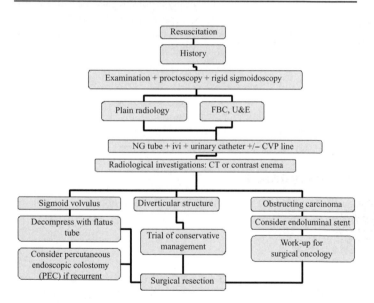

Ultimate surgical treatment may involve one of the following procedures: segmental resection and anastomosis +/− on-table lavage +/− defunctioning ileostomy; Hartmann's procedure or subtotal colectomy. Management of pseudo-obstruction is supportive.

■ Investigations

Diagnosis is usually made clinically and investigations are used to confirm clinical suspicion and localize the level of obstruction and cause if not apparent.

Blood tests: normal initially, followed by signs of electrolyte derangement (fluid sequestration), dehydration (raised urea and haematocrit), sepsis (raised WCC/inflammatory markers), raised tumour markers (CEA, CA19-9) in colorectal carcinoma.

Plain radiology: plain X-ray of the abdomen shows dilated large bowel loops (peripheral position in abdomen, haustra do not completely traverse lumen), air-fluid levels, foreign bodies, hernia, absence of gas and faeces distal to the level of obstruction. Erect chest X-ray to rule out perforation.

Contrast radiology: unprepared *water*-soluble enema (e.g. Gastrografin) will demonstrate level of obstruction, features of stricture suggesting cause, and exclude pseudo-obstruction. This is shown in Figure 36.

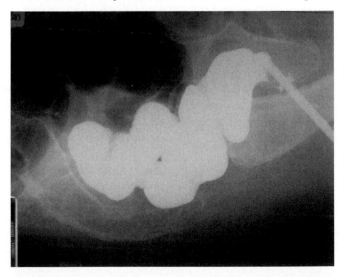

Figure 36

CT (iv with rectal contrast): may help to demonstrate the level of obstruction and frequently the cause of obstruction.

■ Treatment

Resuscitation: treatment of dehydration and electrolyte replacement with crystalloid, with monitoring of fluid status with a urinary catheter (+/− central line). Preoperative optimization and consideration of transfer to HDU. Early anaesthetic review and opinion is useful.

Antibiotics: if signs of peritonitis/sepsis.

Bowel decompression: nil by mouth. Nasogastric tube if small-bowel obstruction secondary to incompetent ileocaecal valve. If closed loop obstruction, early decompression should be instituted due to high risk of strangulation and perforation.

TREATMENT OF CAUSE OF OBSTRUCTION

1. *Carcinoma*: **surgery** is the ultimate treatment (see below) but stent (if such services are available locally) if complete obstruction, for emergency decompression; stage with CT:
   a. Metastatic disease: stent +/− possibility of resection
   b. No metastatic disease: stent (as a bridge to surgery) + resection.
2. *Diverticular disease*: trial of conservative management with bowel rest (nil by mouth), intravenous fluids and antibiotics; proceed to resection if symptoms do not settle or patient has recurrent admissions (see Colorectal disease: colonic diverticular disease Chapter).
3. *Volvulus*: decompression with flatus tube +/− consideration of PEC (percutaneous endoscopic colostomy)/resection.

If the bowel can be decompressed in the acute setting, and surgical resection is planned electively later, then the risk of a stoma can be minimized.

Surgical procedures undertaken for large-bowel obstruction depend on where the obstructing lesion is and include the following (see Figure 37):

1. Anterior resection
2. Hartmann's procedure
3. Left hemicolectomy
4. Right hemicolectomy
5. Subtotal colectomy
6. Segmental resection $+/-$ on-table lavage.

A defunctioning ileostomy may be used with any of the above procedures where primary anastomoses are formed.

DVT prophylaxis: thromboembolic deterrent stockings (TEDS) and low molecular weight heparin.

Nutrition: consider supplemental enteral (or parenteral nutrition), especially in chronic obstruction.

■ Prognosis

The majority of patients with obstructing colorectal carcinoma present at an advanced stage and may require adjuvant chemotherapy. A diverticular stricture secondary to inflammation and bowel spasm may settle with bowel rest and antibiotics. Of those that present with volvulus, 50 % have a further episode, so resection should be considered in patients fit for surgery, and prevention of further episodes with percutaneous mini-colostomy (to fix the sigmoid colon and allow venting of gas) in unfit patients. The overall mortality of large-bowel obstruction is 15 %, and highest in malignant causes of large-bowel obstruction; operative mortality is about twice that of elective resections but is highly dependent on the patient's co-morbidities and how unwell the patient is at the time of surgery.

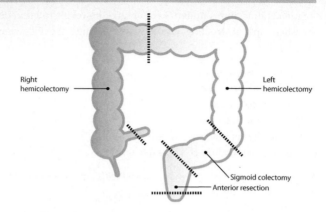

Figure 37 Illustration showing examples of surgical procedures

Small-bowel obstruction

PIERS A. C. GATENBY AND PAWAN MATHUR

■ Introduction

Incidence: this is a common presentation to the general surgeon on call, but the incidence is difficult to estimate: 12–17 % of patients who have previously had abdominal surgery will have subsequent small-bowel obstruction. With increasing elective hernia repair, adhesions (secondary to previous surgery) are now the most common cause of small-bowel obstruction.

Risk factors: related to cause – notably previous surgery resulting in adhesions, hernias, gynaecological malignancy, Crohn's disease.

■ Definition and classification

Definition by site: distal to pylorus, at or proximal to ileocaecal valve.

Causes:

1. Extraluminal

  a. Adhesions (60 %): usually acquired postoperatively, rarely inflammatory or secondary to chemical/starch from surgical gloves.

  b. Hernias (20 %):

    i. Acquired (inguinal, femoral; rarely: obturator, lumbar, spiegelian).

    ii. Secondary incisional, internal postoperative.

  c. Mass lesion: malignant disease (10 %), peritoneal disease from e.g. gynaecological/stomach primary.

Hospital Surgery: Foundations in Surgical Practice, ed. Omer Aziz, Sanjay Purkayastha and Paraskevas Paraskeva. Published by Cambridge University Press. © Cambridge University Press 2009.

2. **Luminal**
   a. Luminal stricture (5 %): Crohn's, radiation enteritis, vasculitis.
   b. Primary tumours: gastrointestinal stromal tumours/carcinoid/ carcinoma (carcinoma of the caecum)/lymphoma; secondary tumours are rare.

3. **Intraluminal**
   a. Bolus obstruction: gallstone ileus, ingested foreign body, bezoar, food bolus; rare: parasites.
   b. Intussusception.

NB A major diagnosis to exclude is paralytic ileus (failure of bowel motility without mechanical obstruction).

■ History

Pain: classically colicky in nature with individual waves lasting a few minutes felt in the centre of the abdomen; pain becomes constant in strangulation or perforation.

Distension: progresses as history lengthens. More marked in more distal site of obstruction.

Vomiting: food and bile, occurs earlier in more proximal obstruction.

Constipation: will become absolute (no flatus or faeces) in complete obstruction after the bowel distal to the obstruction has emptied (often with diarrhoea initially due to increased peristalsis in the early course).

Acute/chronic: patients may have chronic features of worsening obstruction or previous episodes of acute obstruction.

Complete/incomplete: not all patients will have complete bowel obstruction. Complete obstruction is less likely to settle without surgery.

Simple/strangulated: simple = mechanical obstruction, strangulated = compromise of vascular supply.

Time course: initially in time course symptoms and signs increase in severity as the intestinal motility and contractile activity increase, followed later by fatigue and dilation of the bowel. Alternatively the increased intraluminal pressure may result in perforation and peritonitis (especially if the blood supply is compromised e.g. in a strangulated hernia, volvulus, sepsis, hypovolaemia). Large quantities of fluid will be sequestered into the third space (outside of the intracellular and extracellular compartments).

■ Examination

Cardiovascular shock/dehydration secondary to fluid sequestration, systemic inflammatory response or sepsis.

Abdomen:

1. Inspection: distension, visible peristalsis, previous surgical scars, hernia (femoral orifices in females).
2. Palpation: tenderness, peritonism (in the case of perforation), abdominal mass, hernia.
3. Percussion: resonance over gas-filled dilated bowel loops, tender in the case of peritonitis.
4. Auscultation: increase in bowel sound frequency and pitch in earlier stages followed by reduction later in course.
5. Rectum: after bowel emptying may be empty/collapsed (capacious rectum is suggestive of possible large-bowel obstruction (previous chapter); presence of blood would necessitate investigation of large bowel prior to attributing to small-bowel pathology.

■ Investigation

Diagnosis is usually made clinically and investigations are used to confirm clinical suspicion and localize the level of obstruction and cause if not apparent.

Plain radiology: AXR shows dilated small bowel loops (>4 cm, central position in abdomen, valvulae conniventes) as shown in Figure 38. Air-fluid levels as shown in Figure 39. Foreign bodies and occasionally a hernia may be seen. Absence of gas and faeces distal to the level of obstruction.

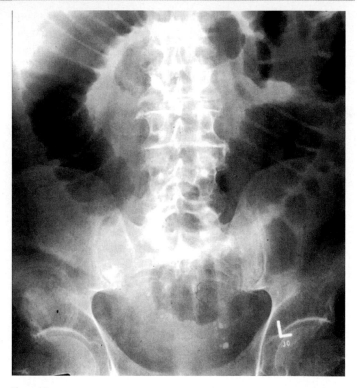

Figure 38

Contrast radiology: small-bowel study (water-soluble contrast orally/ via NG tube) will demonstrate level of obstruction, and osmotic effect may be therapeutic in obstruction secondary to adhesions or extraluminal tumour.

CT +/− contrast: will demonstrate level and frequently the cause of obstruction.

Blood tests: normal initially, followed by signs of electrolyte derangement (fluid sequestration), dehydration (raised urea + haematocrit), sepsis (raised WCC/inflammatory markers).

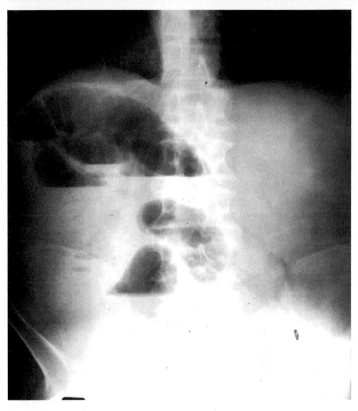

Figure 39

■ Treatment

1. Resuscitation: treatment of dehydration and electrolyte replacement with crystalloid intravenous fluids ('drip'), with monitoring of fluid status with a urinary catheter (+/− central line).
2. Antibiotics: if signs of peritonitis/sepsis.
3. Bowel decompression: with nasogastric tube and NBM ('suck').

4. Surgery: indicated when clinical deterioration/increasing distension on AXR, for hernia repair, bowel strangulation, peritonitis.
5. DVT prophylaxis: thromboembolic deterrent stockings (TEDS) and low molecular weight heparin.
6. Nutrition: consider supplemental enteral (or parenteral nutrition) in chronic obstruction.

As a general principal, conservative management should be reviewed at 24–48 hours with a repeat AXR +/− diagnostic CT, and consider surgery ('do not let the sun go down on a small-bowel obstruction'). Signs of peritonism are an indication for surgery.

Surgical treatment includes division of band adhesions, small-bowel resection and anastomosis, hernia reduction and closure of the defect (Figure 40).

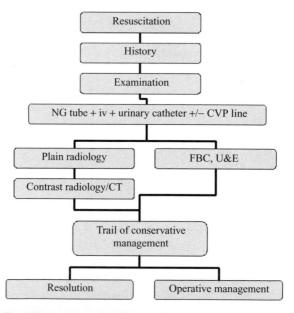

Figure 40 Management algorithm

Methods of adhesion prevention exist (e.g. Adept and use of Seprafilm) but long-term efficacy remains unproven at present.

In advanced malignant disease, palliative management only may be appropriate as surgical bypass has a very poor outcome.

■ Prognosis

60–85 % of patients with partial obstruction settle without surgery.
20–40 % mortality in the presence of strangulation and bowel infarction.

Surgical exploration is indicated early if the patient has not had previous surgery as obstruction secondary to adhesions is unlikely.

Perforated gastro-duodenal ulcer

DANNY YAKOUB AND GEORGE HANNA

A perforated gastro-duodenal ulcer is a surgical emergency requiring urgent assessment and intervention. The incidence of this condition has decreased markedly since the introduction of proton pump inhibitors and *Helicobacter pylori* triple therapy for peptic ulcer disease.

■ Aetiology/predisposing factors

- Chronic benign duodenal ulcer: *Helicobacter pylori* infection is an important predisposing factor (80 % of perforated ulcers).
- Acute ulceration secondary to drugs: steroids, NSAIDs.
- Excessive alcohol consumption.
- Acute ulceration secondary to physiological stressors: burns, trauma, sepsis, chemotherapy and radiotherapy.
- Perforation of a malignant gastric ulcer.

■ Pathogenesis

Ulcer is usually located anteriorly, resulting in the release of gastric contents and air into the peritoneal cavity. Posterior ulcers erode into the gastro-duodenal artery and result in haemorrhage. Anterior perforation may be duodenal, pyloric or gastric and may be **sealed** naturally by omental folds or **open** to the general peritoneum. Release of gastro-duodenal contents induces chemical peritonitis which if untreated results in bacterial peritonitis.

Hospital Surgery: Foundations in Surgical Practice, ed. Omer Aziz, Sanjay Purkayastha and Paraskevas Paraskeva. Published by Cambridge University Press. © Cambridge University Press 2009.

■ Symptoms

History of peptic ulcer disease. Sudden excruciating epigastric pain, haematemesis or melaena. Shoulder pain due to diaphragmatic irritation. Significant vomiting is usually late and due to peritonitis and ileus. Peritoneal soiling may trickle along the right paracolic gutter and localize in the right iliac fossa to mimic appendicitis. Patient may have been on NSAIDs, steroids, heavy drinker, or have other predisposing factors mentioned above.

■ Signs

Severity depends on degree of peritoneal soiling. Upper abdominal tenderness, rebound tenderness and board-like rigidity. Later when ileus ensues abdominal distension, silent abdomen and signs of shock and sepsis.

■ Differential diagnosis

Acute pancreatitis, acute cholecystitis, acute appendicitis, intestinal infarction.

■ Complications

Generalized peritonitis, penetration of the pancreas and pancreatitis, bleeding perforated ulcer and finally sub-diaphragmatic abscess.

■ Investigations

Plain erect chest X-ray or lateral decubitus in very ill patients shows free air under the diaphragm and maybe basal atelectasis in the lung fields (Figure 41). Abdominal X-ray may show fluid levels in the case of general peritonitis and ileus.

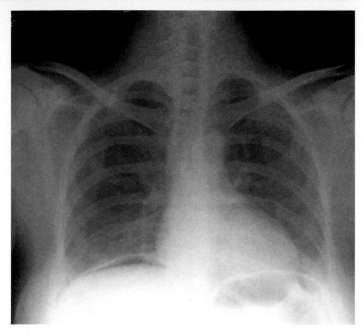

Figure 41

Blood tests: FBC (WCC may be raised), U&E, amylase (raised in up to 20 % of cases), G&S, clotting. **Radiology:** if diagnosis is difficult, a **CT scan**. Investigations for *H. pylori* infection should be done. **Water-soluble contrast** study may differentiate between sealed perforation and that spreading to the lesser sac or general peritoneum.

■ Management

O_2, large-bore iv access and aggressive fluid resuscitation with 0.9 % normal saline to correct hypovolaemia and electrolyte imbalance. An NG tube may be inserted if patient is vomiting profusely. Intravenous anti-emetic and iv proton pump inhibitor. Analgesia im/iv, usually morphine (NOT NSAIDs). Intravenous antibiotics (750 mg cefuroxime and 500 mg metronidazole) should be given while patient waits for further definitive treatment.

Surgery is usually open although this can be done laparoscopically. An upper midline laparotomy is usually performed to gain access to the site of perforation, which is identified and biopsied. Copious **peritoneal lavage** is followed by suture repair of the perforation either by primary closure and omental plug, or by omental plug alone (in cases where tissues are very friable). The patient should be optimized and resuscitated prior to surgery, correcting oliguria and poor peripheral perfusion. This should not, however, delay surgery beyond a few hours from presentation. In cases of perforated gastric ulcer, a biopsy is essential to investigate the presence of malignancy. In these cases a partial gastrectomy with wide margins may be required. In the case of bleeding posterior duodenal ulcers, surgery involves performing an enterotomy and underrunning the ulcer base for haemostasis.

Conservative management of perforated duodenal ulcer may occur in cases where the presentation is delayed with localization of the perforation by the omentum which seals and controls it (Figure 42). This is

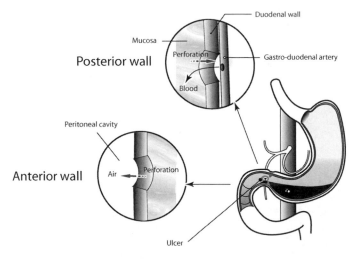

Figure 42

also the case for patients with severe co-morbidity who are not fit for anaesthesia and therefore are not likely to survive an operation. The decision to manage a perforated viscus conservatively must be taken by a senior surgeon and preferably the consultant responsible for the patient. In these cases, intravenous antibiotics and analgesia may help although prognosis remains poor.

■ Prognosis

Immediate surgical management carries excellent prognosis. Long-term inhibition of acid secretion and *H. pylori* eradication is imperative to prevent recurrence. Prognosis worsens with: prolonged period from perforation to admission, hypovolaemia, increased age, and co-morbidity of patients. Patients should complete a course of *H. pylori* eradication triple therapy after surgery.

Volvulus

JAMES KINROSS AND PAUL ZIPRIN

This important condition has a significant morbidity and mortality and therefore requires a high index of suspicion. It can be missed as it often presents in the elderly and infirm.

■ Definition and classification

Volvulus is a rotation of a segment of bowel about its longitudinal mesenteric axis, resulting in occlusion of the proximal section. It most commonly affects the colon (the sigmoid and caecum) although small bowel (usually the lower ileum) or stomach may also be affected. It can be classified as *primary* (i.e. caused by congenital intestinal malrotation, abnormal mesenteric attachments or congenital 'Ladd's' bands), or *secondary* (more common), and can be either *acute* or *chronic*.

■ Incidence

Sigmoid volvulus is the most common type and is responsible for approximately 8 % of all intestinal obstructions. Men are more commonly affected than women, most commonly in the sixth decade of life. Caecal volvulus is more common in women.

■ Aetiology

Associated with increasing age, chronic constipation, a high-roughage diet, lead poisoning, neurological conditions (e.g. Parkinson's disease),

Hospital Surgery: Foundations in Surgical Practice, ed. Omer Aziz, Sanjay Purkayastha and Paraskevas Paraskeva. Published by Cambridge University Press. © Cambridge University Press 2009.

Hirschsprung's disease, patients in nursing homes and mental health facilities. Can be caused by round-worm infection and Chagas disease. Incomplete midgut rotation predisposes to caecal volvulus.

■ Pathology

Macroscopic: volvulus occurs secondary to a narrow mesentery in association with a long redundant sigmoid allowing two segments of bowel to come together and twist around the axis, usually anticlockwise in the case of the sigmoid volvulus, varying from $180°$ (35%) to $540°$ (10%) (Figure 43). Caecal volvulus usually involves clockwise axial rotation of terminal ileum, caecum and ascending colon around ileocolic vessels and mesentery (Figure 44). **Microscopic:** venous congestion and arterial compromise cause ischaemia and infarction. Oedema, bacterial translocation, gangrene and ultimately perforation can occur. Massive volumes of fluid can lie in this pathological third space causing hypovolaemic as well as septic shock. Early reduction is therefore important.

■ History

50 % of patients have had a previous episode. Obstruction may be complete or incomplete. The patient complains of absolute constipation, sudden onset colicky abdominal pain and late vomiting in sigmoid volvulae (early if in a caecal volvulus). Initial obstruction may be intermittent with subsequent passage of large volumes of flatus/stool. Caecal volvulus is often accompanied by small-bowel obstruction.

■ Examination

A distended hypertympanic abdomen with tinkling or absent bowel sounds and an empty rectum are found on examination. If pain is severe with guarding consider perforation. Patients can be shocked and febrile if ischaemia or perforation has ensued. (NB in view of aetiology often serious concomitant systemic diseases are present that need to be con-templated.)

■ Investigations

FBC (leucocytosis), U&E (electrolytes, renal function), G+S (in case of surgical intervention). Arterial blood gas may reveal metabolic acido-sis and raised lactate suggesting ischaemic bowel. Erect CXR (exclude perforation). AXR shows closed double loop of large bowel, haustra may be visible. Classic '*Coffee bean*' sign in 70 %, going from pelvis to RUQ (pointing to left on AXR) in sigmoid volvulus and pelvis to LUQ (point-ing to right on AXR) in caecal volvulus. In caecal volvulus the presence of distended small-bowel loops can make diagnosis difficult. Bowel wall thickening indicates oedema and suggests risk of perforation. Sig-moid volvulus may be confirmed and reduced by Gastrografin enema, demonstrating obstruction at the rectosigmoid junction (contraindi-cated if perforation or evidence of ischaemia). CT scanning confirms diagnosis (identifying other pathology), helps determine bowel wall thickness, and presence of perforated viscus.

■ Treatment

CONSERVATIVE/MEDICAL

Patient should initially be resuscitated with iv fluids and oxygen, catheterized to monitor urine output and decompress abdomen, kept NBM, and NG tube passed if vomiting. Intravenous/im analgesia (mor-phine) with anti-emetic (e.g. cyclizine 50 mg iv) should be given. In cases of sigmoid volvulus (sited at 15–25 cm from anus) where perforation has not occurred, an attempt should be made at reversal and decompres-sion by placement of a long, soft and well-lubricated flatus tube past the site of obstruction during rigid sigmoidoscopy at the bedside. Flex-ible sigmoidoscopy is often a better and easier way of reducing volvulus and should be performed if available or if rigid sigmoidoscopy fails. A

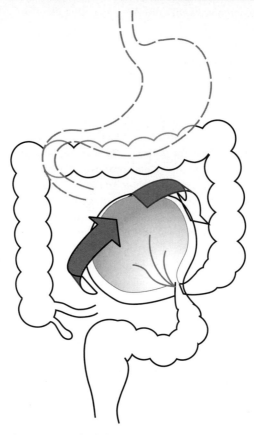

Figure 43 Sigmoid volvulus

successful reduction is indicated by a *hiss* of decompression followed by passage of a large amount of loose stool and secretions occupying the third space. A flatus tube should be connected to a drainage bag, comfortably secured and may be left for 48 hr while oedema resolves. Perforation is a surgical emergency. Recurrent cases require elective surgical treatment. Caecal volvulus should always be treated surgically.

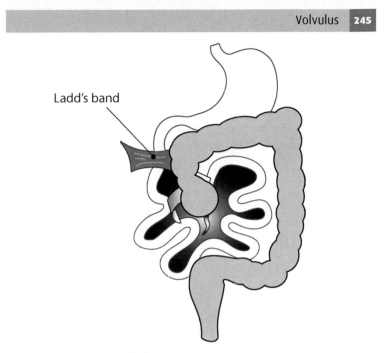

Ladd's band

Figure 44 Caecal volvulus

SURGICAL

Indications for emergency surgery: (1) Failed conservative therapy, (2) Recurrent volvulus, (3) Evidence of perforation/ischaemia, (4) Caecal volvulus. The initial surgery for sigmoid volvulus is a laparotomy with untwisting of the segment, decompression and assessment of bowel viability. Resection (sigmoidectomy) of the compromised segment with primary anastomosis or Hartmann's procedure are often required, though other surgical options exist. In caecal volvulus the same principles apply, with untwisting of the volvulus followed by either resection (right hemicolectomy) or caecopexy performed. Caecostomy or percutaneous drainage are rarely done. Elective procedures follow similar operative principles, can be performed laparoscopically, and are aimed at primary resection and anastomosis.

■ Prognosis

High recurrence rate (60 % at one year) for those managed conservatively. Thirty day mortality is up to 25 % in an emergency due to delayed diagnoses.

Gastrointestinal bleeding

HENRY TILLNEY AND ALEXANDER G. HERIOT

■ Definition

Bleeding from the gastrointestinal tract (GI) is an important surgical emergency that requires urgent evaluation and assessment if major morbidity and mortality is to be avoided. After initial assessment of haemodynamic status and resuscitation, attention should be drawn to trying to determine the site of bleeding as well as potential co-morbidities.

■ Classification

Upper gastrointestinal haemorrhage is defined as bleeding occurring in the GI tract proximal to the ligament of Treitz (duodenojejunal flexure) whereas lower gastrointestinal haemorrhage is defined as bleeding arising in the bowel distal to this.

■ History

Patients commonly present with GI bleeding either to the emergency department, or often during hospital admission for another illness. In most cases the history offers the best clue as to the site of potential haemorrhage:

Bleeding: the mode of bleeding (haematemesis versus rectal bleeding), type (bright red, clotted, altered blood/melaena), and quantity of blood and duration of symptoms offer vital clues. *Melaena* refers to

Hospital Surgery: Foundations in Surgical Practice, ed. Omer Aziz, Sanjay Purkayastha and Paraskevas Paraskeva. Published by Cambridge University Press. © Cambridge University Press 2009.

blood that has been partially digested by enzymes rendering it black and 'tar-like' in appearance and very foul smelling. *Dark clotted blood* usually results from a proximal lower GI bleed, but may be confused with melaena. *Bright red bleeding* usually implies a distal lower GI bleed. Note that a massive upper GI bleed may also present with bright red bleeding although the patient is usually very haemodynamically unstable in this case. *Occult bleeding* refers to a slow and intermittent pattern of blood loss and does not pose an immediate threat though warrants investigation.

Change in bowel habit: may signify underlying pathology.

Pain: may highlight site of bleeding, such as epigastric in peptic ulcer disease (PUD); oesophagitis, lower abdominal crampy pain in Crohn's, ulcerative colitis and diverticulitis.

Past medical history: PUD, alcohol use, severe vomiting, *Helicobacter pylori* infection, previous GI bleeds, inflammatory bowel disease, diverticulosis, polyposis syndromes and trauma.

Medications: anticoagulants (warfarin) are important to note as are other medications such as β blockers, which may result in an abnormally low heart rate, with diuretics and calcium channel blockers resulting in a low blood pressure; also NSAIDs, clopidogrel and steroids.

■ Examination

General status, conscious level, vital signs (BP, HR, RR, oxygen saturation). Orthostatic hypotension (lower BP when standing as compared to lying down). Look for peripheral stigmata of liver disease (jaundice, palmar erythema spider naevi) associated with variceal bleeding. Look in mouth for evidence of blood. Inspect vomitus/stool for type and quantity of blood. Abdominal examination may highlight pathology. **Rectal examination is mandatory** and should be followed by proctoscopy and rigid sigmoidoscopy.

■ Initial management and investigation

Oxygen, large-bore iv access (14–16G), send blood tests for FBC (Hb, Hct and platelets are important), U&E (look for urea rise and renal function), LFT (co-existing liver pathology), clotting, urgent blood crossmatch. Resuscitate with colloids (Gelofusin) and then either normal saline or Hartmann's solution. Pass urinary catheter to monitor output. Nasogastric tube may help differentiate upper and lower GI bleeding. A GCS of <8 due to massive haemorrhage and hypotension is an indication for intubation and urgent transfer to theatre. CXR/AXR may be indicated for perforated/obstructed viscus. Contact anaesthetists early.

■ Further management

The identification of source of bleeding combined with initial therapy is discussed in the following pages on 'Upper GI bleeding' and 'Lower GI bleeding'.

■ Upper GI bleeding

DEFINITION

Bleeding from any source from mouth to ligament of Trietz (suspensory ligament of fourth part of duodenum).

INCIDENCE

50 to 150 per 100 000 per year. Incidence is higher among the lowest socioeconomic groups.

AETIOLOGY

Most common cause in the West is peptic ulceration (*H. pylori* and NSAID associated). Alcoholic cirrhosis resulting in gastric and oesophageal varices is becoming increasingly common. Other aetiologies are listed below.

Cause of upper GI bleed	Frequency (%)
Peptic ulcer	35–50
Varices	5–12
Mallory-Weiss tear	2–5
Oesophagitis	20–30
Duodenitis/gastritis/erosions	10–20
Vascular (Dieulafoy's lesion, angiodysplasia)	2–3
Oesophageal/gastric cancer	2–5
Aortoduodenal fistula	<1
Oesophageal/gastric cancer	<1

■ Lower GI bleeding

DEFINITION AND CLASSIFICATION

Bleeding from source distal to the ligament of Treitz. 'Massive' if >6 unit transfusion in 24 hours. 10–15 % of those with severe bright red rectal bleeding have an upper GI source.

INCIDENCE

Annual incidence approximately 25 per 100 000 adult population. Mean reported age 63–77.

AETIOLOGY

Most common cause of massive lower GI bleeding is diverticular disease (60 %), followed by inflammatory bowel disease (13 %), angiodysplasia and colorectal cancer. Other causes include infective/ischaemic/pseudomembranous colitis, rectal ulcers, radiation colitis, postoperative bleeding (haemorrhoidectomy or polypectomy), aortoenteric fistula, any of the above with co-existing coagulopathy.

■ Upper GI bleeding

SYMPTOMS AND SIGNS

Haematemesis: vomiting of fresh blood or 'coffee grounds' if gastric acid has had time to convert haemoglobin to methaemoglobin.

Melaena: passage of dark, partially digested blood per rectum.

Haematochezia: bright red rectal bleeding in massive upper GI bleed (associated with **cardiovascular instability/shock**).

Co-morbidity: significantly affects outcome.

INVESTIGATION AND INITIAL MANAGEMENT

Resuscitation: $2 \times 14G$ cannulae, IVI, O_2.

Bloods: FBC, U+E, LFTs, clotting, G&S or Crossmatch (four units if melaena on pr and SBP < 100, six units if variceal bleed suspected).

NG tube may be of benefit and aid diagnosis (fresh bleeding, coffee ground).

If GCS < 8 patient is at risk of aspiration and requires **endotracheal intubation**.

Medication: iv proton pump inhibitor.

Urinary catheter for monitoring urine output.

CVP line may be used for monitoring blood volume.

FURTHER MANAGEMENT

OGD: within 24 hours or more acutely if unstable, is both diagnostic and therapeutic. Stigmata of recent haemorrhage and their associated risk of rebleeding include: spurting vessel (80 %); non-bleeding visible vessel (50 %); adherent blood clot (33 %); oozing (10 %); flat spots (7 %); and clean ulcer base (3 %). Note: endotracheal intubation should be considered in large bleeds or in elderly patients with comorbidity who carry a significant risk of aspiration.

Endoscopic treatment: adrenaline injection, laser photocoagulation, heat probe, bipolar diathermy, endo-clip.

Surgical treatment: indicated when (1) Active bleeding cannot be controlled by endoscopic means or (2) Rebleeding after initially successful treatment. (Endoscopic treatment may be repeated once if endoscopist and surgeon believe this to be appropriate.) Surgery involves gastrotomy/duodenotomy with under-running of the ulcer. In very large ulcers resection (gastrectomy) may be required. Combined care (gastroenterologist/surgeon) is optimal. The following criteria may be used to determine need for surgery: **Age < 60 years:** transfusion requirements > 8 units in 24 hr, one or two rebleeds, spurting vessel at OGD not controlled by injection of medication, continued bleeding. **Age > 60 years:** transfusion requirements > 4 units in 24 hr, one rebleed, spurting vessel at OGD, continued bleeding.

PROGNOSIS

The Rockall score is an externally validated risk-assessment tool for patients with upper GI bleeding. The predicted mortality is shown below, followed by the score criteria.

Score	Predicted mortality	
	Initial score (%)	Full score (%)
0	0.20	0.00
1	2.40	0.00
2	5.60	0.20
3	11.00	2.90
4	24.60	5.30
5	39.60	10.80
6	48.90	17.30
7	50.00	27.00
8+	—	41.10

Rockall score criteria	
Initial Rockall score	
Age <60 yrs	0
60–79 yrs	1
>80 yrs	2
Shock None	0
Pulse > 100 and systolic BP > 100	1
Systolic BP <100	2
Co-morbidity None	0
Cardiac failure, IHD, or any major co-morbidity	2
Renal/liver failure or disseminated malignancy	3
Total initial Rockall score (Max 7)	
Full Rockall score after endoscopy	
Endoscopic diagnosis	
M-W tear or no lesion and no sign of bleeding	0
All other diagnoses	1
Malignancy of upper GI tract	2
Major stigmata of recent haemorrhage	
None or dark spot only	0
Blood in upper GI tract, adherent clot, visible or spurting vessel	2
Final Rockall score (Max 11)	

■ Treatment of acute variceal bleeding

Massive haematemesis with variceal bleeding carries a high mortality.

INITIAL MANAGEMENT

Early resuscitation (as above), correction of coagulopathy (with blood products), and airway management. Consider the diagnosis early (e.g. jaundice, liver disease). Poor liver function as indicated by *Child's classification* system results in a much higher risk of mortality. ICU management.

MEDICAL THERAPY

Seek specialist advice. Intravenous infusion of somatostatin analogue (octreotide) decreases splanchnic blood flow, thereby decreasing portal and variceal pressure. Vasopressin may also be used to reduce splanchnic blood flow and portal hypertension.

ENDOSCOPIC TREATMENT

Oesophageal: injection sclerotherapy, banding. Gastric: may be difficult to control endoscopically.

SENGSTAKEN-BLAKEMORE TUBE

If unable to control bleeding endoscopically. Re-endoscope and treat at 24 hours.

TIPSS

Transvenous intrahepatic portosystemic shunts (TIPPS) may be placed to decompress the portal circulation if still persistently bleeding on removal of Sengstaken-Blakemore tube.

SURGICAL TREATMENT

Oesophageal transaction or portosystemic shunt. High morbidity/mortality.

■ Lower GI bleeding

SYMPTOMS AND SIGNS

Haematochezia: passage of bright red blood per rectum (*melaena* – passage of dark/black, partially digested blood – suggests upper GI aetiology).

Shock/haemodynamic instability (rapid thready pulse/hypotension) suggests significant bleed.

Digital rectal examination confirms nature of the blood and excludes a low rectal/anal tumour.

Co-morbidity: significantly affects outcome.

INVESTIGATION AND INITIAL MANAGEMENT

Resuscitation: $2 \times 14G$ cannulae, IVI, O_2 and assessment/investigation in tandem if unstable. Management algorithm is shown in Figure 45. Urgency of investigation is increased with instability.

Bloods: FBC, U&E, LFTs, clotting (beware of anticoagulant medication), crossmatch.

Rigid sigmoidoscopy and proctoscopy: to exclude rectal source.

FURTHER MANAGEMENT

Colonic investigation: elective colonoscopy on prepared colon if bleeding stops. Some advocate acute colonoscopy following rapid cleansing, with adrenaline injection/thermal coagulation of actively bleeding lesions, including diverticula.

OGD: exclude upper GI source (if in doubt).

OTHER INVESTIGATIONS

In the presence of ongoing bleeding where endoscopy and colonoscopy have not yielded a diagnosis, other investigations include:

Mesenteric angiography: requires bleeding rates of >1 ml/min but can be therapeutic with the use of intra-arterial vasopressin or embolization. Vasopressin is associated with a 50 % rebleed rate but even if not therapeutic, arteriography can help to locate the source of bleeding and guide segmental colectomy should surgery be required. Ongoing active bleeding may require diagnostic/therapeutic arteriography/embolization if this is available.

Radionucleotide imaging: can detect rates of bleeding as low as 0.1–0.5 ml/min but accuracy ranges from 24 to 91 %. More useful in haemodynamically stable patients with ongoing bleeding.

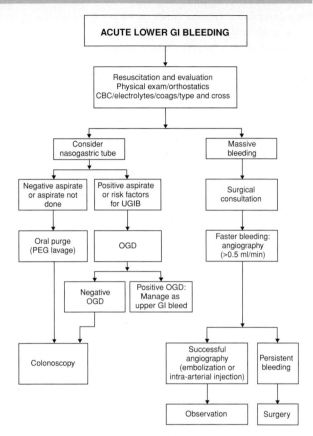

Figure 45 Management algorithm for lower GI bleeding

INDICATIONS FOR SURGERY

If persistent bleeding/shock, >6 U blood transfusion. Surgery includes diagnostic on-table enteroscopy/colonoscopy. Resection of source of bleeding: bowel resection/segmental colectomy if site identified. Sub-total colectomy/end-ileostomy if source not identified.

PROGNOSIS

Overall mortality of 2–4 %. Operative mortality from emergency surgery 10 %. Rebleeding occurs in 14–30 % of patients with a first bleed, and 50 % following a second episode of bleeding.

Mesenteric ischaemia

LAI PUN TONG AND AVRIL CHANG

■ Introduction

DEFINITION AND CLASSIFICATION

Mesenteric ischaemia is the impaired circulation in the mesenteric vessels leading to inadequate perfusion and oxygenation of intestines with possible progression to infarction and necrosis.

May be classified into:

1. *Intermittent or chronic: intestinal angina.* This presents more in an outpatient setting with poorly localized pain often after meals, or weight loss and occasionally with non-specific symptoms such as bloating, or altered bowel habits similar to irritable bowel syndrome. Most of these patients are elderly and have other signs of peripheral vascular disease.
2. *Acute ischaemia*: leading to infarction and necrosis, resulting in acute surgical emergency. This is due to either thrombosis or embolization of the mesenteric arteries, most usually the superior mesenteric artery. Hence the distribution of the ischaemic bowel tends to be jejunum to ileum and may possibly also involve the right colon depending on the extent of arterial occlusion.

■ History

Emergency presentation with moderate to severe acute abdominal pain as main feature. Pain usually generalized or central. Abdominal distension, nausea, vomiting and rectal bleeding commonly occur. Onset of pain may be related to food. Symptoms can be vague. Differential

Hospital Surgery: Foundations in Surgical Practice, ed. Omer Aziz, Sanjay Purkayastha and Paraskevas Paraskeva. Published by Cambridge University Press.
© Cambridge University Press 2009.

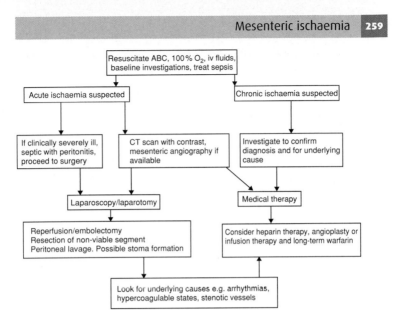

Management algorithm

diagnoses include appendicitis, diverticulitis, acute pancreatitis, ulcerative colitis. Typical patients are >50 years old, with history of peripheral vascular disease or arrhythmias, especially atrial fibrillation. Some patients may have hypercoagulable states or underlying thrombogenic disorders e.g. polycythaemia rubra vera, essential thrombocytosis, protein C and S deficiencies, vasculitides (e.g. polyarteritis nodosa, lupus).

■ Examination

The main feature is the presence of severe abdominal pain, sometimes with very little tenderness or guarding, especially in the early stages; i.e. the abdominal signs may appear out of proportion to the severity of pain experienced by patients. Agitation or restlessness to try and find a comfortable position may be a feature early on. Tachycardia, sweatiness is usually present. With progression of the bowel from ischaemia to necrosis, localized peritonitis from the ischaemic segment will appear.

A tender mass may be palpable. rectal bleeding is common. Sepsis along with widespread peritoneal signs are late signs and may indicate perforation of the ischaemic segment.

■ Investigation

Full blood count, clotting, electrolytes, LFTs, lactate, amylase and CRP. The only abnormality may be a raised WBC count. Arterial blood gases **are mandatory** and may show metabolic acidosis and raised lactat. Chest and abdominal radiograph are mandatory and the findings of small-bowel distension, or later, free intraperitoneal air may occur with perforation. Positive findings appear on 20–30 % of abdominal radiographs but are non-specific; thumb printing can be indicative but not sensitive.

ECG is necessary to exclude atrial fibrillation and other arrhythmias, myocardial infarction causing hypoperfusion etc. as the cause of ischaemia. **NB in the early stages of mesenteric ischaemia, all the above investigations may be normal, and may need to be repeated some hours later.**

CT scan with intravenous contrast is usually the most useful and easily accessible investigation in the acute setting. Note that a negative CT scan does not rule out mesenteric ischaemia, especially in the early stages, but most cases do have positive findings on the CT. A repeat CT scan 24 hours later may be helpful if the patient is suspected of being ischaemic, is treated with anticoagulation and is then followed up. CT angiography specificity can be >90 % depending on the site of the occlusion, and is preferred in most hospitals. Formal mesenteric angiography is the diagnostic gold standard if available. Barium studies are not usually useful in the acute setting but may be used at a later stage to diagnose ischaemic strictures.

■ Treatment

Resuscitation: 100 % oxygen, narcotic analgesic (note that the pain of ischaemia is often poorly relieved with any form of analgesia and this may be diagnostic of the condition), iv hydration with crystalloids. Treat sepsis early with broad-spectrum antibiotics, monitor fluid balance, insert urinary catheter and NG tube, consider central line and ICU/HDU monitoring. Urgent investigations, i.e. CT within the next few hours, not next day.

SURGERY

If infarction/necrosis of bowel is confirmed or strongly suspected (based on clinical signs) then laparotomy (or initial diagnostic laparoscopy in some centres) is mandatory.

Exploratory laparotomy provides the opportunity to identify the segment of ischaemic bowel and decide on the viability of the surrounding tissue, followed by resection or reperfusion therapy if indicated. Occasionally mesenteric ischaemia is caused by strangulation, from a band adhesion, and this may be relieved with division of the band. Depending on the extent of ischaemic bowel, either a resection and primary anastomosis may be performed (if the segment is localized), or a resection with second-look laparotomy, or a stoma and mucus fistula may be brought to the skin. For potentially salvageable bowel consider embolectomy or vascular bypass procedures.

■ Prognosis

Mortality and morbidity rates from acute mesenteric ischaemia are highly dependent on timing of presentation and diagnosis, effectiveness of treatment, extent of intestinal ischaemia and resection and treatment of underlying causes. Mortality has been reported at 45–80 %, averaging at 71 % over the last 15 years. Following bowel resection of more than 50 %, mortality rate reaches up to 80 %. Once bowel wall infarction has occurred, mortality is at 90 %.

One of the specific problems may be short bowel syndrome caused by infarction/resection of most of the small bowel leading to malabsorption. Some of these patients may need long-term total parenteral nutrition (TPN) with all its associated complications.

The underlying cause of mesenteric ischaemia should be sought and treated.

Cases treated non-operatively may be prone to recurrence unless the underlying cause is treated, e.g. with angioplasty or long-term anti-coagulation.

Acute limb ischaemia

CAROLINE D. RODD AND RICHARD GIBBS

■ Definition and classification

A sudden reduction in the perfusion of a limb due to occlusion of an artery or graft resulting in limb ischaemia. The severity of the ischaemia depends on the anatomical site of the occlusion and the extent of existing collateral vessels. The acutely ischaemic limb presents in a variety of forms, as classified by the Society for Vascular Surgery (SVS)/ International Society of Cardiovascular Surgery (ISCVS):

- **Class 1:** a viable leg, without impairment of sensory or motor function and audible Doppler signals.
- **Class 2a:** a potentially threatened limb, with mild sensory loss (usually in the toes) and audible Doppler signals.
- **Class 2b:** limb immediately at risk with marked sensory loss, mild to moderate motor loss and audible Doppler signals.
- **Class 3:** the limb is paralysed, with total sensory loss and irreversible tissue damage. The Doppler signals are absent. (Non-viable limb.)

■ Incidence and outcome

Incidence of 1 in 7000 per year, rising to 1 in 6000 per year when bypass graft occlusions are included. Thirty-day mortality in the UK of 15–30 %, with a limb salvage rate of 75 %.

■ Aetiology

In the UK the vast majority of acutely ischaemic limbs are caused by an *in situ* thrombosis on a pre-existing atherosclerotic plaque in an artery,

Hospital Surgery: Foundations in Surgical Practice, ed. Omer Aziz, Sanjay Purkayastha and Paraskevas Paraskeva. Published by Cambridge University Press.
© Cambridge University Press 2009.

or thromboembolism from a proximal site of intravascular thrombosis. Rarer causes include:

Thrombosis	Atherosclerosis Popliteal aneurysm Bypass graft occlusion Thrombotic conditions
Embolism	Atrial fibrillation (AF) Mural thrombosis Vegetations Proximal aneurysms Atherosclerotic plaque
Other causes	Dissection Trauma External compression Popliteal entrapment Cystic adventitial disease Compartment syndrome

■ Symptoms

A sudden onset painful limb. If they have had a vascular bypass graft, they may have observed that the graft has stopped pulsating. Associated symptoms known as the 6 P's: Paralysis, Paraesthesia, Pain, Pallor (or colour change from blue/purple/white), Pulseless, and Perishingly cold limb.

■ Signs

Earliest signs (30 minutes from onset) are neurological, with sensory deficit followed by motor paresis (in the lower limb look for ankle, foot, and toe paralysis/sensory loss), pain on passive stretching may also occur. From six hours onwards the presence of calf tenderness (particularly the lower limb anterior compartment) indicates muscle ischaemia or necrosis. The acutely ischaemic limb is usually a *marble white* in the early stages, but *mottling* does not occur until 24 hours, and is a late, non-discriminatory sign. If pressure is applied to the mottled skin it will blanch.

■ Differential diagnosis

It is very important to discriminate between the two commonest causes: *in situ* **thrombosis vs. embolism**, as subsequent management depends on the aetiology. A pre-existing history of intermittent claudication, rest pain, well-defined vascular risk factors, and reduced or absent pulses in the contralateral leg suggest the *in situ thrombosis*. AF, recent MI and absence of other peripheral vascular risk factors suggest *embolism*.

■ Investigations

FBC (polycythaemia, thrombocytosis and leukaemia), U&E, clotting (prothombotic state), G&S, ECG (AF, MI), CXR (anticipation of surgery, malignancy). Other general investigations to consider include: cardiac enzymes (MI), digoxin levels (uncontrolled AF), TFT (thyrotoxicosis), thrombophilia screen, and tumour markers. Further specific investigations are determined by the degree of ischaemia. If the limb is Class 2b, then the patient should proceed to surgery, with on-table angiography if required. Performing a departmental angiogram in these circumstances causes unacceptable delay in the treatment of the condition. If the limb is Class 1 or 2a, then urgent angiography or duplex scanning may offer valuable information as to the aetiology and the treatment options.

■ Management

iv resuscitation, O_2, opiate analgesia, AF rate control. Anticoagulation with loading dose of iv 5000 units heparin and initial maintenance of

1000 units/hour with adjustment by measurement of APTT to prevent further propagation of the thrombus. *Class I ischaemia* may resolve with heparinization alone. *Class III ischaemia* requires primary amputation in order to save life. Conservative treatment, i.e. analgesia, may be appropriate especially in the very elderly (poor chance of survival) or those with other life-threatening conditions (malignancy, cardiac failure etc.). Conservative management in such cases usually results in a terminal event and should only occur after close discussion with the patient, family members, and vascular team. In all other cases the limb requires revascularization:

1. **Acute embolic event:** *balloon embolectomy* with a Fogarty catheter under loco-regional anaesthesia.
2. **Arteriopath with an *in situ* thrombosis:** requires diagnostic angiography prior to definitive treatment. *Thrombolysis* is an attractive option in these patients, as it unmasks the culprit lesion and often allows *endoluminal treatment* (transluminal or subintimal angioplasty) in preference to major operative revascularization with a *definitive bypass procedure*. Once the leg is revascularized, *prophylactic fasciotomies* should be considered to avoid the postoperative complication of compartment syndrome secondary to the reperfusion oedema.

Selective local intra-arterial thrombolysis is given by slow infusion or pulsed spray. The drugs used are streptokinase or more commonly tissue plasminogen activator (t-PA). Significant complications include haemorrhage (up to 50 %) and stroke (1.2–2.1 %). Patients must be managed in an HDU and must undergo repeat angiography every 6–12 hours until the thrombus has vanished. This should reveal the underlying atherosclerotic lesion responsible. The treatment tends to be reserved for thrombosis secondary to popliteal aneurysms when the runoff vessels are vulnerable due to chronic embolization and occluded grafts. Thrombolysis is more likely to fail in older patients, females, diabetics and in vein graft occlusion.

■ Summary

The acutely ischaemic limb is a common vascular emergency with significant morbidity and mortality. The management of this condition is complex and multifaceted. The successful outcome is dependent on a careful and thorough assessment of the patient and rapid instigation of treatment.

Leaking abdominal aortic aneurysm

ROBERT BRIGHTWELL AND NICHOLAS CHESHIRE

■ Introduction

Ruptured abdominal aortic aneurysm (AAA) kills 5000 people each year
and is the 15th leading cause of death in the UK. With an incidence of
25–30/100 000 it is implicated in the death of 1.2 % of men and 0.6 % of
women aged over 65 years. In the UK it is the indication for 7500 emergency operations per annum. Despite improved detection and perioperative care it remains a highly lethal pathology.

■ Definition

The presence of blood outside the lumen of an aneurysm affecting the
abdominal aorta. It is usually associated with back, abdominal, flank or
groin pain, in association with haemodynamic instability. The presence
of one or both of these in a patient with an aortic aneurysm is an indication for immediate action.

■ Classification

Many classifications for aneurysms exist. The most frequently encountered are fusiform in shape and atherosclerotic in origin. Anatomi-
cally most are *infrarenal* (90 %), *juxta/supra-renal* (9 %), and *thoraco-
abdominal* (1 %). Other aetiologies include inflammatory, mycotic, and
false or anastomotic. The simplest method of classifying rupture is
retroperitoneal (80 % cases) which is usually to the left side and results in
tamponade of the haematoma, or *free* (intraperitoneal – 20 %) which is

Hospital Surgery: Foundations in Surgical Practice, ed. Omer Aziz, Sanjay
Purkayastha and Paraskevas Paraskeva. Published by Cambridge University Press.
© Cambridge University Press 2009.

in the peritoneal cavity or nearby venous structures and usually results in sudden death or very poor outcome.

■ Management algorithm

Standard resuscitation guidelines should be followed, but with judicious use of colloids (or crystalloids) in maintaining an adequate (but not so high as to cause further bleeding) blood pressure. No single figure should be aimed for; if the patient is conscious and passing urine (0.5 ml/kg/hr minimum) this is sufficient, irrespective of the absolute arterial pressure in mmHg – 100 mmHg systolic is usually more than enough. A quick and accurate diagnosis is vital, with 'door-to-theatre' times of less than 30 minutes being both achievable and desirable. The management protocol is shown below.

■ History

Only 5 % of patients with a ruptured aneurysm have a previous history of AAA. Abdominal, flank or back pain are the most common symptoms in patients with a rapidly expanding or ruptured AAA (70+ %). Some patients may complain of collapse – a feature secondary to sudden haemorrhage (18 %). Less frequently patients may present with vomiting (could be confused with other causes of acute abdomen e.g. bowel obstruction), leg ischaemia (15 %) or neurological deficit.

■ Examination

The signs of ruptured AAA can be very subtle: only 40 % of cases present with the classical triad of pain, hypotension, and pulsatile abdominal mass. 70 % of patients with rupture will have a pulsatile mass, 40 % have abdominal tenderness and few (<10 %) have absent peripheral pulses. Other features to examine for include scars from previous abdominal surgery and pathology in other vascular beds (e.g. heart, carotids). If the diagnosis of ruptured AAA is doubtful then the clinician must be aware of alternative diagnoses and their associated signs (e.g. pancreatitis, perforated duodenal ulcer, myocardial infarction, pulmonary embolus).

■ Investigation

If ruptured AAA is suspected the following tests should be arranged urgently: FBC, U&E, clotting profile, crossmatch 10 units, and arrange for clotting products. Amylase, cardiac enzymes, CRP, liver function tests may be perfomed if other diagnoses are suspected. Bedside ultrasound (USS) equipment can identify an AAA, and suggest the presence of free fluid in the peritoneal cavity, as well as suggesting alternative diagnoses. If the patient is stable, further information can be gained from CT scanning, and this is mandatory if the patient is to have endovascular treatment (see below). The decision to CT scan a patient who is haemodynamically stable with a ruptured AAA (rather than take them straight to theatre) should only ever be at the discretion of a vascular surgeon. CXR can suggest other pathologies (e.g. perforated viscus), and is usually performed during the emergency work-up. AXR may be performed if bowel obstruction is suspected.

■ Treatment

The management summary outlines the treatment that should be instituted prior to the patient arriving in the operating theatre. The operation performed depends on the surgeon and centre, but at the current time will usually be an open operation. An 'inlay' repair technique using a Dacron tube graft is most frequently used. If the iliac vessels are aneurysmal then a bifurcated graft may be used. Some centres now offer endovascular repair of ruptured AAA (EVAR) in selected cases.

■ Prognosis

This remains poor. Over 50 % of patients with ruptured AAA will die in the community; of those that make it to hospital nearly 50 % will die from complications such as uncontrollable intraoperative haemorrhage, ARDS, ARF, SIRS, MI and stroke. Predictors of increased mortality include: advanced age (>80 yrs), preoperative shock, low preoperative haemoglobin, short duration of symptoms prior to A&E arrival and preoperative delay greater than 2–4 hours.

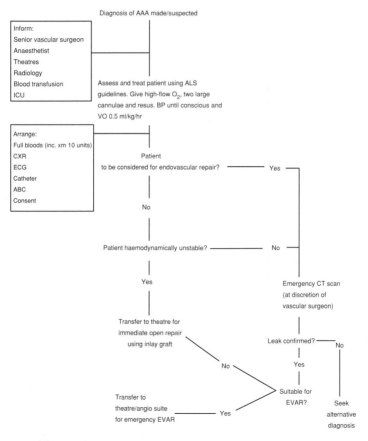

Diagnosis of AAA made/suspected

Inform:
Senior vascular surgeon
Anaesthetist
Theatres
Radiology
Blood transfusion
ICU

Assess and treat patient using ALS guidelines. Give high-flow O_2, two large cannulae and resus. BP until conscious and VO 0.5 ml/kg/hr

Arrange:
Full bloods (inc. xm 10 units)
CXR
ECG
Catheter
ABC
Consent

Patient to be considered for endovascular repair? ———— Yes

No

Patient haemodynamically unstable? ———— No

Yes

Emergency CT scan (at discretion of vascular surgeon)

Transfer to theatre for immediate open repair using inlay graft

Leak confirmed? ——— No

No

Yes

Transfer to theatre/angio suite for emergency EVAR

Yes

Suitable for EVAR?

Seek alternative diagnosis

Protocol for managing AAA

Epistaxis

ANURAG PATEL AND NEIL S. TOLLEY

■ Introduction

The nose cleans, humidifies and warms inspired air. This function is facilitated by a considerable vascular supply.

Vascular anatomy: branches of internal (ICA) and external carotid (ECA) arteries. Most important branch of the ECA is the sphenopalatine (supplies inferior part of the nasal septum). Collaterals of the ECA are the greater palatine and superior labial artery. ICA branches: anterior and posterior ethmoid arteries (supply superior part of the septum). The anterior nasal septum is known as Little's area, which contains a superficial plexus of vessels (Kiesselbach's plexus).

■ Definition and classification

Epistaxis is a nose bleed; classified into anterior or posterior epistaxis. Bi-modal age distribution. Children often anterior septum (small vessels, minor bleeding). Elderly often posterior (medium vessels), can be torrential and life threatening. Arterial epistaxis is far more common than venous epistaxis.

■ Incidence (including predisposition according to sex and geography)

Epistaxis is common and affects all age groups. Prevalence of anterior epistaxis is greatest in children and young adults; posterior epistaxis is more common in adults and the elderly. Childhood epistaxis is more

Hospital Surgery: Foundations in Surgical Practice, ed. Omer Aziz, Sanjay Purkayastha and Paraskevas Paraskeva. Published by Cambridge University Press. © Cambridge University Press 2009.

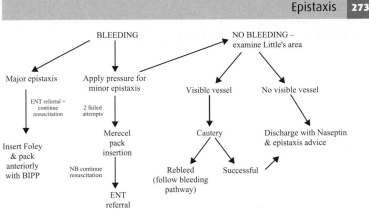

Management algorithm

common in males, elderly have equal sex distribution. More common in the winter months.

■ Aetiology

Idiopathic, trauma including fractured nose and nose picking, post coryzal, bleeding diatheses, drugs, rarely tumours and Osler's disease (hereditary haemorrhagic telangiectasis).

Risk factors include antiplatelet drugs, anticoagulants, rhino-sinusitis, upper respiratory tract infection and fluctuations in temperature and humidity.

■ Pathogenesis (macro/microscopic pathology)

Theories include: small to medium vessel progressive infiltration of collagen in tunica media, and large vessel susceptibility to calcification. May result in propensity to rupture and failure to vasoconstrict adequately.

■ Symptoms and signs

Assess for signs of shock (see Shock Chapter). Bleeding may be visible through the nostrils unilaterally or bilaterally. Examine Little's area with use of pen torch and elevating tip of nose. Assess the posterior oropharyngeal wall for streaks of fresh bleeding or clots with gentle use of a tongue depressor and pen torch. NB aerosolized blood may be present, therefore take barrier precautions (eye, mouth, hand and clothing).

■ Investigation

Blood tests: FBC, clotting and G&S or crossmatch.

■ Treatment

Think 'ABC': resuscitate the patient, establish bleeding site, stop bleeding and treat cause. Specialist advice for haematological replacement therapy. See the management algorithm.

1. **Conservative**: pressure, silver-nitrate cautery or nasal packing:
   a. Pressure: pinch the soft cartilaginous part of nose with patient's head flexed forward. Patient to suck on ice cube and apply ice pack to forehead – aids vasoconstriction.
   b. If vessel(s) visible in Little's area, apply topical local anaesthetic spray then cauterize with silver-nitrate sticks in circle around, then directly on blood vessel. NB avoid contact with skin and tell patient to wipe secretions off skin to prevent burns.
   c. Nasal packing if patient failed two 15 minute trials of pinching. Insert merecel nasal pack along floor of nose (parallel to palate) leaving no residual pack outside nostril. Squirt 5 ml sterile normal saline either side of pack to 'inflate' sponge.
   d. Major epistaxis: insert balloon catheter (e.g. Foley) along floor of nose until just visible below soft palate. Inflate balloon with sterile normal saline until resistance felt (do not use >10 ml).

Draw catheter anteriorly to occlude posterior choanae and secure catheter anteriorly with umbilical clip (to prevent migration of catheter into oropharynx). NB protect skin from ulceration by placement of gauze under plastic umbilical clip. Anterior packing with BIPP (bismuth iodoform paraffin paste) ribbon gauze into nasal cavity (best carried out by ENT team).

e. No bleeding and no packs: apply Naseptin cream (chlorhexidine hydrochloride and neomycin sulphate) to affected nostril three times daily for two weeks. Provide epistaxis advice – sneeze through mouth, no nose blowing, no hot food and drink, no smoking, rest with no exercise for at least 48 hours, nose pinching advice if rebleeds.

2. **Surgical**: septal surgery or vascular ligation by ENT surgeons, or angiography or embolization. If secondary to a fractured nose, the nose often requires reduction to facilitate epistaxis control.

■ Prognosis

Excellent, but there is some associated morbidity and mortality in the elderly.

Inhaled foreign body (FB)

ANURAG PATEL AND NEIL S. TOLLEY

■ Introduction

Airway anatomy: nasal cavity leading to nasopharynx (choanae to above soft palate); Oral cavity (lips to palatoglossal (PG) pillar) leading to oropharynx (PG pillar to superior edge epiglottis). Nasopharynx leads to oropharynx which in turn leads to the hypopharnyx (superior edge epiglottis to cricopharyngeus) (see Figure 46).

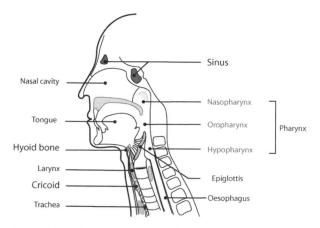

Nasal cavity
Tongue
Hyoid bone
Larynx
Cricoid
Trachea

Sinus
Nasopharynx
Oropharynx
Hypopharynx
Pharynx
Epiglottis
Oesophagus

Figure 46 Sagittal section showing aero-digestive tract

The epiglottis covers and occludes the larynx to allow food to pass into the hypopharynx, travelling down the gutters (pyriform sinuses), which are lateral to the larynx, towards the cricopharyngeus (top of oesophagus) (see Figure 47).

Hospital Surgery: Foundations in Surgical Practice, ed. Omer Aziz, Sanjay Purkayastha and Paraskevas Paraskeva. Published by Cambridge University Press. © Cambridge University Press 2009.

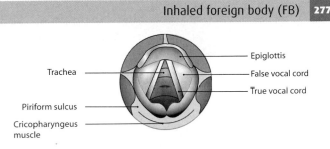

Figure 47 Endoscopic (bird's eye) view of larynx and hypopharynx

Trachea: 10–11 cm long from lower end cricoid cartilage (C6); bifurcation (carina – 'keel of a boat') at T5. Right main bronchus is wider, shorter and more vertical than LMB (left main bronchus).

■ Definition and classification

Types of FB:

1. **Organic:** peas, beans, dried pulses, nuts, paper, cotton wool, rubber, sponge and wood. NB These induce rapid mucosal irritation and swelling by hygroscopic action with rapid inflammatory response – early diagnosis is more important (especially leguminous organic matter).

2. **Inorganic:** washers/nuts, nails, screws, buttons, plasticine, stones, beads, plastic/metal toy pieces and dentures. **NB rough surfaces cause mucosal trauma**.

3. **Animate:** screw worms +/– larvae, maggots, black carpet beetle (usually tropical climates).

■ Incidence (including predisposition according to sex and geography)

Sites of FBs:

Nose – children (especially <3 years old)

Trachea/bronchial tree, much more common than larynx (rare) (see Figure 48)

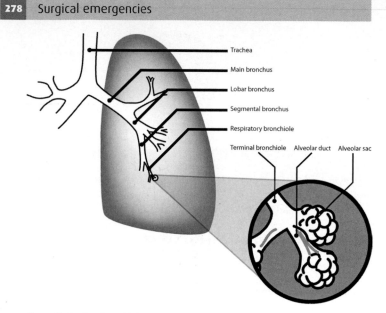

Figure 48 Tracheo-bronchial tree

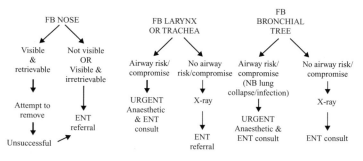

Management algorithm

Right main bronchus > left main bronchus

Overall more common in children (especially < 3 years old).

■ Aetiology

Aspiration risks: sudden fright, laughing, or absent laryngeal sensory innervation.

In adults note predisposition in CNS dysfunction, facial trauma, recent dental procedure, underlying respiratory diseases and patients with learning difficulties. Dentures also important as FB is not sensed and food not chewed so well.

■ Pathogenesis (macro/microscopic pathology)

FBs are irritants and result in an inflammatory reaction and risk of infection (e.g. chemical bronchitis). The resultant increased production of secretion and mucosal oedema increases the risk of airway obstruction. (NB in nose, calcium and magnesium carbonates and phosphates may deposit around an FB to form a rhinolith (needs removal under general anaesthetic).)

■ Symptoms and signs

Nose: symptoms: (1) Mucopurulent +/− blood stained unilateral nasal discharge (unilateral rhinorrhoea in children = FB until proven otherwise!) (2) Unilateral nasal obstruction (3) Other – pain, epistaxis, sneezing.

Signs: unilateral – (1) Reddened congested mucosa (2) Mucopus (3) NB granulations, ulceration and necrosis.

Larynx, trachea and broncial tree: symptoms: (1) Sudden onset choking/coughing +/− vomiting (2) Stabbing pains (3) NB productive cough.

Signs: (1) Respiratory distress (2) Stridor (upper airway and tracheal obstruction) **or** localized wheeze (lower airway bronchial obstruction)

(3) NB whole, lobar, segmental lung collapse dependent on anatomical site of obstruction – tracheal deviations towards side of collapse and decreased breath sounds (4) Productive cough (check for signs of chest infection) +/− systemically unwell (5) Other – clicking sound on respiration (movement of FB in trachea).

■ Investigation

If no signs of respiratory distress:

Nose: none (based on history and examination)
Larynx, trachea and bronchial tree: AP + lateral neck and/or chest.

■ Treatment

Think ABC: if signs of or any risk of airway compromise, seek urgent anaesthetic and ENT consult. If the obstruction is above cricoid cartilage consider Heimlich manoeuvre and if unsuccessful consider cricothyroidotomy.

If no signs of or risk of airway compromise do not attempt to extract FB with digit or instruments (to prevent causing impaction of the FB, and airway compromise). Arrange investigations and prepare patient for removal under GA (see Management algorithm, p. 278).

Visible FB – removal from nose:

Ideally topical local anaesthetic spray application (but not in children as not tolerated), instrument (wax hook), good illumination of nostril, good patient positioning and available suction. Avoid mucosal trauma to prevent epistaxis.

Wax hook: place hook posterior to FB and then gently draw FB anteriorly out through the nostril. NB forceps reduce control (difficult to grip FBs, especially spherical objects, and therefore risk impacting and/or pushing the FB more posteriorly).

Suctioning available: useful for removal of some FBs (NB careful not to push FB more posteriorly) and in the event of epistaxis.

Patient positioning: adults – sitting upright in a chair. Children – sitting on parent's lap with their back against parent's chest, parent crossing legs over their child's legs and hugging child to prevent movement of child's arms, and an assistant to hold child's head steady. Both adults and children: head slightly tilted back to view floor of nose.

CRICOTHYROIDOTOMY

Needle cricothyroidotomy: place 12G cannula into the trachea via the cricothyroid membrane. This allows adequate ventilation for up to 45 minutes (hypercapnoea is the limiting factor). Seek expert airway assistance. This is the preferred technique for children < 12 years.

Formal cricothyroidotomy: immobilize patient's C-spine in neutral position. Prepare, drape and apply local anaesthetic with adrenaline only in the conscious patient with a patent airway (no time in an asphyxiated/dying patient). Stabilize thyroid cartilage and make transverse incision 3 cm long through skin overlying cricothyroid membrane (closer to the cricoid cartilage than the thyroid cartilage). Second pass of the scalpel is through the cricothyroid membrane into the airway. Rotate the blade 90 degrees to face longitudinally. Use artery forceps to take over from the scalpel as the means of holding the incised edges apart. Insert tracheostomy tube into the airway, directed towards the chest; ideal adult size = 6.0.

FB removal under general anaesthetic:

Nose: rigid nasendoscope (e.g. Hopkins rod)
Larynx: rigid laryngoscope +/− endoscope
Tracheobronchial tree: rigid bronchoscopy

All of the above need the use of extraction instruments (e.g. grasping forceps).

■ Prognosis

VQ (ventilation-perfusion) relationship after bronchial FBs may take many months to normalize.

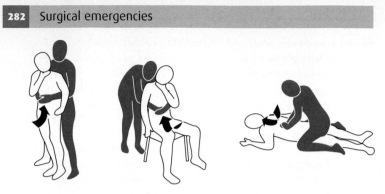

Figure 49 Heimlich manoeuvre shown in three different positions

■ Heimlich manoeuvre

Wrap your arms around the patient while standing posterior to them. Make a fist with only one hand and place your thumb below the xiphisternum. Grasp your fist with your other hand pressing inward and upward into the patient's abdomen. Do not compress the rib cage, confine the force to the thrust of your hands, and don't slap the patient's back as this may cause complete obstruction by the foreign body (see Figure 49).

Urinary retention

ED ROWE, ERIK MAYER AND JUSTIN VALE

■ Introduction

Prompt diagnosis and treatment of this common condition is vital to relieve patient discomfort and hopefully reverse any associated decline in renal function.

■ Definition and classification

Acute retention (AR) is characterized by a sudden inability to void with associated suprapubic pain. Chronic retention (CR) is typically painless, and is subdivided into high or low pressure CR depending on the intravesical pressure at the end of micturition.

■ Incidence (including predisposition according to sex and geography)

The exact incidence is unknown but parallels the increasing incidence of benign prostatic hyperplasia (BPH) in the elderly male population. Approximately 10 % of men in their forties and 90 % of men in their eighties have detectable BPH. Studies have shown an approximate 10 % risk of urinary retention in men with BPH. Retention of urine is relatively uncommon in females.

■ Aetiology

Commonest causes in males: benign prostatic hyperplasia, prostate cancer, urethral strictures and postoperative (secondary to drugs, immobility, constipation, pain and local oedema).

Hospital Surgery: Foundations in Surgical Practice, ed. Omer Aziz, Sanjay Purkayastha and Paraskevas Paraskeva. Published by Cambridge University Press. © Cambridge University Press 2009.

Commonest causes in females: retroverted gravid uterus, atrophic urethritis, fibroid uterus.

Other causes: faecal impaction, drugs (e.g. anti-cholinergics, alcohol, anti-histamines), blood clot (clot retention), urethral calculus, traumatic rupture of the urethra, infection (urethritis, prostatitis) and phimosis.

■ Pathogenesis (macro/microscopic pathology)

BPH occurs due to enlargement of glandular component of the transition zone of the prostate under the influence of the male hormone testosterone. This represents the commonest cause in men.

■ Symptoms and signs

In acute retention the patient classically presents with an inability to pass urine with suprapubic bladder discomfort.

There may be a history of lower urinary tract symptoms (LUTS), which suggest bladder outflow obstruction (BOO), such as a poor urinary stream, frequency, hesitancy, and nocturia. Preceding urinary tract infections may be a sign of incomplete bladder emptying. Previous urethral trauma, sexually transmitted disease (STD) or UTI may precede stricture formation. Headaches, anorexia, vomiting and mental disturbance may be a sign of post-renal (obstructive) renal failure.

May be pyrexial secondary to urinary sepsis. Examination reveals an enlarged bladder (tender in AR), which is dull to percussion. Digital rectal examination (DRE) to check for constipation and prostate pathology. Neurological assessment (lower limb power and reflexes, perianal tone and sensation) to exclude a cauda equina lesion.

■ Investigation

FBC, U+E, renal ultrasound (exclude hydronephrosis), and CSU for MC&S. Consider urodynamic assessment. PSA may be relevant if prostate feels malignant, but acute retention and catheterization themselves raise PSA.

■ Treatment

Aseptic urethral catheterization (see Urethral Catheterization Chapter). If the catheter does not pass easily first time consult an urologist or consider suprapubic catheterization. **Note residual urine volume**. Haematuria following decompression of the bladder is not uncommon and usually clears spontaneously.

Observe for post-obstructive diuresis ($\geq$200 ml of urine/hour), especially if residual volume is $\geq$800 ml. This is potentially fatal if not managed promptly. If diuresis occurs, replace volume with normal saline adjusting the rate as necessary on an hourly basis. Early central venous pressure monitoring is advised. Repeat U&E, and ABG. Patient may require temporary dialysis.

Trial without catheter (TWOC) if: predisposing cause removed (e.g. constipation), no renal impairment, no preceding LUTS, residual <800 ml. Drugs such as α blockers can improve the chances of a successful TWOC.

Consider bladder outflow surgery (e.g. transurethral resection of prostate – TURP) if there were preceding LUTS, residual >800 ml, high-pressure chronic retention and/or renal impairment.

Low-pressure chronic retention (bladder detrusor failure) may require clean intermittent self-catheterization.

■ Prognosis

Approximately 30 % of men will undergo a successful TWOC, which increases to over 50 % with the help of an α blocker (tamsulosin). Approximately one-third will have a further episode of retention within one year. The risk of further episodes of AR may be reduced by the addition of a 5-α reductase inhibitor (finasteride).

TURP or retropubic prostatectomy (if the gland exceeds 80 to 100 g) has a high success rate (>90 %). Side-effects include impotence (10 %), retrograde ejaculation (nearly 100 %), bleeding (5 % risk of transfusion) and infection (need antibiotic prophylaxis).

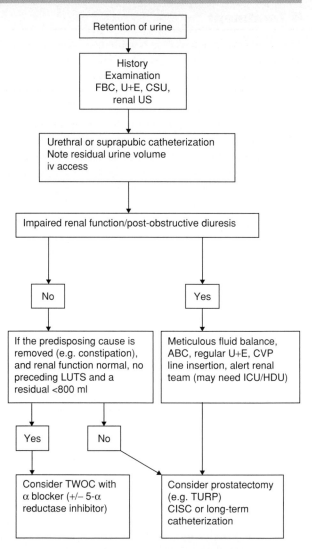

Management algorithm (CISC – clean intermittent self catheterization)

Gross haematuria

ERIK MAYER, ED ROWE AND JUSTIN VALE

■ Introduction

If a patient is experiencing frank haematuria with the passage of clots, the most immediate risk is of **clot retention**, which may be difficult to resolve. It is extremely rare for haematuria to present to such a degree that it becomes acutely life threatening from exsanguination, although those on anticoagulant medication are at more risk. Gross haematuria is significant in the setting of genitourinary trauma.

■ Definition and classification

There is no absolute definition for massive haematuria. Haematuria is divided into **microscopic** and **macroscopic** (gross/frank) and then further divided into **painless** or **painful**. Initial painless macroscopic haematuria may become painful with the passage of clots or impending clot retention.

■ History

A good history and examination will indicate the likely source of haematuria. Initial simple classifications, as above, will include/exclude multiple causes. It is always important to take a full urological history including:

- Previous urological procedures
- History of UTIs/STDs
- Lower urinary tract symptoms (LUTS)

Hospital Surgery: Foundations in Surgical Practice, ed. Omer Aziz, Sanjay Purkayastha and Paraskevas Paraskeva. Published by Cambridge University Press. © Cambridge University Press 2009.

- Risk factors for urinary tract malignancies (smoking/occupational risks/family history)
- Preceding trauma.

A thorough past medical and drug history will also highlight diagnosis and treatments associated with haematuria, such as anticoagulant/antiplatelet agents.

■ Examination

In the presence of extreme haematuria, the patient should be resuscitated with regards to their **airway, breathing and circulation**. This may well be in the setting of advanced trauma life support (ATLS) if trauma has been a precipitating cause. Once **intravenous access** and **fluid resuscitation** have been initiated, examination can be directed towards identifying a cause for haematuria. A full **abdominal system examination**, including **external genitalia** in both men and women and **digital rectal examination (DRE)** in men is thus performed. Particular attention must be paid to identifying the presence of a palpable bladder with the inability to void, and signs which would indicate trauma:

- Evidence of penetrating trauma
- Flank bruising (with or without rib fractures)
- Perineal bruising
- Unstable pelvis
- Blood seen at the external urethral meatus
- High-riding prostate on DRE.

■ Investigation

Blood tests: FBC, U&E, LFTs, bone profile, clotting, G&S or crossmatch if there is a suspicion of significant anaemia. **Urine** is sent to microbiology for microscopy, culture and sensitivity (MC&S) and cytology. A plain kidneys, ureters, bladder (**KUB**) radiograph will indicate the presence of calcified lesions within the urinary tract. An intravenous urogram (**IVU**) will identify filling defects in the urinary tract indicating probable tumours. **CT** (with intravenous contrast) is the gold standard for investigating the kidneys in trauma. Bedside **ultrasound** may have to be employed for an unstable patient, but provides no information about important factors such as kidney function and urinary extravasation.

■ Management

- Fluid resuscitation to stabilize the patient haemodynamically.
- Urethral catheterization should be attempted using a large-bore three-way catheter. This will allow subsequent bladder irrigation with normal saline to prevent clot retention. Catheterization in the presence of perineal trauma is always hotly debated. Current guidelines indicate that a single gentle attempt at urethral catheterization is unlikely to convert a partial urethral tear into a complete tear and is thus acceptable.
- Often a period of bladder irrigation with regular manual bladder washouts will suffice to ensure continuing bladder drainage while haemorrhage ceases.
- Consideration should be given to the correction of clotting abnormalities, which may be secondary to pharmacological agents or ensue from allogeneic blood transfusion.
- In the unlikely event of a significant arterial bleed, angiographic studies and attempted therapeutic embolization may be required.
- A cystoscopy under GA may be required if bleeding is unremitting and the likely source is in the lower urinary tract.

■ Prognosis

Gross haematuria usually settles with bed rest and a period of resuscitative management as outlined above. A patient should then be formally investigated to identify aetiology.

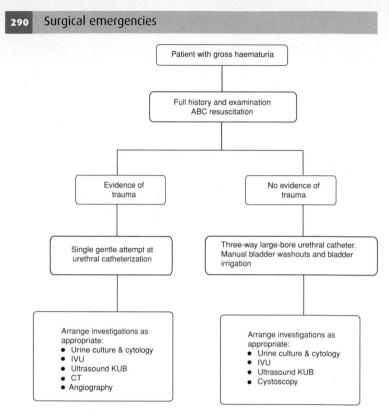

Management algorithm

Renal colic

ED ROWE, ERIK MAYER AND JUSTIN VALE

■ Introduction

Renal colic is common, and generally regarded as one of the most painful surgical conditions. It can be life threatening when there is associated urinary sepsis. Exclude a ruptured abdominal aortic aneurysm (AAA) which can have a similar presentation.

■ Definition and classification

Renal colic most commonly results from the presence of a calculus in the upper urinary tract. Interference with normal cyclical peristalsis leads to the classic symptoms of intense colicky pain, stabbing in nature, often with nausea and vomiting.

■ Incidence (including predisposition according to sex and geography)

The incidence of stone disease is approximately 0.1 to 0.3 %. Male to female ratio 3:1. Prevalence 2–3 %. Peak incidence 20–40 years. More common in mountainous, desert and tropical areas.

■ Aetiology

The most common cause of renal colic is a ureteric stone. Other causes include blood clots (clot colic), and a sloughed renal papilla (associated with diabetes, sickle-cell disease). Partially obstructing ureteric transitional cell carcinomas can present with similar symptoms.

Hospital Surgery: Foundations in Surgical Practice, ed. Omer Aziz, Sanjay Purkayastha and Paraskevas Paraskeva. Published by Cambridge University Press. © Cambridge University Press 2009.

■ Pathogenesis (macro/microscopic pathology)

For stones to form, urine must be supersaturated with the salt that can then form crystals and ultimately the stone. Hypercalciuria (secondary to hypercalcaemia e.g. hyperparathyroidism, immobility), hyperoxaluria and hyperuricaemia may predispose to stone formation. Foreign bodies (e.g. ureteric stents) and certain proteins may form a framework for crystal deposition. The commonest types of stone are: calcium (oxalate, phosphate and mixed) 70 %, infection stones (magnesium ammonium phosphate or struvite stones, associated with urease splitting organisms such as Proteus, leading to a high urinary pH and occasionally staghorn calculi) 15–20 %, uric acid 5–10 %, cystine 1–5 % (autosomal recessive inheritance). Typically stones form in the renal pelvis and pass into the ureter where they become impacted at its narrowest parts i.e. pelviureteric junction, pelvic brim and ureterovesical junction. Natural inhibitors of stone formation in the urine (e.g. urinary citrate) may be reduced.

The pain in renal colic is usually caused by the distension of the ureter or collecting system, while non colicky (constant) renal pain is caused by stretching renal capsule.

■ Symptoms and signs

Severe intermittent colicky loin pain which radiates to the groin. Often associated with nausea and vomiting. Unrelated to movement. May present as UTI, penile or testicular pain, haematuria, or renal failure. Past medical history (PMH) may include previous renal colic, medullary sponge kidney, or hyperparathyroidism. There may be a family history of familial renal tubular acidosis, cystinuria or xanthinuria. Abdominal examination is normal except for some loin tenderness. (NB check for AAA which may have a similar presentation. Pyrexia and rigors suggest associated infection and require urgent treatment.)

■ Investigation

FBC, U&E, serum calcium and uric acid, blood and urine cultures if evidence of sepsis. Urinalysis confirms microscopic haematuria in 90 % of cases. Urinary β-HCG to exclude pregnancy prior to imaging. Urinary pH (pH < 5.5 suggestive of uric acid stone, pH > 8 suggestive of infective stone). Imaging – plain KUB (90 % of stones are radio-opaque, uric acid stones are radiolucent) then IVU or CT KUB (the latter has the greatest sensitivity).

■ Treatment

Analgesia (opioid or NSAID with anti-emetic). Beware of urinary sepsis associated with an obstructing calculus because of the risk of fatal gram negative septicaemia. These patients require urgent iv antibiotics, iv fluid resuscitation, ultrasound and immediate discussion with on-call Urology specialist registrar (SpR)/Consultant for consideration of nephrostomy or ureteric stent insertion.

If the pain is controlled, there are no signs of sepsis (WBC count can be raised in renal colic without infection) and renal function is normal then the patient can be discharged with advice to return if they develop further pain or a fever. Follow up in the local stone clinic is required (approximately two weeks with a KUB) according to local policy. If these criteria are not satisfied the patient requires admission.

Stones that will not pass spontaneously can be treated as follows:

1. Proximal ureteric stone: ESWL (extracorporeal shockwave lithotripsy); if >1 cm consider PCNL (percutaneous nephrolithotomy).
2. Mid ureteric stone: ESWL or ureteroscopy and lithoclast/basket retrieval.
3. Lower ureteric stone: ESWL or ureteroscopy and lithoclast/basket retrieval.

Advise the patient to maintain a higher fluid intake to keep the urine dilute. Dietary modifications such as reduced tea, chocolate, nuts, spinach and leafy vegetables which are high in oxalates may be of benefit. Calcium-restricted diets are controversial.

■ Prognosis

Approximately 90 % of stones ≤ 4 mm, 50 % of stones 4–5.9 mm, and 20 % of stones ≥ 6 mm will pass spontaneously. Stones in the proximal ureter are less likely to pass (25 % chance) than those in the distal ureter (75 % chance). There is a 50 % lifetime risk of further attacks of renal colic following the first presentation.

■ Renal colic management algorithm

Suspect ureteric colic: loin to groin pain $+/-$ haematuria.

NB: AAA may have a similar presentation (microscopic haematuria can be present)

1. Analgesia:

    2.5–5 mg morphine iv/im $+/-$ anti-emetic (cyclizine 50 mg)

    Paracetamol 1 gm iv

    Or Voltarol (diclofenac) im/pr if no renal impairment (age < 60)

    Pethidine 50–100 mg

    (Local guidelines may vary.)

2. Basic investigations: FBC/U&E, calcium, uric acid, urine dipstick, β-HCG (♀).

3. Radiological investigations: plain KUB film and either CT KUB or IVU. (May need to discuss with on-call radiologist.)

4. Tamsulosin (400 μg) is an α blocker that can act as smooth-muscle relaxant to the ureter and vesico-ureteric junction (VUJ), aiding passage of stones.

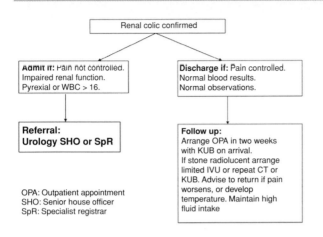

Management algorithm

(NB Patients with ureteric obstruction and infection (pyonephritis) are at risk of fatal gram negative septicaemia and require urgent imaging, iv antibiotics, iv fluid resuscitation and immediate discussion with on-call urologist for nephrostomy insertion.)

Testicular pain

ERIK MAYER, ED ROWE AND JUSTIN VALE

■ Introduction

Testicular pain is common and causes much anguish for patients and doctors alike. As a rule, if testicular torsion cannot be confidently excluded, urgent surgical exploration is necessary.

■ Definition and classification

Torsion is typically 'intravaginal' (the testis and cord twist inside the tunica vaginalis). In newborns the tunica vaginalis is not yet adherent to the dartos fascia and hence the testis and tunica vaginalis twist together resulting in 'extravaginal' torsion (Figure 50). The annual incidence of torsion is 1 in 4000 males below the age of 25 years, and accounts for 90 % of acutely painful scrotums between the ages of 13 and 21 years. Other causes of testicular pain include infection (epididymo-orchitis, scrotal abscess, Fournier's gangrene, tuberculosis, mumps orchitis), torsion of the appendix testis (most common cause of pain in prepubertal boys, accounting for approximately 50 % of cases), testis tumour, idiopathic scrotal oedema, hernia, and hydrocoele; rarely, renal colic with a stone in the lower ureter can cause testicular pain.

■ History

Suspect torsion when there is a sudden onset of pain in the testicle. The left testis is more commonly affected than the right. It occurs most commonly in adolescent males (peak incidence 14–16 years), but can occur at any age. Pain in the testicle may be exacerbated by movement or

Hospital Surgery: Foundations in Surgical Practice, ed. Omer Aziz, Sanjay Purkayastha and Paraskevas Paraskeva. Published by Cambridge University Press. © Cambridge University Press 2009.

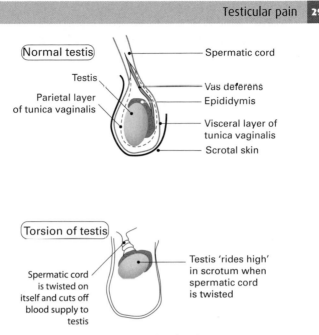

Figure 50 Diagrammatic representation of torsion

pressure. Referred pain to the abdomen, along with nausea and vomiting are not uncommon. Torsion of the testis can be intermittent with previous attacks of pain that resolve spontaneously. Note, pain may be minimal or absent initially in young children. Exercise or exposure to cold weather prior to the onset of torsion is not uncommon. A recent history of urinary infection, STD/urethral discharge or trauma may be present to indicate other causes of pain, but does not exclude torsion. Epididymo-orchitis tends to have a more gradual onset.

■ Examination

Fever is suggestive of an infective aetiology. The testis may be swollen, tender, erythematous and hot in both torsion and epididymo-orchitis.

Classically a torted testis tends to lie high in the scrotum in a horizontal position (bell-clapper testis). The cremasteric reflex is often absent. A lump in the testis may represent a tumour (10 % present with pain). The 'blue dot' sign (bluish lump at the superior pole of the testis) may be present in up to 20 % of cases when the appendix testis (hydatid cyst of Morgagni) undergoes torsion. Following trauma, a tender scrotal haematoma may be present. Check for inguinal hernia.

■ Investigation

FBC, U&E, urinalysis, MSU for MC&S, blood cultures. Ultrasound scan (USS) if tumour or epididymo-orchitis is suspected (but NB do not get an ultrasound if a torsion is suspected, it wastes valuable time and is unreliable).

When testicular USS confirms a tumour arrange a staging CT, and tumour markers. Doppler USS can identify hypervascularity in an acute epididymo-orchitis. Scrotal USS in testicular trauma is also useful to identify testicular rupture.

■ Treatment

If torsion cannot be excluded the patient should be taken to theatre immediately (within 4–6 hours of the onset of pain) for emergency scrotal exploration. Consent for bilateral orchidopexy (three point fixation with a fine non-absorbable suture) and possible orchidectomy if the testis is non viable. Extravaginal torsion (newborns) requires formation of a dartos pouch.

If there are obvious signs of infection treat with antibiotics (e.g. quinolone or aminoglycoside). If septic the patient will require admission for iv antibiotics and fluids. In men under 35 years of age, *Chlamydia trachomatis* and *Neisseria gonorrhoea* account for most cases of epididymo-orchitis, unlike older men in whom coliforms (e.g.

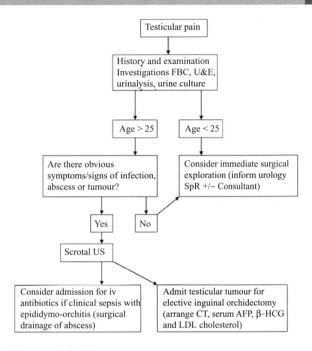

Management algorithm

Escherichia coli) are commonest, and often related to bladder outflow obstruction. Scrotal abscess and *Fournier's gangrene* (necrotizing infection usually affecting the male genitals) requires surgical drainage, and urgent debridement, respectively.

Torsion of the appendix testis is best treated by surgical excision, but can be managed conservatively.

Confirmed testicular tumours require inguinal orchidectomy +/− insertion of a prosthesis.

Testicular rupture or scrotal haematoma is best managed with scrotal exploration.

■ Prognosis

If testicular torsion is taken to theatre within 4–6 hours of the onset of pain, the testis is usually salvaged. Bilateral orchidopexy prevents future episodes of torsion. Follow-up studies have revealed reduced semen quality following unilateral adolescent torsion. Epididymo-orchitis resolves with a prolonged course of antibiotics (14–21 days). Recurrent infections can be due to bladder outflow obstruction or a partially treated earlier episode and may need further evaluation. In testicular rupture the testis is usually salvaged.

Priapism

ED ROWE, ERIK MAYER AND JUSTIN VALE

■ Introduction

The term priapism is derived from Priapus, the Greek god of fertility. If left untreated it may lead to irreversible penile ischaemia, necrosis and scarring of the intracavernosal erectile tissue.

■ Definition and classification

Penile erection that persists beyond, or is unrelated to sexual activity. Typically specialists have tried to define a time beyond which an erection is no longer 'physiological'; four hours has been accepted in many definitions. It is classified as ischaemic (low flow) or non-ischaemic (high flow).

■ History

The peak incidence is bi-modal, occurring between 5 to 10 and 20 to 50 years.

Ischaemic priapism: the patient complains of a painful erection (pain may not be present in the first few hours). Fifty per cent of cases are idiopathic. Pharmacological causes include Viagra (sildenafil), the use of intracavernosal therapy (e.g. alprostadil), antipsychotics (e.g. chlorpromazine), antihypertensives (e.g. prazosin), anticoagulants (e.g. intravenous heparin), some antidepressants (e.g. trazodone), and recreational drugs (e.g. cocaine). Haematological diseases such as sickle-cell disease (or trait) and leukaemia are the commonest causes in the young.

Hospital Surgery: Foundations in Surgical Practice, ed. Omer Aziz, Sanjay Purkayastha and Paraskevas Paraskeva. Published by Cambridge University Press. © Cambridge University Press 2009.

Rarer aetiologies include cerebrovascular disease, lumbar disk disease, and infiltrating prostate and bladder cancer.

Non-ischaemic priapism is less common and generally not associated with severe pain. Presentation may be delayed by days or months. Typically it is related to trauma to the penis, perineum or pelvis resulting in injury to the cavernosal artery, leading to increased arteriolar inflow of oxygenated blood.

■ Examination

In ischaemic priapism the patient will have a rigid painful erection, unlike a non-ischaemic priapism in which the penis is typically semi-erect and non painful. Perineal bruising may be indicative of trauma.

■ Investigations

FBC, U&E and sickle screen. Cavernosal blood gas (pH < 7.25 usually ischaemic, pH > 7.3 usually non-ischaemic). Doppler ultrasound (no cavernosal arterial flow found in ischaemic priapism). Consider urine toxicology for recreational drugs.

■ Treatment

Treat the underlying cause where possible.

Ischaemic priapism: analgesia. Evacuate old blood from the corporal bodies using a 19 or 21 gauge butterfly needle. If unsuccessful inject a diluted α agonist into the corporal space (500 μg of phenylephrine) and observe for 3 to 5 min. Monitor pulse and blood pressure during treatment. Repeat if necessary. If this fails then surgical treatment such as the formation of a glans-cavernosal shunt is necessary (consultation with a specialist centre is recommended). Early insertion of a penile implant, before scar tissue has formed, should be considered.

Non-ischaemic priapism: treatments range from conservative (fistula may close spontaneously), to angiographic embolization or open surgical ligation of the damaged artery.

■ Prognosis

In ischaemic priapism smooth muscle necrosis occurs after 24 to 48 hours. If untreated, detumescence occurs over 2–4 weeks as the

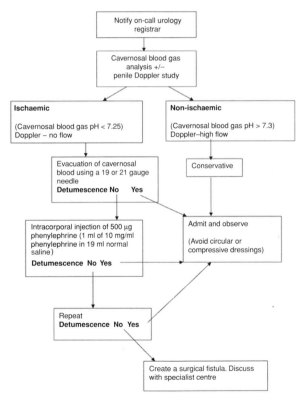

Management algorithm

smooth muscle is replaced by fibrous tissue. Up to 50 % of patients will have some form of erectile dysfunction regardless of treatment.

Recurrent (stuttering) priapism has an unknown aetiology, and is typically seen in men with sickle-cell disease or trait. Therapies include procyclidine, baclofen, anti-androgens and gonadotrophin-releasing hormone agonists.

Paraphimosis

ED ROWE, ERIK MAYER AND JUSTIN VALE

■ Introduction

Always ensure the foreskin is correctly replaced after insertion of a urethral catheter. Failure to do so may result in a paraphimosis.

■ Definition and classification

A condition in which the retracted foreskin becomes oedematous and thereby difficult to manoeuvre to its correct position.

■ History

Often there is a history of urethral catheterization in which the foreskin was not adequately replaced or later slipped back. Occasionally men forget to replace their foreskin and present as an emergency. There may be a history of earlier episodes.

■ Examination

Below the corona of the glans there is an oedematous area of foreskin (often circumferential). Proximal to the oedematous area there is a tight ring of skin. This 'constriction ring' leads to venous congestion and exacerbates the oedema of the foreskin and glans. As the condition progresses arterial occlusion and necrosis may occur.

Hospital Surgery: Foundations in Surgical Practice, ed. Omer Aziz, Sanjay Purkayastha and Paraskevas Paraskeva. Published by Cambridge University Press. © Cambridge University Press 2009.

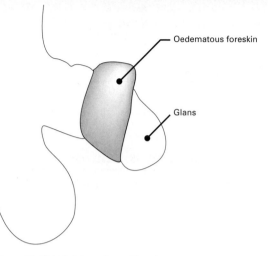

Oedematous foreskin

Glans

Figure 51 Clinical picture of paraphimosis

■ Treatment

In the early stages gentle retraction of the foreskin is enough to reduce the foreskin. Firmly squeezing the glans for five minutes prior to reduction helps to reduce the oedema. It is important that the 'tight band' in the foreskin is brought over the glans of the penis during reduction. Once the paraphimosis is established, however, it is too tender and swollen to reduce without anaesthetic. This can be achieved through a general or local anaesthetic (occasionally topical local anaesthetic cream/gel is used, but this makes gripping the foreskin more difficult). A penile ring block using 10 ml of plain 1 % lidocaine (**never** use adrenaline) is usually sufficient. First the oedema is reduced by gentle squeezing or superficially stabbing the foreskin several times with a 22 gauge needle and then applying pressure over a swab to release the oedema. Occasionally the constricting ring of skin requires incision or dorsal slit. Prophylactic antibiotics are recommended (Figures 51, 52).

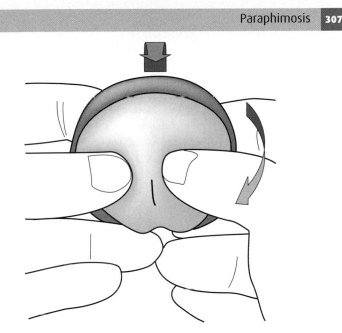

Figure 52 Manual reduction of paraphimosis

■ Prognosis

The condition is likely to recur, and therefore the patient is best advised to have a circumcision once the inflammation has settled.

Necrotizing fasciitis

BEN ARDEHALI AND UMRAZ KHAN

In necrotizing fasciitis prompt diagnosis and early surgical debridement saves lives. The unwary doctor can get caught out by not considering this surgical emergency as part of their differential when presented with a soft-tissue infection post surgery, trauma or apparent spontaneous manifestation. The patient is more unwell than expected with a simple wound infection. A 24-hour delay in diagnosis and treatment may result in a mortality rate of up to 50%.

■ Definition

Necrotizing fasciitis is a progressive, rapidly spreading microbial soft-tissue infection, which spreads along the superficial and deep fascial planes with secondary necrosis of subcutaneous tissues and ensuing sepsis.

■ Classification

- **Type I:** polymicrobial necrotizing fasciitis mainly occurs after recent surgery or trauma. Anaerobic and facultative bacteria work synergistically (one potentiates the growth of the other). Much more common than mono-microbial necrotizing fasciitis (Type II).
- **Type II:** group A streptococcus infection necrotizing fasciitis. Mono-microbial haemolytic streptococci infection. Rapid development of erythema over 24 hours with subsequent blue discolouration bullae and superficial gangrene over the ensuing days. *Streptococcal toxic shock syndrome*: caused by *Streptococcus pyogenes*. The systemic pathogenesis is induced by the superantigen M proteins which lead to

Hospital Surgery: Foundations in Surgical Practice, ed. Omer Aziz, Sanjay Purkayastha and Paraskevas Paraskeva. Published by Cambridge University Press. © Cambridge University Press 2009.

release of tumour necrosis factor, interleukins 1 and 6. The rapid systemic response leads to fever, shock and organ failure.

- **Type III:** clostridial necrotizing fasciitis, mainly *Clostridium perfringens* A decrease in local oxygen tension results in spore activation. Gram staining reveals gram positive rods. It is associated with myonecrosis and gas gangrene.

■ Epidemiology

Incidence: 500 new cases per year in the UK.

Sex: the male-to-female ratio is 2–3:1.

Age: the mean age of a patient with necrotizing fasciitis is 38–44 years. This disease rarely occurs in children. Paediatric cases have been reported from countries where poor hygiene is prevalent.

■ Risk factors

- Impaired host defence: immunosuppression (transplant patients on medication, HIV/AIDS patients)
- Chronic systemic illnesses: diabetes, alcoholism, chronic renal failure, peripheral vascular disease and cancer
- Intravenous drug use
- Age > 60
- Obesity
- History of: blunt or penetrating trauma, recent surgery, burns, soft-tissue infection and child birth.

■ Pathogenesis

Bacterial replication is promoted in the presence of a micro-aerobic wound milieu. This leads to further decrease in local tissue oxygen which allows the anaerobic organisms to thrive. The synthesis and release of proteolytic enzymes expedite the extent of spread. The ensuing thrombosis of nutrient vessels to the skin and subcutaneous vessels further exacerbates local ischaemia. Features include liquifactive necrosis of subcutaneous fat, air tracking along deep fascial planes and vascular thrombosis with resultant skin changes (see Figure 53).

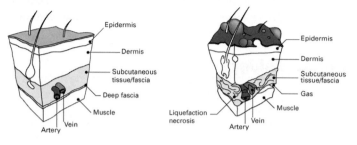

■ History

Patient may give a history of recent trauma or surgery to the area of concern. Presence of constitutional symptoms, such as fever and rigors. Pain and swelling around the area involved. Idiopathic cases are not uncommon.

■ Physical examination

Low grade pyrexia and early sepsis, presence of oedema beyond the extent of erythema, dusky or purplish skin discolouration, skin vesicles or bullae, crepitus, anaesthesia of involved skin caused by thrombosis of small subcutaneous vessels leading to necrosis of sensory nerve fibres. Late signs include septic shock and multi-organ failure.

■ Investigation

Should be used as adjuncts to help diagnosis but should not delay treatment which largely remains surgical. *Laboratory tests*: FBC (leucocytosis), U&E (renal impairment), LFTs (hypoalbuminaemia), raised lactate, raised CRP, clotting screen (coagulopathy), and G&S. *Imaging*: plain radiograph may show soft-tissue gas, CT and MRI delineate the extent of the disease and presence of gas. *Incisional biopsy*: for histological confirmation of disease and microbiological assessment for identification of pathogens involved (**but should not delay definitive treatment**).

■ Treatment

Surgery: early radical surgical debridement of the necrotic tissue extending to viable tissue is the definitive treatment. Repeat exploration is necessary 24 to 48 hours later to excise further involved tissue. Postoperative care in intensive or high dependency unit with invasive monitoring and aggressive resuscitation is essential.

Antibiotics: broad coverage essential until identity of microbe(s) involved is established. Gram positive and gram negative organisms should be covered by penicillin and gentamicin respectively. Clindamycin and/or metronidazole for anaerobic cover. It is important to realize that antibiotics alone are not enough and surgical debridement of the infected area is imperative.

Immunotherapy: patients with streptococcal toxic shock syndrome should be given intravenous immunoglobulin to neutralize the bacterial exotoxin.

Hyperbaric oxygen (HBO) therapy: current evidence does not support the efficacy of this treatment. Robust randomized controlled trials are needed in this area of treatment.

■ Prognosis

The overall morbidity and mortality ranges from 25–75 %. The mean age of survivors is 35 years and non-survivors is 49 years. The disease is rare in children. One main reason for high morbidity and mortality is the delay in proper diagnosis.

Principles of fracture classification and management

RAVI SASTRY, JAI RELWANI AND SUDIPTA PURKAYASTHA

■ Introduction

A fracture is defined as a disruption in the integrity of living bone. It involves injury to bone marrow, periosteum, and adjacent soft tissues. Fractures can be classified as closed or open. In closed fractures the enveloping skin and soft tissue are intact but the area may be bruised and swollen. When fractures are classified as open, the integrity of the skin is lost and the fracture haematoma communicates with the external environment. In a complete fracture, the bone is broken completely into two or more fragments. In an incomplete fracture, the bone is divided but with periosteal continuity remaining. In a greenstick fracture, seen most commonly in children, the bone is buckled or bent. Intra-articular fractures are those where the fracture line involves the joint.

Fractures are also described in terms of the fracture patterns, such as transverse, oblique, or spiral. In comminuted fractures there are more than two broken fragments. Compressive forces may result in impacted or crush fractures; avulsion fractures are caused by traction forces, and spiral or oblique fractures are due to rotational forces. Fracture segments are defined by looking for displacement (described as: translation, angulation or tilt, and finally rotation). If a trivial force was needed to produce the injury then a pathological fracture must be ruled out as the bone may be diseased with osteoporosis, Paget's disease or malignancy (primary or secondary).

Hospital Surgery: Foundations in Surgical Practice, ed. Omer Aziz, Sanjay Purkayastha and Paraskevas Paraskeva. Published by Cambridge University Press. © Cambridge University Press 2009.

■ Fracture healing

Occurs in four different stages (Figure 54):

1. Haematoma formation
2. Granulation tissue and soft callus formation
3. Bony callus
4. Bone remodelling.

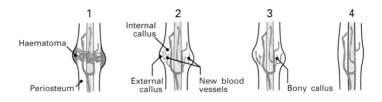

Figure 54

■ Risk factors

Road traffic accidents (high-energy trauma), contact sports in the young, and osteoporosis in the elderly.

Causes: falls, road traffic accidents, direct blow, child abuse, repeated stress.

■ Symptoms

A comprehensive history is essential so as to distinguish between trauma-related and non-traumatic causes.

Pain, swelling, bleeding and bruising around the fracture site, dependent upon extent of injury, as are deformity and loss of function.

■ X-rays

Standard AP and lateral radiographs are essential. Never forget to include the joint proximal and distal to the fracture. Radiographs show the exact pattern of the fracture and the amount of displacement. In children, injuries involving the growth plate (epiphysis) are very common.

■ Salter–Harris classification of epiphyseal injuries in children

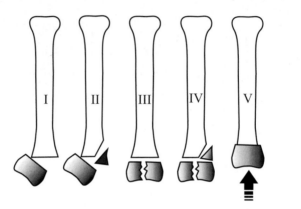

Figure 55 Salter–Harris classification

Type I – fracture through the growth plate
Type II – fracture through the growth plate and metaphysis
Type III – fracture through the growth plate and epiphysis
Type IV – fracture through the growth plate, epiphysis and metaphysis
Type V – crush or compression injury of the growth plate.

This classification helps us to assess the severity of the injury. Type I and Type II have good prognosis, whereas Types III, IV and V can lead to growth deformities. Hence accurate identification and appropriate treatment at the initial presentation is extremely important. A mnemonic that may help to remember this classification is 'SALT-Crush':

I: S – separation

II: A – across physis

III: L – lower (metaphysic not involved)

IV: T together (epiphysis and metaphysic involved)

V: Crush – compression fracture.

■ Treatment

The ideal objective of fracture treatment is to completely rehabilitate the patient as quickly as possible.

■ Resuscitation

Follow the ATLS protocol of airway/breathing/circulation with in-line cervical spine stabilization. Correct shock with crystalloids/colloid +/− blood. Stop any active points of bleeding.

■ Immobilization

Analgesia may require opiates such as morphine. Cover any open wounds with Betadine (povidone-iodine) soaked dressings. Use antibiotics for open fractures according to local guidelines and consider tetanus cover if necessary.

■ Open fractures are assessed based on Gustilo's classification

Type I: small laceration (<1 cm) from inside to outside.

Type II: laceration more than 1 cm long +/− minimal soft-tissue injury.

Type IIIA: crush injury component; adequate soft-tissue coverage.

Type IIIB: inadequate (loss of sufficient) soft tissue to cover bone and close wound.

Type IIIC: arterial injury.

■ Definitive care

Fracture management can be divided into non-operative and operative methods.

There are four basic principles that can be applied to every fracture and the appropriate management planned:

1. Reduce the fracture
2. Hold the reduction
3. Treat the soft tissues
4. Rehabilitate the patient.

1. **Reduction:** to correct the deformity and restore alignment. This can be carried out by either open or closed methods. Extra-articular fractures need accurate alignment alone. Intra–articular fractures need anatomical reduction to restore the joint surfaces, followed by early mobilization to avoid stiffness and early-onset osteoarthritis.

2. **Hold the reduction:** *external aids*: (a) Plaster cast (b) Functional cast bracing (c) Traction (d) External and internal fixation. *Internal aids*: intramedullary (IM) device e.g. IM nail or extra-medullary devices e.g. plates and screws and K-wires.

   a. Plaster cast offers three-point fixation across the fracture site. Ideally immobilize the joint above and joint below to prevent any rotation. Disadvantages include prolonged immobilization leading to muscle wasting, joint stiffness and osteoporosis. Casts offer stability and pain relief and they can be used in conjunction with internal fixation devices such as K-wires. Swelling and subsequent pressure beneath the cast can lead to serious consequences, including compartment syndrome, therefore elevation of the limb after cast application is essential.

   b. Functional cast bracing is a method of treating fractures conservatively, which permits functioning of the joints and muscles while immobilizing the fracture. The basic principle of cast bracing is to induce physiologically controlled motion, which is shown to promote osteogenesis. Joint stiffness is avoided in cast bracing.

c. Traction splints are used to regain alignment of a fracture by applying appropriate force. This also overcomes muscle spasm and reduces pain while the bone is healing. However, advances in surgical techniques have resulted in a steady decline in the use of traction.

   Types of traction: skin or skeletal. One should be aware of the risks and precautions to be taken while using any type of traction. Indications: e.g. fractures of shaft of femur, tibial plateau fractures, acetabular fractures.

d. **External fixation**: provides stabilization of a fracture at a distance from the fracture site without interfering with the soft-tissue structures that are near the fracture. This provides stability for the extremity and maintains length, alignment and rotation without requiring casting. It also allows for inspection of the soft-tissue structures vital for fracture healing (Figure 56).

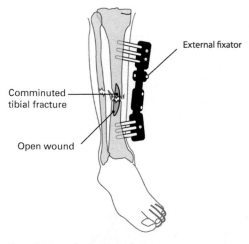

External fixator

Comminuted tibial fracture

Open wound

Figure 56 Example of external fixator

Indications for external fixation: open fractures, comminuted and unstable fractures, fractures with extensive soft-tissue injury, acetabular and pelvic fractures, limb-lengthening procedures and in non-union of fractures.

Internal fixation: can be achieved after reduction of the fracture by either closed or open methods.

Indications for internal fixation: intra-articular fractures, fractures associated with nerve or artery injury, multiple fractures, failure of conservative management, pathological fractures.

Closed reduction and internal fixation with K-wires is adequate for small fragments in metaphyseal and epiphyseal regions, especially in fractures of the distal foot, wrist and hand, such as Colles' fractures, and in displaced metacarpal and phalangeal fractures.

K-wires may be inserted percutaneously. K-wires can maintain alignment but cannot resist rotational or torque forces.

Open reduction and internal fixation (ORIF): The objective is to expose the fracture haematoma and reduce the fracture under direct vision. Fixation can be achieved by using plates and screws (Figures 57 and 58).

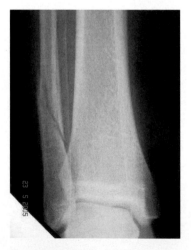

Figure 57 Preoperative

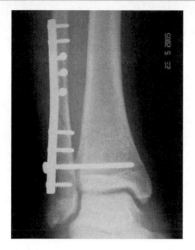

Figure 58 Postoperative

■ Complications

Early: infection, nerve and artery injuries, tendon injuries, compartmental syndrome, thromboembolic events, reflex dystrophy.

Late: delayed union, mal-union, non-union, avascular necrosis, myositis ossificans, stiffness, Sudeck's osteodystrophy.

Compartment syndrome

STEPHEN WARD AND SUDIPTA PURKAYASTHA

■ Introduction

Compartment syndrome is a life and limb threatening condition that occurs when an increase in pressure develops in a closed anatomical compartment. This increase in pressure can be caused by either restriction of the compartment size, by bandaging and casts for example, or from an accumulation of compartmental fluid or blood. Accumulation of compartmental fluid may result from haemorrhage, fractures, soft-tissue injuries, burns and swelling from both ischaemia and reperfusion. As the compartment pressure rises, so does venous pressure within the compartment. Once venous pressure exceeds capillary perfusion pressure, hypoxia of the tissues ensues.

Consequences of failure to decompress a compartment syndrome and relieve tissue hypoxia are: muscle necrosis and loss of function, renal failure, shock, septicaemia and death.

A compartment syndrome can develop in any closed osteofascial space in the upper and lower limbs. It most commonly occurs in the leg, involving the lateral compartment more frequently than the anterior or posterior compartments (see Figure 59). An abdominal compartment syndrome has also been described, caused by an increase in intra-abdominal pressure.

■ Definitions and classification

A collection of symptoms and signs associated with an increased pressure in a closed anatomical compartment that threatens tissue perfusion and viability.

Hospital Surgery: Foundations in Surgical Practice, ed. Omer Aziz, Sanjay Purkayastha and Paraskevas Paraskeva. Published by Cambridge University Press. © Cambridge University Press 2009.

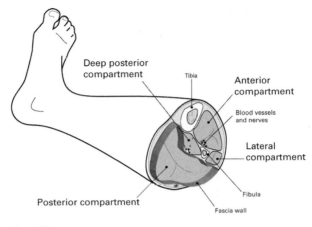

Figure 59

Acute compartment syndrome: rise in compartment pressure to the extent and duration that necessitates urgent decompression to prevent muscle necrosis.

Chronic (exertional) compartment syndrome: exercise-induced pain which subsides at rest usually in the anterior or lateral compartments of the lower leg, related to oedematous swelling of the muscles due to overuse.

Volkman's ischaemic contracture: a flexion deformity of the wrist and fingers caused by brachial artery injury at the elbow or a compartment syndrome of the forearm.

■ History and examination

Nature of the injury: fracture (tibial and radial fractures most at risk), high-energy trauma, crush injury. Anticipate a compartment syndrome following reperfusion of an ischaemic limb.

- *Pain* is the most important symptom, said to be excessive or out of proportion to the injury, although this is subjective.

- *Pain on passive stretching* of the muscle, felt in the affected compartment.
- *Persistent swelling* and tenderness of the compartment.
- *Paraesthesia* occurs late in the syndrome and is associated with poor outcome following fasciotomy.

The 6 P's of acute ischaemia are not directly applicable to the compartment syndrome (pale, pulseless, painful, paraesthesia, paralysis, perishing cold), as pallor, coldness, pulselessness and paralysis are very late signs and are associated with a limb that is beyond salvage.

It is important to realize that capillary refill, skin colour and pulses can all be normal while muscle viability is threatened.

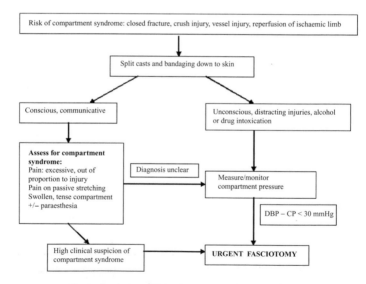

Management algorithm (DBP = diastolic blood pressure; CP = compartment pressure)

■ Investigations

Blood tests: U&E to monitor renal function; creatine kinase for extent of rhabdomyolisis.

Compartment pressure monitoring: in patients who are unconscious, unable to respond to pain or who demonstrate only some features of the compartment syndrome, it is useful to measure compartment pressures to decide on the need for fasciotomy. Handheld needle devices are available for measurement of compartment pressure, which should be performed at or close to the fracture site or where the compartment appears most swollen. A pressure difference between diastolic pressure and compartment pressure of <30 mmHg is an indication for urgent fasciotomy. Ultimately the suspicion of compartment syndrome from the history is imperative.

■ Treatment

Frequent assessment and evaluation is the key to diagnosis and prevention. The limb should be supported on a pillow at heart level and if a developing compartment syndrome is suspected, casts and bandages must be split down to the skin.

Urgent fasciotomy to open the compartment and debride necrosed tissue is required as soon as a possible diagnosis of compartment syndrome has been made. The wounds can then be inspected 4–5 days later and assessed to see if further debridement is necessary or if the wound can be closed. Skin grafting may be required. Intravenous fluid therapy is necessary as part of the treatment of a compartment syndrome to prevent the development of renal failure.

■ Prognosis

Prognosis is excellent if diagnosed and treated early. Delayed diagnosis and treatment may result in significant disability or even death.

Acute abdominal pain in pregnancy

OMER AZIZ AND TEO TEO

Any cause for an acute abdomen can occur coincident with pregnancy, while others are specific to pregnancy.

■ History

- *Time of onset, duration, intensity* and *character* of abdominal pain during pregnancy and *associated symptoms* need to be established.
- *Evaluation of gestational age* is essential as aetiologies change with gestational age, and fetal viability also depends on this.

■ Examination

- *Peritoneal signs are often absent* in pregnancy due to lifting and stretching of the anterior abdominal wall. Underlying inflammation has no direct contact with the parietal peritoneum, which precludes any expected muscular response such as guarding.
- The *uterus can obstruct and inhibit movement of the omentum* to an area of inflammation, distorting the clinical picture.
- Examination of patient in the right or left decubitus position may help distinguish extra-uterine tenderness from uterine tenderness.
- Due to the gravid abdomen, the *location of intra-abdominal contents will vary at different gestations.*

■ Investigations

- *Blood tests* are dependent on the suspected pathology. Some laboratory tests have altered reference ranges in pregnancy. For example,

Hospital Surgery: Foundations in Surgical Practice, ed. Omer Aziz, Sanjay Purkayastha and Paraskevas Paraskeva. Published by Cambridge University Press. © Cambridge University Press 2009.

pregnancy can produce white blood cell counts of 6000–16000/mm^3 in the second and third trimesters and 20000–30000/mm^3 in early labour.

- *Ultrasound* is the most frequently used non-invasive investigation for evaluating the pregnant abdomen.

Physiological changes in pregnancy	
System	Physiological adaptation in pregnancy
Cardiovascular	Increased stroke volume and heart rate Increased cardiac output, 50 % by 30 weeks Reduced systemic peripheral resistance Reduced diastolic pressure in third trimester
Pulmonary	Raised tidal volume by 40 % 15 % increase in respiratory rate Reduced functional residual capacity Total lung volume unaltered
Gastrointestinal	Relaxation of lower oesophageal sphincter Reduced motility, delayed gastric emptying Reduced pH of gastric juices
Renal	Renal plasma flow up by 30–50 % 50 % increase in GFR
Haematological	Plasma volume increased by 50 % Increased red cell mass by 20–30 % Average Hct 33 % (physiological anaemia) Increased WBC

■ Differential diagnoses related to pregnancy

Early pregnancy complications such as ectopic pregnancy or miscarriage. Consider rare possibility of a heterotopic pregnancy (1:7000–1:30 000).

Acute urinary retention due to retroverted uterus.

Uterine leiomyomas are common (0.5–5 %). In approximately 10 % of women, uterine myomas can cause severe abdominal pain due to red degeneration (haemorrhagic infarction related to inadequacy of blood supply during pregnancy) or due to torsion of a pedunculated fibroid. Pain and tenderness are usually localized and can be associated with low-grade fever and leucocytosis. Most cases settle with bed rest and analgesia and rarely require laparotomy.

Placental abruption occurs in 0.5–1 % of pregnancies. Onset of pain is sudden, with or without bleeding and uterine irritability. Back pain may be predominant in those with posterior placenta. On examination, the uterus can be tender and fetal parts difficult to palpate. Diagnosis is clinical as an ultrasound finding of a retro placental clot is often a late finding. Abruption can lead to coagulopathy (33–50 % of severe cases) and fetal death (up to 60 %). Postpartum haemorrhage is also common.

Acute fatty liver of pregnancy (1:15 000) often in third trimester: symptoms include sudden abdominal pain, nausea, vomiting and jaundice. Serum bilirubin levels raised with abnormal LFTs, leucocytosis, thrombocytopaenia, hypoglycaemia and coagulopathy. Correction of fluid, electrolyte and coagulation abnormalities and prompt delivery are mandatory.

Chorioamnionitis: pre-labour rupture of membranes usually precedes chorioamnionitis, but antecedent infection may result in abdominal pain.

Uterine rupture: rupture of gravid uterus is rare (1:1500). It usually occurs during labour but can present before onset. A high fetal mortality rate (30 %) and significant maternal morbidity (5 %) are associated with this. Most cases arise from rupture of caesarean section scar but can also occur in pregnancy that developed in a rudimentary horn, with excessive oxytocin use, in obstructed labour, high parity and following surgical trauma such as perforation or previous myomectomy scars. Continuous abdominal pain, tenderness, fresh vaginal bleeding and fetal distress with or without maternal shock are common presentations. Prompt resuscitation, laparotomy and delivery by caesarean section and repair of the uterus or hysterectomy are mandatory.

Severe uterine torsion: the uterus usually rotates axially 30–40° to the right in 80 % of pregnancies. If rotation extends beyond 90°, it causes severe abdominal pain, a tense uterus and urinary retention in the latter half of the pregnancy, leading to vasovagal shock and fetal distress. Predisposing factors include fibroid, congenital uterine anomaly, adnexal mass or pelvic adhesions. Conservative measures (bed rest, analgesia and altering the maternal position) can be used to produce spontaneous correction of the uterus. However laparotomy and caesarean section may be necessary.

Ovarian pathology: rupture, haemorrhage and torsion of ovarian cyst can cause severe abdominal pain. There is potential for any adnexal mass (corpus luteum, simple cysts, dermoid and neoplasm) to undergo torsion. Torsion presents as intermittent lower-quadrant pain with nausea, vomiting as well as tachycardia, mild pyrexia and leucocytosis. Laparotomy is effective treatment in cases of a suspected torsion. Oophorectomy is carried out in cases of necrosis or a cystectomy if the adnexa are viable.

Severe pre-eclampsia and HELLP (haemolysis, elevated liver enzymes and low platelets): liver involvement occurs in 10 % of women with severe pre-eclampsia. Women present in late second and third trimester with right hypochondrial and epigastric pain with nausea and vomiting due to distension or haemorrhage stretching of the liver capsule. Delivery is the only cure. Induction of labour or delivery by caesarean section depends on the clinical picture. Stabilize blood pressure and aim for mean arterial pressure less than 125 mmHg. Magnesium sulphate should be used for the prevention of eclampsia. Strict fluid management is paramount to avoid pulmonary oedema and acute adult respiratory distress.

■ Differential diagnoses unrelated to pregnancy

Acute appendicitis (1:1000 pregnancies): the caecum and appendix are displaced upwards and to the right with advancing gestation, therefore location of the pain may be in the right lower quadrant, lumbar or flank region. Delay in diagnosis and treatment leads to increased incidence of perforation (15–20 %), peritonitis and sepsis. Perforation is associated with high maternal (17 %) and fetal (43 %) mortality (compared to 5–10 % without perforation).

Intestinal obstruction: up to 60 % of cases are due to adhesions and previous surgery. Other causes include volvulus, intussusception, hernias, complications of Crohn's disease and neoplasm. An erect and supine abdominal X-ray will demonstrate dilated loops of bowel with fluid levels. High maternal (10–20 %) and fetal (30–50 %) mortality reported when obstruction is complicated by strangulation, perforation or fluid and electrolyte imbalance.

Acute cholecystitis and cholelithiasis: decreased gallbladder motility during pregnancy and delayed emptying result in acalculous cholelithiasis in 3.5 % of pregnant women. Conservative management (analgesia, intravenous fluids and antibiotics) recommended. Preferable to defer surgery until after puerperium.

Crohn's disease: pregnancy does not adversely affect the disease. Presentation with abdominal pain, diarrhoea, anaemia and weight loss as well as rectal bleeding and passage of mucus.

Acute pancreatitis: although rare it can present late in pregnancy or soon after delivery with central and/or upper abdominal pain, often radiating to the back. Raised serum amylase will confirm the diagnosis.

Acute pyelonephritis (1–2 % of pregnancies): features include fever, loin tenderness, urinary frequency and a positive midstream urine culture. Renal ultrasound may demonstrate hydronephrosis.

Urolithiasis (0.3–0.5 %): sudden-onset abdominal pain with co-existing urinary tract infection and haematuria warrant admission. Ultrasound findings of hydronephrosis or a calcified area are suggestive of renal calculi. Intravenous urography is not contraindicated in pregnancy.

Sickle-cell crises: may present in pregnancy with acute abdominal pain, and is often not initially suspected.

■ General management considerations

1. Consult early with senior obstetrician and surgeon.
2. Resuscitate the pregnant patient, as fetal life is dependent on maternal condition.
3. Oxygen consumption is increased in pregnancy, maintain adequate oxygenation.
4. Maintain effective circulating volume (owing to raised plasma volume, signs of hypovolaemia may occur late).
5. Uterine compression of the vena cava may reduce venous return to the heart, aggravating shock – evaluate the pregnant patient on the left side.
6. Continuous fetal monitoring after 20–24 weeks may be performed using CTG to look for signs of fetal distress.

Paediatric surgical emergencies

ALEX C. H. LEE AND MUNTHER HADDAD

■ Introduction

Paediatric surgery encompasses a wide range of surgical pathologies based on the age of the patient (newborn to <16 years). Children <4 years old or with complicated pathologies and major medical
co-morbidities are best managed in tertiary centres. Older paediatric
patients with surgical conditions can be managed locally with medical
paediatric advice. In children with a progressing surgical illness physiological derangement occurs rapidly and often without sufficient warning. Paediatric input is particularly important when managing the very
ill and the very young. This applies particularly to newborns prior to
referral/transfer to a tertiary surgical unit, who require cannulation etc.
Inform the paediatric team early; their experience and practical skills
will be invaluable. In the case of transfer to paediatric surgery tertiary
referral units, clear communication is imperative to ensure they are adequately prepared for the child. Paediatric escort may be needed for safe
transfer.

■ The parent

Can usually give important clues about a child's illness, especially the
subtle changes of its early course. Children often give valuable clinical
information which should not be ignored. History taking and examination in children requires patience, may not be in the usual order, and
is best done with the parent and a paediatric nurse present. Consent
for examination and procedures may be given by the mother or father

Hospital Surgery: Foundations in Surgical Practice, ed. Omer Aziz, Sanjay
Purkayastha and Paraskevas Paraskeva. Published by Cambridge University Press.
© Cambridge University Press 2009.

(legally married) or a legal guardian. Further details on this are dealt with in the Consent and medico-legal considerations Chapter.

■ Fluid management

Careful fluid management is essential. Basic maintenance fluid requirements for infants and children can be calculated as below. Discuss with the paediatrician/senior staff for neonates, infants <10 kg, postoperatively or those needing prolonged fluid replacement. The fluid of choice for short-term use in most units is 0.18 % NaCl with 5 % dextrose with 20 mmol K per litre. The following can be used to calculate the maintenance regime for a child:

Neonates	150 ml/kg/24 hr
Infants (up to 10 kg)	120 ml/kg/24 hr
Children (10–50 kg)	4 ml/kg/hr for 1st 10 kg 2 ml/kg/hr for next 10 kg 1 ml/kg/hr for the rest

EXAMPLE

8 kg infant = $(120 \times 8) / 24 = 96$ ml/hr
16 kg child = $(4 \times 10) + (2 \times 6) = 52$ ml/hr
25 kg child = $(4 \times 10) + (2 \times 10) + (1 \times 5) = 65$ ml/hr.

Electrolyte requirement varies with age but as a general guide: Na 3 mmol/kg/24 hr, K 2 mmol/kg/24 hr, Ca 1 mmol/kg/24 hr.

■ Common paediatric presentations

Trauma: the leading cause of death in children, with car accidents accounting for majority of cases.

Bilious vomiting: always requires early identification and investigation, especially as dehydration and aspiration may ensue. Differential diagnoses include intussusception, incarcerated inguinal hernia, malrotation $+/-$ volvulus, intra-abdominal bands (vitellointestinal duct), Hirschsprung's disease, and atresias. Medical causes (including sepsis) need to be excluded. Surgical causes ($+/-$ intestinal obstruction) may lead to intestinal infarction and warrant prompt resuscitation and referral.

Acute abdominal pain: as in adults, history taking from the parent or child and active observation is the most important management strategy. Try to avoid over-investigating a child. Blood tests should not be routinely taken from a child. However, beware of the quiet toddler who is refusing examination. Although >50 % of cases turn out to have 'non-specific abdominal pain' (NSAP), this is only a diagnosis of exclusion. Sometimes a perforated appendix can be misinterpreted as NSAP by the unwary. If surgical pathology is suspected, refer promptly to surgical team for further management. Beware of atypical presentations in young children as well as medical causes for abdominal pain in children (pneumonia, HSP, etc.). If sinister pathology is ruled out and NSAP suspected, simple analgesia may be useful.

Acute scrotum: testicular torsion must be considered in any male child with unilateral scrotal pain. Abdominal pain or vomiting may be the presenting complaint. Testicular viability reduces after six hours, therefore prompt surgical exploration is mandatory. Refer to paediatric surgery or urology immediately. Other important differential diagnoses include: torsion of hydatid of Morgagni, idiopathic scrotal oedema, and inflammatory causes (rare).

Undescended testes: up to 2 % of boys have undescended testes in the first year of life, but by three months most have descended spontaneously. The testicle may or may not be palpable in the inguinal canal, and may be associated with an ipsilateral inguinal hernia. Differentiate *true undescended testes* where testicle cannot be manipulated into the scrotum, from a *retractile testis* where it can be delivered into the scrotum. Retractile testes do not normally require further therapy beyond parental reassurance, while undescended testes increase the risk of infertility and malignancy. Refer to specialist for further treatment involving orchidopexy $+/-$ hernia repair. A non-palpable

(pain may be similar to appendicitis) and intussusception. Often diagnosed at surgery (appendicectomy), but also using Meckel's scan (above). Surgery with wedge/segmental resection and anastomosis together with appendicectomy should be performed. Remember 'rule of 2s': 2% incidence, symptomatic in 2%, 2 feet from ileocaecal valve, 2 inches long, 2 types of mucosa, 2 times more common in men, 20% present before 2 years of age (Figure 60).

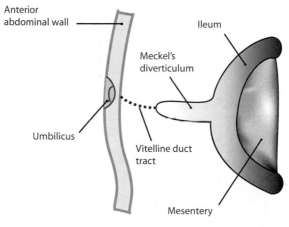

Anterior
abdominal wall

Ileum

Meckel's
diverticulum

Umbilicus

Vitelline duct
tract

Mesentery

Figure 60

HIRSCHSPRUNG'S DISEASE

Neurogenic abnormality associated with muscular spasm of the distal colon resulting in a functional obstruction. Caused by absence of parasympathetic ganglion cells (in Auerbach's myenteric, and Meissner's submucosal plexus). The abnormal bowel (distal) contracted and normal bowel (proximal) dilated.

INFANTILE HYPERTROPHIC PYLORIC STENOSIS

Circular pylorus muscle hypertrophy results in constriction and gastric outlet obstruction, leading to non-bilious, projectile vomiting, and loss of gastric HCl. Metabolic derangement with hypochloraemic, metabolic alkalosis, and ultimate dehydration is common.

Clinical features: typically occurs in a first born male (M:F = 4:1), presenting at 3–6 weeks of age with non-bilious vomiting. Baby is hungry after vomiting and may be dehydrated. Visible gastric peristalsis and RUQ/epigastric olive-shaped mass may be palpable (easiest with an empty stomach during a test feed).

Investigations: U&E; capillary gases typically show low Na, K, Cl and metabolic alkalosis. USS useful in equivocal cases (e.g. good history but impalpable mass).

Management: intravenous fluid/electrolyte replacement is essential and may take 2–3 days before the baby is ready for surgery. NG tube is passed on free drainage and initial hourly aspiration. One to two boluses of 20 ml/kg of 0.9 % NaCl may be needed (some units use HAS (human albumin solution)). *Maintenance fluids:* 150 ml/kg/24 hours with 0.45 % NaCl + 5 % dextrose and potassium (if K $\geq$ 3.8 add 20 mmol per litre; if K $\leq$ 3.8 add 40 mmol per litre). Replace NG losses ml for ml with 0.9 % NaCl. Recheck U&E and capillary gas 12–24 hourly and proceed to surgery when normalized. *Surgery:* Ramstedt pyloromyotomy (standard, peri-umbilical or laparoscopic approach). The thickened pyloric muscle is incised (cut across) without breaching the mucosa. Commencement of feeding according to surgeon's preference and may be started as early as four hours postoperation. Initial postoperative vomiting not uncommon.

INTUSSUSCEPTION

Intestinal invagination into adjacent distal intestine typically in the ileocolic region. These patients can be extremely ill and senior staff/paediatric team should be alerted early.

Clinical features: typically 3–12 months old with colicky pain, drawing up knees, episodic inconsolable cries and may be completely well in between times. Late presenters may be dehydrated/shocked and moribund. 'Red currant jelly' stools are a late sign. A sausage-shaped mass may be palpable in the upper abdomen.

Investigations: FBC, U&E, G&S. AXR then USS will show intussuscepting bowel.

Management: iv access, fluid resuscitation and pass NG tube for free drainage and aspiration. Intravenous analgesia (e.g. morphine) as required. Several fluid boluses of 0.9 % NaCl or HAS may be needed for replacement in addition to maintenance fluid. Air enema reduction by an experienced radiologist. Consent for possible perforation and laparotomy. Intussusception not reduced by air enema can be reduced surgically by open or laparoscopic approaches with broad-spectrum antibiotics cover. Resection may be required in the presence of bowel infarction. *Postoperatively*: oral fluid and feed can be commenced after eight hours. Parents should be warned that recurrence is possible (<5 %) regardless of the reduction method used. Suspect underlying pathology (e.g. polyp, Meckel's) as lead point in recurrent cases (usually older children).

MECONIUM ILEUS

Obstruction of distal ileum in the newborn with meconium represents the earliest clinical manifestation of cystic fibrosis (15 % of cases). Progressive abdominal distension and failure to pass meconium noted, with obstruction seen on AXR. Water-soluble contrast enema reveals microcolon and plugs of meconium and may be therapeutic. Surgery indicated if this fails or if perforation/peritonitis present.

NECROTIZING ENTEROCOLITIS

Most common gastrointestinal emergency in the neonatal period, with prematurity the biggest single risk factor. Often non-specific and unpredictable presentation with irritability, pyrexia or poor feeding. Eventually leads to abdominal distension, vomiting, passage of a bloody stool, apnoea and bradycardia. Initial management with nasogastric tube (bowel rest) fluids, antibiotics and parenteral nutrition. Surgery indicated if these measures fail to resolve the situation.

Acute hand injuries

MARIOS NICOLAOU AND DAVID FLOYD

■ History and examination

HISTORY TAKING

Record the patient's age, occupation, dominant hand and any special hobbies e.g. piano player.

HPC: when did it happen?How did it happen?Posture of hand at time of injury. Tetanus toxoid status.

PMH: relevant co-morbidity, anaesthetic risks, past hand trauma/disease/surgery.

Other: record medications and allergies. The events leading to hand injuries frequently result in litigation cases so ensure that the notes are accurate and complete.

HAND EXAMINATION

General examination is important to exclude other injuries and significant co-morbidity. On the hand:

Look: for obvious wounds, colour changes, asymmetry, deformities, and previous scars.

Feel: checking for adequate *perfusion*, look for capillary refill by pressing the nail bed. Check for any *sensory deficit* (see Figure 61) using a blunted needle or paper clip. The 'Bic biro' test can also be performed by running a pen along each digit. Lack of hydrosis due to nerve damage results in decreased frictional force.

Hospital Surgery: Foundations in Surgical Practice, ed. Omer Aziz, Sanjay Purkayastha and Paraskevas Paraskeva. Published by Cambridge University Press. © Cambridge University Press 2009.

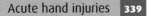

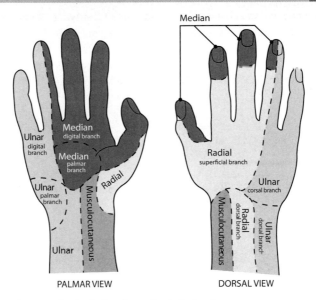

Figure 61 The distribution of sensation in the hand

Move: check for any *tendon-injury* by tendon-specific tests (see Figure 62). Pain on motion against resistance is indicative of a partial tendon injury and should be noted. Check for *joint stability* and *bony tenderness* suggestive of a fracture.

INVESTIGATIONS

Consider X-ray of the injured hand in cases of suspected fracture(s) or foreign bodies and all glass injuries. Minimum two views required e.g. AP, lateral ($+/-$ oblique).

MANAGEMENT

Always manage life-threatening injuries first. Have a high level of suspicion for occult injuries. Control arterial or venous bleeding by compression and elevation (avoid clamping or tying off vessels if possible as this may compromise surgical repair). Only explore a wound when there is no clinical evidence of underlying damage that would require surgical exploration by a hand surgeon. Uncontrolled exploration may create more damage. Irrigate wounds thoroughly and dress with non-adherent dressings.

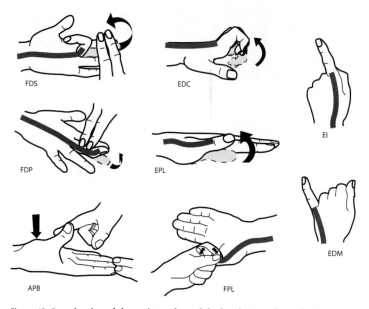

Figure 62 **Examination of the main tendons of the hand:** FDP = flexor digitorum profundus, FDS = flexor digitorum superficialis, EDC = extensor digitorum communis, EI = extensor indicis, EDM = extensor digiti minimi, FPL = flexor pollicis longus, APB = abductor pollicis brevis, EPL = extensor pollicis longus

■ Closed fractures

The most common fractures in humans, regardless of sex, age and ethnic origin. *All hand fractures should be referred to the hand clinic.* Open

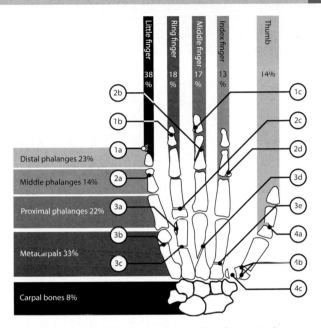

Figure 63 Common hand fractures with their relative frequencies (as a percentage of all hand fractures) by bone and digit. Numbers refer to fractures in the text

fractures pose a risk of osteomyelitis and need immediate referral to a hand surgeon and commencement of antibiotics. Some common closed fractures are indicated in Figure 63.

Distal phalanx fractures: **1a** **1b** **1c** often result from a crush injury. Associated nailbed injuries should be repaired and a mallet finger identified and splinted appropriately (see below). Evacuate large subungual haematomas by trephining. Immobilize in a Zimmer splint. Intraarticular fractures **1c** involving >30 % of joint may need ORIF.

Proximal and middle phalanx fractures: **2a** **2b** **2c** **2d** examine for rotational deformity (Figure 66). Undisplaced, non-rotated stable fractures may be treated with 2.5 cm buddy strapping (Figure 65) and require

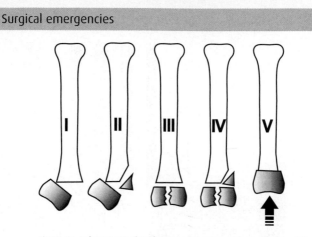

Figure 64 Salter–Harris classification of epiphyseal fractures. Type II is most common

repeat X-ray in seven days. Unstable ②ⓐ, displaced or rotated fractures may require ORIF. Treat with ulnar/radial gutter splints up to affected digit's distal phalanx and refer to fracture clinic. Treat intra-articular fractures ②ⓓ with splinting in *safe position* (Figure 67) and refer for fixation. Hand elevation reduces swelling.

Metacarpal (MC) fractures: fractures of the MC head ③ⓐ are often comminuted and intra-articular and should be splinted in the safe position (Figure 67) and referred for expert management. Fractures of the MC neck (Boxer's fracture) ③ⓑ usually result from a punch, are extremely common (especially in the little finger) and can be rotated and angulated. Up to 15° angulation for the index and middle fingers and 40° for ring and little fingers can be accepted with no loss of function. Treat with a dorsal slab with buddy strapping. MC fractures of the shaft ③ⓒ ③ⓓ are less common and may be associated with an overlying tendon injury. Displaced, angulated or rotated fractures may need fixation. Immobilization can be achieved with a Colles'-type slab. MC base fractures ③ⓔ are rare except of the little finger, which can be associated with subluxation of the MC-hamate joint. Treat with a gutter splint and refer to hand surgeon.

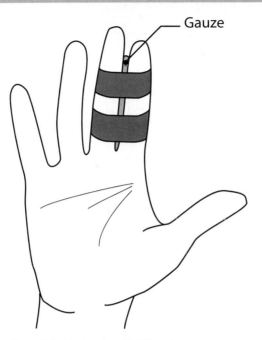

Gauze

Figure 65 Buddy strapping with 205 cm tape

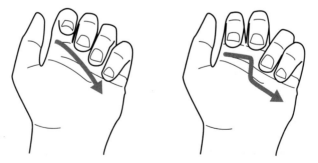

Figure 66 Assessing for any rotational deformity: all digits should point to the scaphoid and be parallel

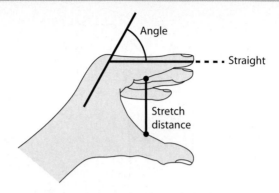

Figure 67 The safe position for splinting the hand. In this position the collateral ligaments at the MCP joint are stretched, resulting in minimal fibrosis, preparing the joints for mobilization

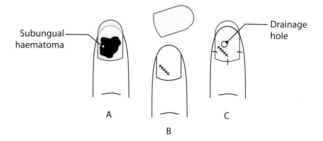

Figure 68 Nailbed repair: (A) Remove the nail using scissors, (B) Clean and repair the defect using 6-0 Vicryl, (C) Cut a small window on the nail to prevent haematoma formation, replace the nail and suture it *in situ*

Thumb fractures: the commonest fracture of the thumb is an intra-articular fracture-dislocation at the base of the metacarpal (Bennett's) **4c**. Rolando's fracture is similar but there is a dorsal fragment creating a T or Y at the base of the MC **4b**. In both cases, immobilize in a thumb spica and refer for surgery to a hand surgeon. Phalangeal fractures **4a** of the thumb are potentially unstable and require K-wire fixation.

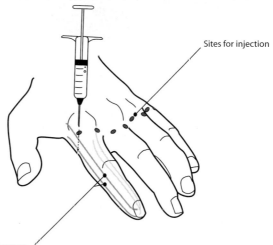

Sites for injection

Digital nerves

Figure 69 Digital block: inject approximately 4 ml of a mixture of 1 %
lidocaine and 0.25 % bupivacaine over the extensor tendon into each web
space and wait 5–10 minutes. Do not use epinephrine

Game keeper's thumb: also known as skier's thumb, results from an injury to the ulnar collateral ligament by forceful radial deviation. Pain over the ligament and laxity on radial stress is characteristic. X-ray may show avulsion fracture. Partial tears are treated with a thumb spica, complete tears usually need surgical repair and should be referred.

Mallet finger: closed extensor tendon rupture of the insertion of the tendon onto the distal phalanx. Often results from a forceful flexion of the extended fingertip. X-ray is indicated to exclude large avulsion fracture. Treatment of a simple injury is by a correctly sized mallet splint for six weeks (Figure 70). The patient should be taught how to reposition the splint if necessary, maintaining distal interphalangeal (DIP) joint extension at all times.

'Rugby jersey' injury (closed flexor digitorum profundus (FDP) avulsion): occurs when finger is violently extended while flexed at the

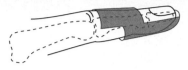

Figure 70 Mallet splint

DIP joint e.g. while footballer grabs a player's jersey. This is commonly missed and a proper examination necessary for diagnosis. Digit should be immobilized in current position and the patient should be referred for surgical repair.

Dislocation: commonly occurs after hand injury. Interphalangeal joint dislocations can usually be reduced with traction after a digital nerve block. Difficult to reduce interphalangeal (IP) joint and metacarpophalangeal (MCP) joint dislocations should be promptly referred for expert management.

Hand fractures in children: these are rare and should raise suspicion of non-accidental injury. Fractures in children heal twice as fast and the epiphyseal growth may correct for angular but not rotational deformities. Apart from the fractures described above, children can also sustain five types of epiphyseal fractures (Figure 64). A hand surgeon's opinion should be sought in most cases.

■ Open injuries

Nailbed injuries: usually follow crush injuries of the fingertip. Fifty per cent associated with an underlying distal phalangeal fracture **1a**, hence an X-ray may be useful. The middle and distal thirds of the nail most frequently affected. A large subungual haematoma requires the nail to be removed using the blades of iris scissors. A simple laceration is carefully repaired using 6-0 absorbable suture e.g. Vicryl. The nail is then replaced and sutured *in situ* to protect the repair (see Figure 68). More complicated lacerations or skin loss should be referred for expert reconstruction. The wound should be checked at 3–5 days and the nail will fall off as the new one grows. Warn the patient of the possibility of nail deformity.

Hand lacerations: this is one of the commonest presentations to A&E. A small wound may hide a serious underlying injury, so careful history taking and a well-documented examination is necessary. Any clinical evidence of an underlying tendon, nerve or vessel injury should be referred for surgical exploration. In these cases, the wound should **not** be explored in the A&E department. Consider an X-ray if a foreign body such as glass or a fracture are suspected. Human or animal bite wounds should not be primarily closed, and require copious irrigation and antibiotics. If no underlying injury is suspected, a non-contaminated wound after adequate irrigation can be sutured using 4-0 or 5-0 non-absorbable sutures which are removed after 14 days. The hand should be elevated to reduce any swelling and minimize the risk of further bleeding.

Flexor/extensor tendon injuries: lacerations to the flexor/extensor tendons usually follow a penetrating injury and poor treatment may result in serious disability. A careful examination is indicated especially noting any associated nerve or vascular injuries. Nearly all flexor and most extensor tendon lacerations require surgical exploration and repair, so refer all tendon lacerations/injuries to the hand specialist within 24–48 hours. Special attention should be paid to lacerated extensor tendons over the MCP joint which often occur from a punch. The MCP joint may be penetrated by a tooth with a high risk of wound infection and septic arthritis. Copious irrigation of the wound is required and referral for joint washout. The hand can be temporarily dressed in the safe position (see Figure 67), and elevated.

High-pressure injection injuries: an occupational hazard, commonly involving the non-dominant hand. The small entry wound can be misleading as the underlying damage can be very severe and result in digital amputation. An X-ray can show the extent of the damage. Antibiotics should be commenced and the patient should be referred for urgent surgical exploration and debridement.

Ring avulsion injuries: this occurs when the ring is caught while the hand is moving and can cause partial to complete degloving of the digit, often compromising its blood supply. This is a surgical emergency and the patient should be promptly referred to a hand surgeon for exploration and revascularization.

Amputations: these need urgent surgical referral. Bleeding can usually be controlled with pressure and elevation. Patient should be adequately resuscitated before transfer. Keep all amputated parts (however small or damaged) and transport with the patient in a sealed plastic bag wrapped in saline-soaked gauze. The bag is then placed on ice.

■ Infection

Acute infections of the hand are common and the causes include trauma (60 %), human bites (25 %), animal bites (10 %) and others (5 %). Common organisms include *Staphylococcus aureus* and β-haemolytic streptococci although gram negative bacilli such as *E. coli* and *Proteus* can cause infection in contaminated wounds. Human/animal bites can result in severe infections and should be treated with oral antibiotics (covering both aerobes and anaerobes e.g. co-amoxiclav, erythromycin). It is important to identify the presence of a collection of pus and promptly drain it, as the infection can rapidly extend and threaten the limb. Patients with simple cellulitis can be treated with oral antibiotics and sent home, whereas all other hand infections need surgical referral and drainage. Initial investigation, such as X-rays, blood tests (FBC, CRP, blood cultures) and ample microbiological samples, should be taken before commencing antibiotic treatment.

Cellulitis (35 %): this usually presents with erythema, pain and swelling but no pus. Simple localized cellulitis can be treated with oral antibiotics (e.g. flucloxacillin and penicillin V), but larger areas and ascending lymphangitis usually require high dose iv antibiotics (flucloxacillin and penicillin or a cephalosporin), hand rest in an elevated splint and close observation. Failure to improve after 24–48 hours may require incision and drainage of a collection.

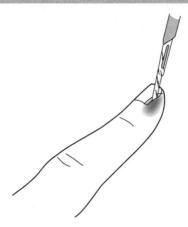

Figure 71 Drainage of paronychia

Paronychia (35 %): this involves abscess formation along the side of a fingernail secondary to trauma. Usually caused by *Staphylococcus aureus*. Treat by draining the abscess using a blade directed away from the nailbed and matrix (with or without ring block local anaesthesia) (Figure 71). The resultant cavity is irrigated and packed with saline-soaked gauze changed every other day, and oral antibiotics (flucloxacillin) continued for five days. A digital nerve block may be used for this (Figure 69).

Pulp-space infection (felon) (15 %): a subcutaneous abscess in the tight space created by the multiple septa of the distal pulp of a digit. Prompt diagnosis is required to avoid extension of the infection to the bone and tendon sheath. Treatment consists of a longitudinal incision over the abscess (in the midline of the digit to avoid the digital nerve and artery), and drainage. The wound is packed for 48 hours and oral or iv antibiotics are instituted.

Tenosynovitis (10 %): usually a penetrating injury of the palm precedes this infection. The classic presentation follows *Kanavel's four cardinal signs*: flexed finger posture, symmetrical finger swelling, tenderness along the tendon sheath and pain on passive extension.

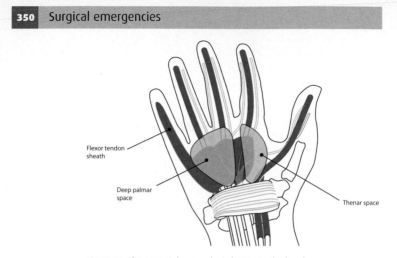

Flexor tendon sheath

Deep palmar space

Thenar space

Figure 72 The potential spaces for infection in the hands

This is a dangerous infection which can easily spread along the tendon sheath and may lead to adhesions and tendon necrosis. An urgent referral for surgical exploration is thus required, followed by high doses of iv antibiotics, elevation and splinting. Infection can also collect in two potential spaces: the thenar and deep palmar space (see Figure 72). Urgent surgical drainage is required to prevent extensive tendon and muscle damage.

Septic arthritis (2%): this is common after a penetrating injury e.g. caused by a tooth after a punch, and is characterized by erythema, swelling over a joint and pain on movement. It may lead to joint destruction, so surgical exploration and irrigation is required, followed by iv antibiotics, splinting but early mobilization.

Hernias

SANJAY PURKAYASTHA AND PARASKEVAS PARASKEVA

Definition: the protrusion of all or part of a viscus, through the wall of the cavity in which it is normally contained, taking with it its covering layers.

■ Types

a. **Abdominal**
   1. Inguinal (Figure 73) – via the inguinal canal: indirect (passing through the deep ring and into the inguinal canal, lateral to the inferior epigastric vessels); direct (not passing through the deep ring, but a weakness in the posterior wall of the inguinal canal and medial to the inferior epigastric vessels) and pantaloon (has components of indirect and direct).
   2. Femoral: via the femoral canal (Figures 75 and 76).
   3. Incisional: through previous abdominal incisions.
   4. Umbilical: true umbilical through a defect in the cicatrix of the umbilicus.
   5. Paraumbilical: a weakness around the umbilicus.
   6. Epigastric: between the xiphisternum and the umbilicus.
   7. Sphegelian: protrudes from linea semilunaris.
   8. Lumbar (Petit's) via lumbar triangle (iliac crest, external oblique and latissimus dorsi).
   9. Littre's: contains Meckel's diverticulum.
   10. Maydl's: 'W' shaped loop of small bowel lies in the hernia sac.
   11. Gluteal: through greater sciatic foramen.

Hospital Surgery: Foundations in Surgical Practice, ed. Omer Aziz, Sanjay Purkayastha and Paraskevas Paraskeva. Published by Cambridge University Press.
© Cambridge University Press 2009.

12. Sciatic: through lesser sciatic foramen.
13. Obturator: passing through the obturator canal.
14. Perineal: herniation through the perineum, usually postoperatively when pelvic organs have been removed.
15. Richter's: just one wall involved ('knuckle' of bowel).
16. Hiatus: herniation of the fundus of the stomach through the diaphragm ('sliding' and 'rolling').
17. Paraduodenal: herniation, usually of the small bowel into one of the paraduodenal spaces i.e. this is internal herniation.
18. Sliding (hernia en glissade): sac wall is composed in part by retroperitoneal viscus, e.g. caecum.
19. Amyand's hernia: one that contains the appendix.

b. **Cranial**
1. Tentorial.
2. Uncal.
3. Brainstem.

c. **Intervertebral disk**
1. Disk prolapse: nucleus pulposus into annulus fibrosus.

■ Incidence of inguinal hernia

Males > females.

Inguinal > femoral (even in women).

Right commoner than left. Femoral hernia has a greater risk of strangulating and three sides of the femoral ring are rigid.

■ 'Must know' hernia terms

Incarceration: means irreducible i.e. cannot be pushed back into the original anatomical position.

Reducible: can be pushed back into its original anatomical position.

Strangulation: when a hernia gets stuck passing through the defect and the structures lose their blood supply.

Reduction en masse: reduction of hernial sac and contents, so that intestinal obstruction is still present.

■ Risk factors

Age; smoking; chronic cough; increased intra-abdominal pressure e.g. BPH, constipation etc.; connective-tissue disorders e.g. Ehlers-Danlos/Marfan's.

■ History

Lump +/– pain – worse with: standing, coughing, straining. Possibility of scrotal involvement.

Reducibility: symptoms of strangulation, obstruction or peritonism. Evidence of risk factors.

Co-morbidities for an operation/anaesthetic risks.

■ Examination

Position – if the neck of the hernia is above and medial to pubic tubercle: inguinal, if below and lateral to pubic tubercle then it is a femoral hernia.

Scrotal involvement: examine lying and standing. Ask patient to reduce hernia for you as he will know it best! Is it tender? Are there bowel sounds? Is it reducible? Is there skin erythema or a cough impulse?

Inguinal canal contents (three arteries, three veins, three nerves and three other structures):

a. **Spermatic cord: external spermatic fascia, cremasteric fascia, internal spermatic fascia.**
   1. Vas deferens
   2. Testicular artery
   3. Testicular vein (pampiniform plexus)

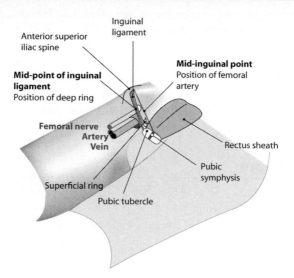

Figure 73 Basic inguinal anatomical landmarks: inguinal ligament runs from the ASIS (anterior superior iliac spine) to the pubic tubercle

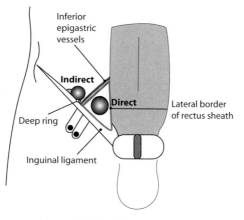

Figure 74 Hasselbach's triangle

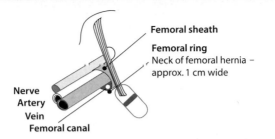

Figure 75 Basic femoral anatomy: N – femoral nerve; A – femoral artery; V – femoral vein; E – empty space; L – lymphatics

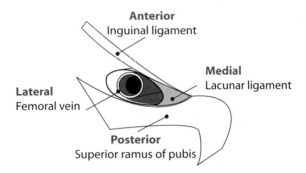

Figure 76 Visualizing the femoral ring from above

4. Lymphatics
5. Cremasteric artery
6. Cremasteric vein
7. Genital branch of genitofemoral nerve
8. Sympathetic nerves
9. Artery to the vas
10. Vein to the vas.

b. **Fatty tissue**.
c. **Ilioinguinal nerve**.

Remember that the testis starts off in the abdomen and then descends into its final space.

■ Management

1. **Conservative**
   Watch and wait. That is, don't operate on a 101-year-old with multiple
       medical problems because of a lump in the groin.
   Truss if it offers symptomatic relief.

2. **Medical**
   Sort out risk factors and medical problems.

3. **Surgical**
   Tension free repair – now mesh is standard (Lichtenstein).
   Open versus laparoscopic (especially for fit and well patients, partic-
       ularly bilateral).
   Mesh versus no mesh.
   Elective versus emergent.

■ Complications of repair

Wound: bleeding, haematoma, seroma, sepsis, sinus.

Scrotal: ischaemic orchitis, testicular atrophy, hydrocoele, genital
   oedema, damage to vas and vessels.

Special complications: nerve injury, persistent postoperative chronic
   pain, compression of femoral vessels, urinary retention, impotence.

DIFFERENTIAL DIAGNOSES

Lymph node
Saphena varix
Lipoma
Skin lump
Maldescended testis
Vascular lesion.

Dysphagia: gastro-oesophageal reflux disease (GORD)

DANNY YAKOUB AND GEORGE HANNA

■ Definition

Reflux of gastro-duodenal contents into the oesophagus, causing symptoms that are sufficient to interfere with quality of life.

■ Incidence

20 to 25% of population have symptoms of GORD, oesophagitis is detected in 25 to 40% of gastroscopies performed on symptomatic patients. It is thought to be predisposed to by obesity, smoking and alcohol. Dietary factors such as excess fat, caffeine and citrus fruits; drugs such as atropine, calcium channel blockers and anti-histamines, various hormones and prostaglandins have also been described.

■ Aetiology and pathophysiology

Incompetence of lower oesophageal sphincter (LOS) due to predisposing factors or distortion of the acute angle of His as in hiatal hernia as well as absence of adequate length of intra-abdominal segment of oesophagus (<2 cm), destroyed mucosal rosette and deficient diaphragmatic crural mechanism. Finally, diminished oesophageal clearance by peristalsis and lowered mucosal resistance, normally maintained by its histological and biochemical properties; all these factors lead to reflux of gastric secretions into lower oesophagus exposing the mucosa to harmful gastric acid.

Hospital Surgery: Foundations in Surgical Practice, ed. Omer Aziz, Sanjay Purkayastha and Paraskevas Paraskeva. Published by Cambridge University Press. © Cambridge University Press 2009.

■ Natural history

90 % asymptomatic. 10 % of asymptomatic individuals develop complications such as reflux oesophagitis, ulceration and peri-oesophagitis; strictures and webs (Shatski's ring), which if severe can cause intermittent total obstruction (Steakhouse syndrome); columnar metaplasia (Barrett's oesophagus), where 10 % of these progress to dysplasia which is precancerous.

■ Symptoms

Heartburn, regurgitation, water brash and dysphagia. Symptoms are aggravated with posture and are greater at night. Severity can be assessed by DeMeester scoring system which grades each of heartburn, regurgitation and dysphagia 0–3 according to severity. Clinical examination is usually performed to exclude other pathologies. Infrequently patients may present with mild epigastric tenderness.

■ Differential diagnosis

Cardiac pain, biliary colic, gastric and oesophageal carcinoma, irritable bowel syndrome, motility disorders and peptic ulcer disease.

■ Investigations

Endoscopy: biopsy followed by oesophageal pH assessment. Oesophageal manometry. *Contrast radiology*: also provides information on hiatal hernia or short oesophagus.

■ Classifications

Los Angeles classification grades severity of oesophagitis detected on upper gastrointestinal endoscopy: Grade A (mucosal breaks < 5 mm) up to D (circumferential breaks in the oesophageal mucosa). Alternatively, Savary–Miller classification can be used (Grade I: linear, non-confluent erosions, to Grade IV: severe ulceration or stricture).

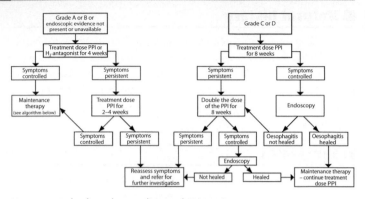

Management plan for endoscopy-diagnosed GORD patients

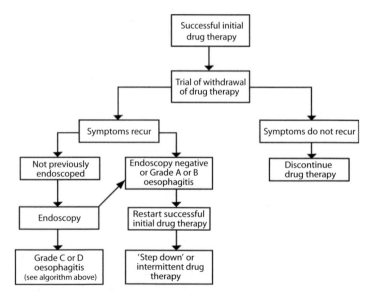

Maintenance management of GORD grades A and B

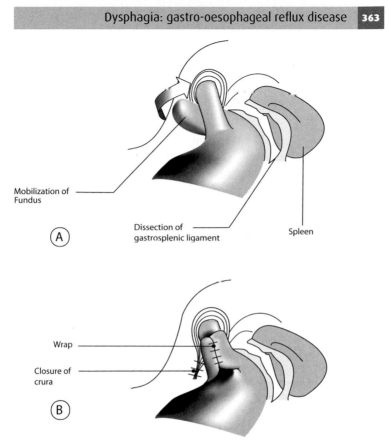

Figure 77 Laparoscopic fundoplication

■ Management

Conservative: frequent small meals and sleeping with the head of the bed raised. Medical: antacids, H_2 antagonists and proton pump inhibitors. Surgical: laparoscopic fundoplication (Figure 77) with or without hiatal hernia repair; postoperative complications include tight wrap and recurrence. New endoscopic procedures are emerging for the reconstruction of lower oesophageal sphincter.

■ Prognosis

Up to 80 % of patients relapse once medication is discontinued. Therefore, many people require surgery. Endoscopy-negative reflux disease usually remains stable and those with severe oesophagitis may develop complications such as oesophageal strictures or Barrett's oesophagus.

Dysphagia: oesophageal neoplasia

DANNY YAKOUB AND GEORGE HANNA

■ Incidence

Oesophageal cancers arise in up to 10–20 per 10^5 of the population. It is more common in patients >60 years of age. M:F ratio of 5:1. Recently, incidence has increased in 30–50 yrs age group with M:F ratio decreasing. Adenocarcinoma is becoming more common in western white men predisposed by Barrett's oesophagitis.

■ Aetiology

Predisposed by excess alcohol intake (acts as a promoter), smoking (acts as direct carcinogen), low 'protective' vitamin and trace element intake in vegetables and fruits, achalasia, strictures; some genetic conditions such as *Tylosis* Type A and *Plummer – Vinson syndrome*.

■ Pathophysiology

Benign: most common is leiomyoma. Malignant: 90 % are squamous cell carcinomas; 1–2 % are adenocarcinomas. Tumours are commonly polypoid, but may be stenosing or ulcerative. Gastro-oesophageal junction tumours are the main type in western countries and are mostly adeno-carcinomas. They may be extending from oesophagus, true cardial, or extending from stomach (Types I, II, III respectively).

■ Natural history

Spread is by direct invasion followed by lymph node and haemato-genous spread. Longitudinal submucosal spread and skip lesions are not

Hospital Surgery: Foundations in Surgical Practice, ed. Omer Aziz, Sanjay Purkayastha and Paraskevas Paraskeva. Published by Cambridge University Press. © Cambridge University Press 2009.

uncommon. Dysphagia might not be apparent until two-thirds of the oesophagus is occluded.

■ Presentation

Progressive dysphagia, regurgitation and weight loss. Rarely pain due to local invasion, and 25–30 % of patients present with symptoms of distant metastases e.g. cervical lymph nodes, jaundice, bony aches, chest manifestations, vocal cord and phrenic nerve paralysis, which are indicators of inoperability.

■ Investigations

Blood tests: nutritional anaemia. *Contrast radiology:* 'Rat tail' appearance with mild proximal dilatation in the oesophagus. *Endoscopy and biopsy* is the gold standard for diagnosis. *Endoscopic ultrasound* and *CT scan* of chest and abdomen have accuracy of up to 90 % in local T and N staging. *Positron emission tomography scan* is done to detect regional and distant metastasis. *Bronchoscopy* should be done for proximal tumours to exclude bronchial involvement.

■ Management

Surgery: is the gold standard for resectable disease (80–90 % of T1 – T2) aiming at cure for early-detected cases in the form of trans-thoracic (Ivor Lewis or Mckeown) or trans-hiatal, open or thoracoscopic, partial or total oesophagectomy with replacement using stomach, colon or jejunum; together with radical excision of regional lymph nodes according to site of tumour (Japanese surgeons tend to do lymphadenectomy of abdomen, mediastinum and neck, i.e. three fields, in most of their cases (Figure 78)); surgery may be preceded or followed by chemotherapy. Postoperative mortality is 5–10 % in specialized centres. Main postoperative complications include pulmonary infections, anastomotic and thoracic duct leakage. *Endoscopic mucosal resection,* laser and photodynamic therapy may be considered for selected early cases. *Palliative therapy:* (1) Palliative surgery may be done to alleviate dysphagia. (2) Chemoradiotherapy in advanced cases (>Stage III), generally squamous carcinoma is more sensitive to this treatment than adenocarcinoma. (3) Stenting and intubation e.g. Mousseau-Barbin or Celestin tube to traverse the obstructing segment. (4) Laser fulgration or electro-coagulation as a temporary measure to create a lumen inside the tumour.

■ Prognosis

Five-year survival for Stages I and IIa is 25–40 %. Higher numbers have been reported in Japanese studies. Advanced cases have five-year survival of less than 5 %. Prognostic indices identified are age, tumour size, stage, number of positive lymph nodes, histological lymphatic and vascular invasion.

■ TNM staging of oesophageal tumours

PRIMARY TUMOUR (T)

TX: Primary tumour cannot be assessed
T0: No evidence of primary tumour
Tis: Carcinoma in situ
T1a,b: Tumour invades lamina propria, submucosa
T2: Tumour invades muscularis propria
T3: Tumour invades adventitia
T4: Tumour invades adjacent structures.

REGIONAL LYMPH NODES (N)

NX: Regional lymph nodes cannot be assessed
N0: No regional lymph node metastasis
N1: Regional lymph node metastasis.

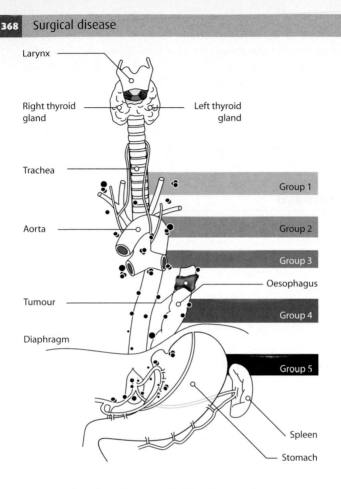

Lymph node groups draining the oesophagus

Group 1: Cervical
Group 2: Superior mediastinal
Group 3: Mid mediastinal
Group 4: Inferior mediastinal
Group 5: Abdominal

Figure 78 Lymph node groups draining the oesophagus

DISTANT METASTASIS (M)

MX: Distant metastasis cannot be assessed

M0: No distant metastasis.

M1: Evidence of distant metastasis.

STAGE

Stage 0:	Tis	N0	M0	**Stage I:**	T1	N0	M0
Stage IIa:	T2	N0	M0	**Stage IIb:**	T1	N1	M0
	T3	N0	M0		T2	N1	M0
Stage III:	T3	N1	M0	**Stage IV:**	Any T	Any N	M1
	T4	any N	M0				

(Adapted from the American Joint Committee on Cancer 1998.)

Dysphagia: oesophageal dysmotility syndromes

DANNY YAKOUB AND GEORGE HANNA

■ Classification

Primary: specific, such as achalasia, diffuse oesophageal spasm and nutcracker oesophagus; non-specific with symptoms and manometric changes not fitting to one of the above. Secondary: much less common as an association with progressive systemic sclerosis and scleroderma.

■ Achalasia

Aetiology and pathophysiology: there is decrease or loss of ganglion cells in the myenteric plexus of nerves (Figure 79) leading to incomplete relaxation of the LES and loss of propulsive peristalsis in the proximal oesophagus with dilation and regurgitation of contents. It is either idiopathic or as part of Chagas disease (mega-oesophagus associated with *Trypanosoma cruzi* infection endemic in Latin America). Prevalence is up to 8 per 100 000.

Presentation: gradual development of dysphagia mainly for solid food, regurgitation of previous day's meals, halitosis and chest pain. Recurrent chest infection.

Natural history: may take up to two years to develop, mostly accidentally discovered on chest radiography or endoscopy. Stasis of food and secretions predispose to complications such as oesophageal ulceration and strictures; regurgitation leads to chest complications such as pneumonia, bronchiectasis and lung abscess. Long-standing achalasia increases risk of oesophageal cancer development.

Hospital Surgery: Foundations in Surgical Practice, ed. Omer Aziz, Sanjay Purkayastha and Paraskevas Paraskeva. Published by Cambridge University Press. © Cambridge University Press 2009.

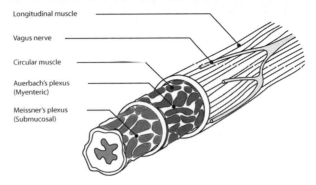

Figure 79 Neuromuscular anatomy of the oesophagus

■ Diffuse oesophageal spasm

Multiple spontaneous or swallow-induced, simultaneous contractions of the oesophagus of large amplitude and long duration alternating with periods of normal peristalsis. Mostly occurs in emotional persons; yet, aetiology is still unknown.

Pathophysiology: thought to be due to sensitivity to cholinergic and olfactory stimuli and to some emotional states.

Presentation: dysphagia for solids and liquids alike, odynophagia and retrosternal chest pain often confused with IHD pain. No weight loss or obstructive episodes. In up to 50 % of cases, symptoms of irritable bowel syndrome are present.

■ Nutcracker oesophagus

Characterized by high amplitude (more than 140 mmHg) peristaltic contractions throughout the lower or whole oesophagus. It is associated with smooth muscle hypertrophy. Aetiology and pathophysiology are unclear.

Presentation: non-cardiac chest pain rather than dysphagia.

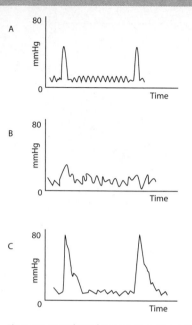

Figure 80 Oesophageal manometry patterns (A) Normal (B) Diffuse oesophageal spasm (note simultaneous contractions) (C) Nutcracker oesophagus (note high amplitude peristalsis)

Investigations: *blood tests:* may show nutritional anaemia or hypovitaminosis. *Contrast radiology:* usually diagnostic according to abnormality shown. *Endoscopy:* done to confirm diagnosis and exclude malignant dysphagia. *Oesophageal manometry:* is the gold standard for diagnosis and shows characteristic pattern for each syndrome (Figure 80). *Radionucleotide transit studies:* may be done to augment diagnosis.

Management: medical: to relax the smooth muscles as Ca^{2+} channel blockers and nitrates. Endoscopic balloon dilation and recently endoscopic *Botulinum* toxin injection (neurotoxin to paralyse smooth muscle). Surgical: extramucosal smooth muscle division at the cardia and proximal stomach (Heller's cardiomyotomy, Figure 81) combined with anti-reflux procedure (e.g. Dor or Toupet fundoplication) is commonly used for treatment of achalasia, with a laparoscopic approach now commonplace.

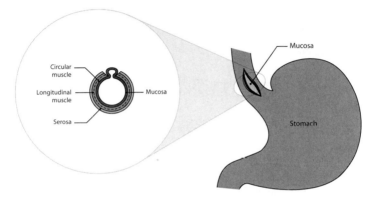

Figure 81 Heller's cardiomyotomy

Gastric disease: peptic ulcer disease (PUD)

SANJAY PURKAYASTHA AND GEORGE HANNA

Definitions: peptic = pertaining to digestion or the enzyme pepsin i.e. areas where pepsin may be present. Ulcer = an area of tissue erosion, for example of the skin or lining of the gastrointestinal (GI) tract. Due to the erosion, an ulcer is concave. It is always depressed below the level of the surrounding tissue.

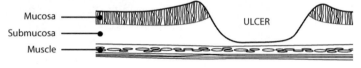

Figure 82

Prevalence and incidence: the annual age-standardized period prevalence of peptic ulceration in the UK is approximately 1.5/1000 for men and 1/1000 for women. Current trends are for a decreasing incidence in young men and an increasing number in older women. Internationally, the frequency of PUD is decreasing in the developed world but increasing in developing countries. PUD is twice as common in men compared to women.

Aetiology: the mechanisms involved that lead to PUD are probably due to an imbalance between erosive factors, such as gastric acid and pepsin production, and protective factors, such as mucus production, bicarbonate, and blood flow.

Stress, alcohol consumption, bile, smoking and non-steroidal anti-inflammatory drugs (NSAIDs) are all known to increase gastric acid production. More recently the presence of *Helicobacter pylori* in the gastric mucosa has been demonstrated as the most important cause of PUD.

Hospital Surgery: Foundations in Surgical Practice, ed. Omer Aziz, Sanjay Purkayastha and Paraskevas Paraskeva. Published by Cambridge University Press. © Cambridge University Press 2009.

Complications of PUD include: malignancy, haemorrhage, perforation, obstruction.

Symptoms: classically, epigastric and left upper quadrant pain that radiates to the back. May be worse with food (gastric ulcer) or better with food (duodenal ulcer). Heartburn and vomiting may also be the presenting complaint. It may present with upper GI bleeding (haematemesis or melaena), both acutely and insidiously with anaemia and its related symptoms. PUD occasionally presents following an acute perforation of the stomach or duodenum, with shock, peritonitis and subsequent systemic inflammatory response syndrome.

Examination: depends on the type of presentation, which may range from haemodynamic instability following a massive upper GI bleed or perforated viscus to mild epigastric pain and tenderness (see above). Rectal examination may demonstrate melaena.

Differential diagnosis: pancreatitis, GORD, bilary colic, AAA, MI, amongst others.

Investigations: *blood tests:* FBC, clotting, G&S or crossmatch may be needed if haemorrhage is evident, U&E, amylase, LFTs, CRP; in the elective setting serology for *H. pylori* and biochemical tests for pepsin-secreting tumours may be sent if the presentation is suspicious.

X-rays: erect CXR (note 10–15 % of perforations do not present with free air). *Abdominal CT:* if patient is stable and perforation is queried but there is no free air on the erect CXR. For individuals that present through outpatients, urea breath tests and elective OGD (see chapter on OGD) and biopsies for CLO (*Campylobacter*-like organism) may be used.

Management: treat the acute presentation i.e. upper GI bleed (see Gastrointestinal bleeding Chapter) or perforation (See Perforated gastroduodenal ulcer chapter). If patient has clinical or radiological signs of perforation they must be seen immediately by a senior member of the surgical team. In the interim the patient needs aggressive resuscitation and optimization, to be NBM, if vomiting an NG tube to be inserted, a urinary catheter +/– central line for careful fluid balance monitoring, iv antibiotics (1.5 mg cefuroxime and 500 mg metronidazole), iv PPI (40 mg pantoprazole), analgesia, anaesthetic review and consent for an emergency laparotomy. Surgical treatment of perforated PUD includes laparotomy with repair of the ulcer using an omental patch. If the ulcer macroscopically is suggestive of malignancy, then partial or total gastrectomy may be considered depending on the extent of disease.

■ Outpatient treatment

Lifestyle changes: change in diet: less fatty or spicy food, cessation of smoking and alcohol intake.

Medical therapy:

Stop NSAIDs, steroids and other drugs that may erode the gastric mucosa.

Antacids: alginates such as gaviscon for symptomatic relief.

H_2 receptor blockers such as ranitidine.

Proton pump inhibitors (PPIs) such as omeprazole.

Direct mucosal protection: e.g. sucralfate.

H. pylori eradication: one week triple therapy that includes a PPI, antibiotics (amoxicillin and either clarithromycin or metronidazole).

Following medical eradication, patient should have a repeat breath test or OGD + CLO.

Surgical treatment: this has in the past included vagotomies, antrectomies, partial and total gastrectomies. With the advent of H_2 blockers, PPIs and triple therapy, such operations are performed less and less frequently, although if surgery is necessary then a laparoscopic approach may be adopted even for cases suspicious of malignancy.

Gastric disease: gastric neoplasia

DANNY YAKOUB AND GEORGE HANNA

■ Gastric adenocarcinoma

Incidence: 10 per 100 000. More common in men (M:F = 2:1). Incidence increases with age > 50 (peak age = 70), and is highest in Asia (80 times more common in Japan).

RISK FACTORS

- *Diet* – high nitrate content foods (smoked, salted, and dried foods), low protein/fat consumption, high complex carbohydrate consumption
- *Occupational hazards* – heavy metals, asbestos, rubber
- *Low socioeconomic class* (except in Japan)
- *Cigarette smoking*
- *Alcohol consumption*
- *Genetic* – blood group A, family history and black race.

ASSOCIATED CONDITIONS

- *Pernicious anaemia*
- *Previous gastrectomy* (for benign disease)
- *Polyps*
- *Atrophic or hypertrophic gastritis*
- *Chronic peptic ulcer disease*
- *Barrett's oesophagus*
- Helicobacter pylori *infection.*

Hospital Surgery: Foundations in Surgical Practice, ed. Omer Aziz, Sanjay Purkayastha and Paraskevas Paraskeva. Published by Cambridge University Press. © Cambridge University Press 2009.

PATHOPHYSIOLOGY

90–95 % of gastric cancers are **adenocarcinomas** (cellular types include pylorocardiac, signet ring, intestinal and anaplastic). 5 % are benign tumours, lymphomas and sarcomas. Most common sites include: pyloric canal (37 %), cardia (30 %), body (20 %), and entire stomach – *linitis plastica* (12 %) (see Figure 83). Appearance and distribution may be classified during endoscopy according to **Borrmann's classification** (see Figure 84) as *Type 1*: polypoid, non-ulcerated, *Type 2*: ulcerated, well circumscribed, *Type 3*: ulcerated, not well circumscribed, and *Type 4*: diffuse, infiltrating (+/– ulceration), *linitis plastica, Type V*: does not fit into any of the other groups.

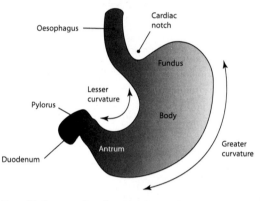

Figure 83 Common sites of gastric adenocarcinoma

NATURAL HISTORY

Insidious onset. **Diagnosis often delayed** as symptoms are initially managed as gastritis. The tumour metastasizes by *direct invasion, lymphatic spread* (regional, supraclavicular – Virchow's, and umbilical – Sister Mary Joseph's nodes), *peritoneal spread* to ovaries (Krukenburg tumours), and *haematogenous spread* may occur via portal system to liver or to systemic circulation.

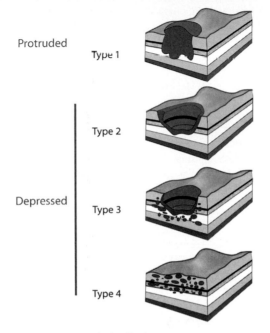

Figure 84 Borrmann's classification

SYMPTOMS AND SIGNS (NON-SPECIFIC IN EARLY DISEASE)

Weight loss, abdominal pain, anorexia, nausea, dysphagia, melaena, anaemia, abdominal mass, early satiety, manifestations of metastases (lymphadenopathy, ascites and pleural effusion). Dyspepsia – should be differentiated from gastritis and benign gastric ulcers.

INVESTIGATIONS

Blood tests: FBC (anaemia), serological markers such as CEA and CA 72-4 are of prognostic value.

Radiology: *barium meal* – may show the ulcer crater/mass lesion. *CT* and *radionucleotide (PET) scans* may be combined with *endoscopic ultrasound* for cancer staging with accuracy of up to 90 %.

Endoscopy and biopsy: has up to 95 % accuracy in diagnosing gastric cancer.

STAGING

The system currently in use worldwide is the AJCC TNM staging system. It is based on depth of primary tumour invasion through the gastric wall (T), number of lymph nodes involved (N), and the presence/absence of metastasis (M) as shown below:

PRIMARY TUMOUR (T)	
TX	Primary tumour cannot be assessed
T0	No evidence of primary tumour
Tis	Carcinoma in situ: intra-epithelial tumour without invasion of the lamina propria
T1	Tumour invades lamina propria or submucosa
T2	Tumour invades muscularis propria or subserosa
T2a	Tumour invades muscularis propria
T2b	Tumour invades subserosa
T3	Tumour penetrates serosa (visceral peritoneum) without invasion of adjacent structures
T4	Tumour invades adjacent structures
REGIONAL LYMPH NODES (N)	
NX	Regional lymph node(s) cannot be assessed
N0	No regional lymph node metastasis
N1	Metastasis in 1 to 6 regional lymph nodes
N2	Metastasis in 7 to 15 regional lymph nodes
N3	Metastasis in more than 15 regional lymph nodes
DISTANT METASTASIS (M)	
MX	Distant metastasis cannot be assessed
M0	No distant metastasis
M1	Distant metastasis

Based on this an overall stage grouping is assigned:

STAGE GROUPING			
Stage 0	Tis	N0	M0
Stage 1A	T1	N0	M0
Stage 1B	T1	N1	M0
	T2a/b	N0	M0
Stage II	T1	N2	M0
	T2a/b	N1	M0
	T3	N1	M0
Stage IIIA	T2a/b	N2	M0
	T3	N1	M0
	T4	N0	M0
Stage IIIB	T3	N2	M0
Stage IV	T4	N1–3	M0
	T1–3	N3	M0
	Any T	Any N	M1

MANAGEMENT

For **curable disease** surgical resection entails **subtotal or total gastrectomy** with various extents of **radical lymphadenectomy** (D1, D2, and D3) according to tumour stage, where D refers to extent of lymphadenectomy (Figures 85 and 86).

The aim is to have a resection with no residual tumour. D2 resection has been shown to improve staging in randomized controlled trials; however, survival benefit is yet to be proved in trials with standard surgical technique. The lymph node stations as described by the **Japanese classification for gastric carcinoma (JCGC)** staging system are shown in Figure 87.

Neoadjuvant chemotherapy is currently under investigation and has shown some promising early results.

Advanced cancer is treated with palliative chemotherapy and radiotherapy, with the option of palliative surgical bypass.

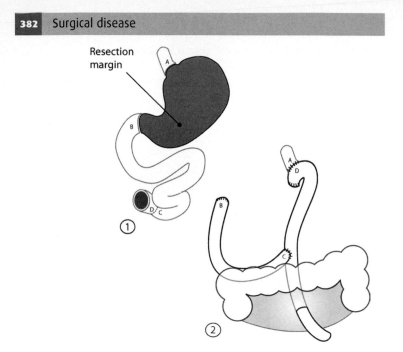

Resection margin

Figure 85 Total gastrectomy and Roux-en-Y anastomosis

GASTRECTOMY COMPLICATIONS

These must be looked out for in the postoperative period and include: immediate – postoperative haemorrhage; early – anastomotic leakage, reactive haemorrhage and ileus. Late complications include tumour recurrence and post-gastrectomy syndromes:

- **Early postprandial dumping** – rapid emptying of hyperosmolar gastric contents results in intravascular fluid shifts. Symptoms occur within minutes of a meal and may be vasomotor (flushing, palpitations and dizziness) or gastrointestinal (abdominal pain, fullness, vomiting and diarrhoea) in origin. Symptoms may be controlled by more frequent, smaller meals with higher protein and lower

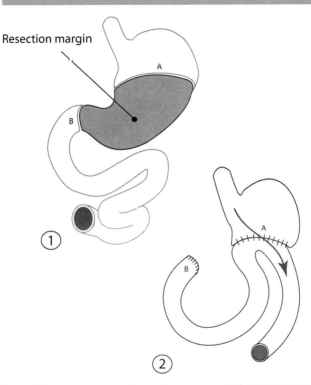

Resection margin

Figure 86 Subtotal gastrectomy (gastrojejunostomy) and Billroth II anastomosis

carbohydrate component. If severe and unresolved this may require surgical correction.

■ **Late postprandial dumping** – large amounts of carbohydrates reaching the small intestine stimulate insulin release, producing a reactive hypoglycaemia a few hours after the meal. Symptoms include tachycardia, dizziness and sweating 1–2 hours after eating. Treatment includes smaller meals and the ingestion of carbohydrates when the reactive hypoglycaemia starts. Ultimately surgical re-intervention may be needed if symptoms fail to resolve.

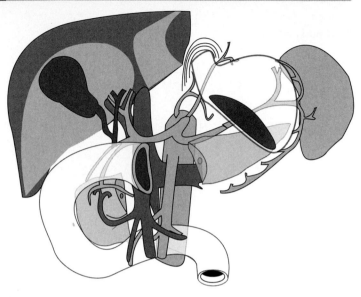

Figure 87

PROGNOSIS

Five-year survival after surgical resection for Stages I, II, III, IV is 40%, 29%, 13%, and 3% in the UK, while it is up to 90%, 71%, 44% and 9%, respectively, in Japan. Prognostic indicators include age, TNM stage, vascular invasion, lymphatic invasion, peritoneal cytology. **Overall five-year survival in the Western World for gastric adenocarcinoma is poor at 10–20%.**

■ Gastric lymphoma

The most common type of gastrointestinal lymphoma. Clinical presentation is similar to that of gastric adenocarcinoma. Often diagnosed on endoscopy and biopsy with brush cytology. Usually resectable with surgery, usually in the form of subtotal gastrectomy, followed by chemotherapy (+/− radiotherapy for bulky tumours). Two-thirds of cases are resectable. Prognosis is better than with adenocarcinoma. Five-year survival is 25–50 %. Microscopic positive margins do not affect survival.

GASTROINTESTINAL STROMAL TUMOURS (GISTs)

GISTs are non-epithelial, connective-tissue tumours (sarcomas). 70 % occur in the stomach. Treatment is subtotal gastrectomy +/− chemotherapy.

■ Gastric leiomyosarcoma

Usually present with haemorrhage, weight loss and pain. Endoscopic examination reveals bulky intraluminal mass with central area of necrosis; biopsy/brush cytology confirms diagnosis. Surgical resection is only curative treatment. Five-year survival 30–50 %.

■ Benign gastric tumours

The presentation varies and depends on size of tumour. Common aetiologies include:

■ Hyperplastic polyps
■ Adenoma
■ Leiomyoma
■ Heterotopic pancreas.

These may be managed by either endoscopic or surgical (laparoscopic or open) excision.

Hepatobiliary disease: jaundice

OMER AZIZ AND MARK THURSZ

■ Definition

Jaundice (icterus) refers to the yellow pigmentation of skin, sclerae and mucosae due to raised plasma bilirubin (>35 mmol/l).

■ Pathophysiology

Bilirubin is a normal breakdown product of haemoglobin produced in the reticuloendothelial system following destruction of old red blood cells. The resulting *unconjugated bilirubin* is insoluble and carried to the liver bound to albumin. In the liver, the enzyme uridine diphosphate-glucuronyl transferase conjugates this with glucuronic acid into water-soluble *conjugated bilirubin*. This is then secreted into bile canaliculi, and ultimately enters the duodenum. Bilirubin is converted into uro-bilinogen in the terminal ileum and colon, of which up to 20 % is reabsorbed into the portal circulation. This is then either re-excreted back into the bile or excreted by the kidneys into the urine. Increased production, failure of uptake, or conjugation all result in unconjugated bilirubinaemia and jaundice.

■ Classification

Pre-hepatic: excess unconjugated bilirubin production (from red blood cells) exhausts the liver's capacity to conjugate e.g. haemolytic anaemias (hereditary spherocytosis, sickle-cell disease, hypersplenism).

Hospital Surgery: Foundations in Surgical Practice, ed. Omer Aziz, Sanjay Purkayastha and Paraskevas Paraskeva. Published by Cambridge University Press. © Cambridge University Press 2009.

Hepatic: unconjugated hyperbilirubinaemia due to inborn failure of conjugation (Crigler Najjar syndrome) and inborn failure of bilirubin uptake (Gilbert's syndrome). Hepatocellular causes include cirrhosis, viruses (hepatitis A, B, C, E; Epstein-Barr), autoimmune diseases, drugs (paracetamol, halothane).

Post-hepatic: obstructive conjugated hyperbilirubinaemia may be due to *intrahepatic obstruction* (primary biliary cirrhosis, some hepatocellular disease) or *extrahepatic obstruction* (gallstones, carcinoma of the head of pancreas, cholangiocarcinoma, portal lymphadenopathy, and sclerosing cholangitis).

■ Symptoms

Pain, typically RUQ biliary colic, occurs when there is choledocholithiasis. Dull persistent pain may be present with acute hepatitis or bulky tumours in the liver. **Pruritis** usually signifies post-hepatic jaundice due to the accumulation of bile acids. **Risk factors for viral hepatitis** (travel, sexual history and blood transfusion) should be sought. **Drugs and alcohol** history are essential. Obstructive jaundice presents with history of **pale stools,** difficult to flush (steatorrhoea) and **dark urine.**

■ Examination

Look for jaundice (skin, sclera, mucus membranes), stigmata of chronic liver disease (spider angiomas, palmar erythema, asterixis, clubbing, caput medusae, ascites, encephalopathy) and bruising indicating coagulopathy. Weight loss or a palpable gallbladder usually indicates extrahepatic biliary obstruction due to a tumour. **Courvoisier's law** states that a palpable gallbladder in the presence of jaundice is unlikely to be due to gallstones. Typically caused by a neoplastic stricture obstructing the common bile duct.

■ Investigations

Blood tests include FBC, LFTs, prothrombin time (PT). **Urinalysis** with dipsticks for urobilinogen/bilirubin. **Ultrasound scan** (USS) to look for biliary pathology. Derangement of LFTs may help with diagnosis, with elevated transaminases (ALT, AST) indicating hepatocellular injury, and ALP indicating ductal injury/obstruction. See the table below. PT derangement indicates failure of synthesis of clotting factors (V, VII and X). Further investigations depend on the initial results (see algorithm).

Fluid balance: ensure adequate hydration to prevent *hepatorenal syndrome*; preoperative diuresis may reduce incidence (administer 5% dextrose/saline for 12 hours preoperatively +/– loop diuretic at time of induction). Note: hypoalbuminaemia may lead to fluid retention in jaundice patients; catheterize and monitor accurate input/output chart.

Treat hypokalaemia: secondary hyperaldosteronism leads to Na^+ retention and K^+ depletion.

Blood test	Pre-hepatic jaundice	Hepatic jaundice	Post-hepatic jaundice
Unconjugated bilirubin	↑↑	↔ / ↑	↑
Conjugated bilirubin	↔	↑	↑↑↑
Urinary bilirubin	↔ / ↑	↑	↑↑↑
Urinary urobilinogen	↔ / ↑	↓	↓↓↓
ALP	↔	↑	↑↑↑
γ GT	↔	↑	↑↑↑
ALT	↔	↑↑↑	↑
LDH	↔	↑↑↑	↑
Reticulocytes	> 2%	↔	↔

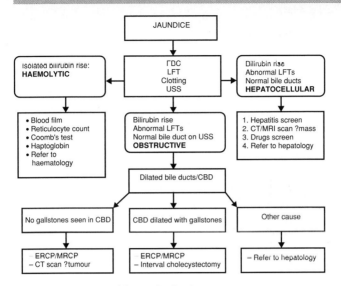

Algorithm: management of the jaundiced patient

Clotting: decreased vitamin K absorption in cholestatic jaundice leads to reduced synthesis of factors II, VII, IX and X, leading to a prolonged prothrombin time (PT). Intramuscular injection of phytomeniadione (10–20 mg) will reverse the clotting deficiency within 1–3 days. If more urgent correction is required use fresh frozen plasma (FFP) within 1–2 hours of the procedure.

Wound infection: greater risk of postoperative wound infection; consider prophylactic broad-spectrum antibiotics to avoid cholangitis.

Relieve jaundice prior to surgery if possible: endoscopic sphincterotomy to relieve CBD obstruction and remove common bile duct stones. Note: liver failure may be encountered in patients with prolonged CBD obstruction or with preoperative hepatocellular disease. If jaundice is severe (>150 mmol/l), a period of decompression is required prior to surgery, via endoscopic stenting or sphincterotomy.

Hepatobiliary disease: gallstones and biliary colic

OMER AZIZ AND ARA DARZI

■ Gallstones

Incidence: 8 % M, 17 % F. Predisposed by obesity, multiparity, diabetes mellitus, cirrhosis, pancreatitis, chronic haemolytic states, malabsorption, inflammatory bowel disease, genetic factors (Pima Indians).

Aetiology: bile contains bile salts (cholic and chenodeoxycolic acids), phospholipids (lecithin), and cholesterol in soluble micelles. Gallstones form with failure to maintain these components in a soluble state either due to nidus (centre) formation or as a result of lithogenic bile (Figure 88). Biliary 'sludge' consists of cholesterol crystals, calcium bilirubinate granules, and a mucin gel matrix, and predisposes to gallstones.

Pathophysiology: three types: *mixed* (80 %), multiple; *cholesterol* (10 %), solitary, large, round; *pigment* (10 %), contain unconjugated bilirubin and calcium, usually multiple, smaller black or brown in colour, and associated with haemolytic states.

Natural history: 80 % asymptomatic. 2 % per year of asymptomatic individuals develop complications and 2 % require cholecystectomy. The longer stones remain quiescent, the less likely symptoms are to develop. Biliary colic is the most common presentation, but may also present as acute cholecystitis, pancreatitis, cholangitis, or other complications of these conditions.

Complications: *in the gallbladder* (biliary colic, acute cholecystitis, mucocoele, empyema, gangrene, perforation, carcinoma), *in the biliary tree* (choledocholithiasis, obstructive jaundice, cholangitis, pancreatitis, strictures, biliary cirrhosis) or *outside the gallbladder and biliary tree* (cholecystenteric fistula, gallstone ileus). In the case of gallstone ileus,

Hospital Surgery: Foundations in Surgical Practice, ed. Omer Aziz, Sanjay Purkayastha and Paraskevas Paraskeva. Published by Cambridge University Press. © Cambridge University Press 2009.

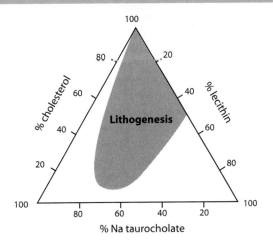

Figure 88 Triangular phase diagram with axes plotted in percent cholesterol, lecithin (phospholipid) and the bile salt sodium taurocholate. Outside shaded area, cholesterol is maintained in solution in micelles. Inside shaded area the solid line, bile is supersaturated with cholesterol and precipitation of cholesterol crystals can occur

repeated attacks of cholecystitis result in formation of a fistula between the gallbladder and most commonly the duodenum. Gallstones may pass through this, causing intermittent small-bowel obstruction most commonly at the ileocaecal junction. Air is seen in the biliary tree in approximately 40 % of these cases on AXR.

■ Biliary colic

Definition: pain arising from the gallbladder without evidence of infection (different to acute cholecystitis). Due to transient obstruction of the cystic duct by a gallstone.

Symptoms: constant RUQ and epigastric pain lasting minutes to hours (differs from other 'colics'). Can radiate to back or to right scapula. May be exacerbated by fatty foods or begin following meals. Sometimes difficult to differentiate from acute gastritis. Other associated symptoms are nausea, vomiting and bloating.

Examination: some RUQ tenderness, no peritonism. Gallbladder usually not palpable.

Differential diagnosis: PUD, pancreatitis, GORD, hepatomegaly, and pneumonia.

Investigations: *blood tests:* ALP may be elevated but WBC, LFTs, and amylase often normal. *X-rays:* AXR often normal (only 15 % of gallstones contain enough calcium to be radio-opaque). *Ultrasound:* diagnostic procedure of choice, able to identify stones, gallbladder wall thickening, comment on duct dilation, liver, pancreatic head, masses and fluid collections. Sensitivity 95 %, specificity 90 %. *Radionucleotide HIDA scan:* diagnoses acute cholecystitis with 95 % sensitivity. *Abdominal CT:* Only identifies calcified gallstones in 50 % of patients, but can diagnose acute cholecystitis.

Management: asymptomatic stones do not require further management. Symptomatic patients should be offered laparoscopic cholecystectomy.

Prognosis: 70 % of patients with biliary colic will have further painful episodes within the following year. Delay in laparoscopic cholecystectomy may result in gallstone-related complications, increased morbidity, and ultimately a more difficult operation.

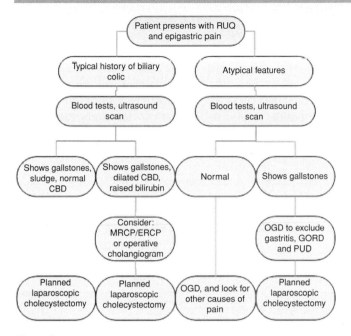

Biliary colic management summary

Hepatobiliary disease: pancreatic cancer

ANDREW J. HEALEY AND LONG R. JIAO

Incidence: sixth most common type of cancer death in UK (fourth in USA). Peak ages 65–75 yrs (M = F). Very poor five-year survival rates, so incidence ≈ mortality (USA 2003: 30 700 new patients, 30 000 deaths).

Aetiology: positive familial background in 5–10 % cases. Risk factors: smoking, chronic pancreatitis, cassava root. Possible small minority genetic component e.g. germline mutations in BRCA2, $p16^{INK}$ familial syndromes.

Pathology: pancreatic ductal adenocarcinoma 85 %, others include: papillary, mucinous, carcinoid, acinar (note: endocrine tumours 1 %). 80–90 % found in head of gland.

Direct spread common and majority present with advanced disease. Metastatic spread (in decreasing order): lymph nodes (multiple nodes and multiple groups), perineural, vascular. Common sites of metastases: liver, peritoneum and (of extraperitoneal) lung.

Union Internationale Contre le Cancer staging of pancreatic cancer (2002)			
Stage	T	N	M
0	Tis	0	0
IA	T1	0	0
IB	T2	0	0
IIA	T3	0	0
IIB	T1–3	N1	0
III	T4	Any	0
IV	Any	Any	M1

Tis, carcinoma in situ; T1, tumour limited to pancreas <2 cm; T2, tumour limited to pancreas >2 cm; T3, tumour extending beyond the pancreas but not involving coeliac/SM arteries; T4, tumour involving the coeliac/SM arteries; N0, no regional lymph nodal metastasis; N1, regional lymph node metastasis; M0, no distant metastasis; M1, distant metastasis

Hospital Surgery: Foundations in Surgical Practice, ed. Omer Aziz, Sanjay Purkayastha and Paraskevas Paraskeva. Published by Cambridge University Press. © Cambridge University Press 2009.

Symptoms/signs: painless obstructive jaundice (in up to 85%) from mainly pancreatic head cancer, depending on the location of cancer (see Figure 89), otherwise non-specific symptoms, weight loss, back or epigastric pain, anorexia, abdominal mass, ascites; (more rarely) unexplained acute pancreatitis or late-onset diabetes.

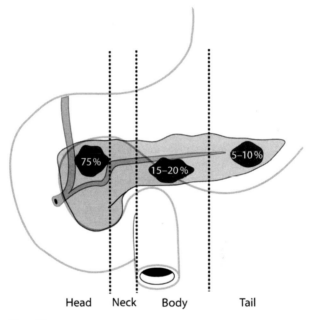

Head   Neck   Body   Tail

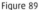
Figure 89

Examination: evidence of weight loss, palpable liver, palpable gallbladder (Courvoisier's law), metastatic lymph nodes (e.g. neck/supraclavicular), Trousseau's sign.

Investigations: *blood tests:* LFTs to assess jaundice, amylase (in acute pancreatitic presentation), FBC (anaemia of chronic disease), CA19-9 (sensitive tumour marker in normobilirubinaemia, but not specific). *X-rays:* AXR usually normal, if there is history of chronic pancreatitis there may be some pancreatic calcification. *Ultrasound*: initial procedure of choice, able to identify extra-hepatic duct dilation +/– pancreatic head masses (depending on amount of overlying bowel and body habitus), liver metastases and fluid collections. *ERCP*: for direct visualization and biopsy of periampullary tumours, although increasingly replaced by *MRCP* and *endoscopic ultrasound (EUS)*. *Abdominal CT* (multislice with arterial and portal venous phases): gold standard for clinical staging; 80–90 % accuracy at predicting resectability in large tumours, but less accurate in small.

Management: is tumour resectable? (Stages I and II, see table.) Factors contraindicating resection include: liver peritoneal or other metastases, distant lymph node metastases (note: positive lymph nodes within the operative field are not a contraindication), major venous or arterial (coeliac, superior mesenteric or hepatic) encasement, as well as major co-morbidities.

Curative surgery: often preceded by biliary drainage endoscopically with plastic stent (no clear evidence-based effect on surgical outcome). Operations: standard Kausch–Whipple procedure (or the variant), pylorus-preserving proximal pancreaticoduodenectomy. Distal pancreatectomy indicated for lesions in body or tail (involvement of splenic artery or vein not itself a contraindication to resection). Adjuvant chemotherapy standard (ESPAC-1 trial, 2001), two adjuvant regimens currently being studied (ESPAC-3); 5-FU and folinic acid for 24 weeks vs. gemcitabine for 24 weeks vs. surgery alone, target 990 patients (330 randomized to each group). Note: localized adjuvant intra-arterial chemotherapy with radiotherapy also under investigation (ESPAC-2, target 220 patients, due to finish 2007).

Postoperative complications: mortality 1–4 %, intra-abdominal abscess 1–12 % (managed with CT-guided drainage), haemorrhage 2–15 %, in first 24 hr either due to insufficient intraoperative haemostasis or anastomotic bleed (stress ulceraton rare). Secondary bleeds, 1–3 wks postoperatively, carry higher mortality and might include erosion of retroperitoneal vasculature or pseudoaneurysm; pancreatic fistula 2–24 % (rates vary widely – no standardized definition). Meta-analysis of pre/perioperative somatostatin analogues, e.g. octreotide, suggests role in reducing postoperative complications.

Palliation treatment: majority of patients not amenable to resection at presentation. Biliary drainage: (1) Stent (endoscopic or radiological); <3 cm approximate primary size needs metallic stent, >3 cm primary needs plastic/metallic. (2) Surgical bypass (Roux-en-Y hepatojejunostomy) for those without co-morbidities; maximizes amount of remaining time spent at home without readmission for recurrent jaundice (stents can occlude or migrate), however there is a risk of surgical complications (e.g. cholangitis and biliary leak). Stent vs. bypass: no significant difference in survival or procedure-related death.

Prognosis: late presentation means overall median survival < 6 months. Pancreatic resection in 10–15 %, with median survival 11–20 months and five-year survival 10–25 %. Irresectable locally advanced non-metastatic disease median survival 6–11 months, metastatic 2–6 months. Majority of patients develop disease recurrence within two years after resection with liver metastases presenting earlier (5–11 months) than local recurrence (13 months). Overall five-year survival 0.4 %.

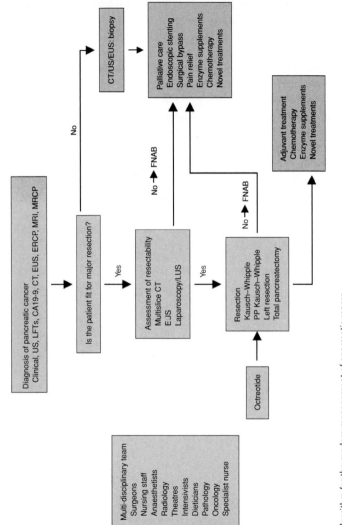

Algorithm for the modern management of pancreatic cancer.

CT, computed tomography; ERCP, endoscopic retrograde cholangio-pancreatography; EUS, endoluminal ultrasonography; FNAB, fine needle aspiration biopsy for cytology; LFTs, liver function tests; LUS, laparoscopic ultrasonography; MRCP, magnetic resonance cholangio-pancreatography; MRI, magnetic resonance imaging; PP, pylorus preserving; US, ultrasonography

Hepatobiliary disease: liver tumours

OMER AZIZ AND MARK THURSZ

Liver tumours may present with clinical symptoms but are increasingly presenting at a pre-clinical stage due to surveillance in patients with cirrhosis. This has led to a significant change in the 'natural history' of liver tumours and provides an opportunity to alter prognosis in what has been a uniformly dismal diagnosis.

■ Definition and classification

Liver tumours may be benign or malignant, primary or secondary. The two 'common' primary tumours are hepatocellular carcinoma (HCC) or cholangiocarcinoma. Rarer tumours include haemangiosarcoma and hepatoblastoma. Secondary tumours are the most common cause of liver malignancy and may arise from any organ but most commonly from the stomach, colon, pancreas, breast and ovary. Benign tumours of the liver include haemangiomas, focal nodular hyperplasia and hepatic adenomas.

■ Incidence

In patients with cirrhosis and chronic viral hepatitis HCC occurs at a rate of 1–4 % per year. Incidence is higher in males and those over the age of 40. HCC is a common malignancy in China, South-East Asia and Sub-Saharan Africa. The incidence of HCC is increasing in Europe and the USA due to hepatitis C virus infection. The incidence of cholangiocarcinoma is increasing rapidly in developed countries.

Hospital Surgery: Foundations in Surgical Practice, ed. Omer Aziz, Sanjay Purkayastha and Paraskevas Paraskeva. Published by Cambridge University Press. © Cambridge University Press 2009.

■ Aetiology

Almost all HCCs arise from a background of cirrhosis. All causes of cirrhosis may cause HCC but viral hepatitis, haemochromatosis and alcohol are the most important aetiologies. Exposure to aflatoxin increases the risk of HCC particularly in populations where hepatitis B virus infection is common. In developed countries the risk factors for cholangiocarcinoma are primary sclerosing cholangitis and inflammatory bowel disease. In tropical countries the tumour is associated with chronic liver fluke infection.

■ Pathophysiology

HCC invariably develops from a background of cirrhosis, with high cell turnover and failure of apoptosis in genetically damaged cells implicated. Free radical damage to the genome and insertional mutagenesis with hepatitis B virus have also been postulated. Large and small cell dysplasia are often found in patients with cirrhosis. Small cell dysplasia is found in up to 50 % of patients with HCC and when discovered at biopsy should be carefully investigated. HCC may be multifocal and often metastasizes within the liver. Distal metastases in the abdominal cavity and lung are usually late-stage events. Cholangiocarcinoma usually occurs in the context of chronic inflammation in the biliary system, with 20 % of patients with primary sclerosing cholangitis developing a tumour. Often this is slow growing and death may occur as a result of prolonged or recurrent biliary sepsis where biliary drainage is poor. Invasion of the portal vein leading to thrombosis and portal hypertension are common complications of both HCC and cholangiocarcinoma. The most common site for cholangiocarcinoma is the hilum but tumours may occur more distally in the common bile duct or may be peripheral in the liver parenchyma.

■ Symptoms

HCC may present as RUQ pain or mass, abdominal distension, weight loss or decompensated liver disease. Variceal bleeding may occur particularly when the portal vein is obstructed or thrombosed. Peripheral cholangiocarcinoma may present in a similar way to HCC but the most frequent presentation is with obstructive jaundice. Secondary carcinoid tumours in the liver may present with hormonal symptoms such as flushing, diarrhoea or attacks of hypotension.

■ Examination

Many patients will have stigmata of chronic liver disease and a palpable mass at the time of presentation. HCC often presents at a very late stage when therapy is futile. Ultrasound screening, while of controversial benefit, is successful at identifying tumours at a treatable stage.

■ Investigations

USS is successful at identifying tumours at a treatable stage. Features suggestive of HCC may be present on triple phase CT or MRI scanning. Definitive diagnosis may depend on the mass increasing in size on sequential scans or association with a raised α-fetoprotein level (>400 ng/l). Biopsy should be avoided as track seeding is a recognized complication particularly when transplantation is being considered. However, where the diagnostic criteria above are not met, CT/US-guided biopsy may be necessary. Cholangiocarcinoma is usually diagnosed by cholangiography. A biliary stricture associated with a mass lesion on cross sectional imaging is usually sufficient to make a diagnosis. Biliary cytology is helpful in only about 50 % of cases and attempts to biopsy the tumour at ERCP are rarely successful due to the dense fibrous stroma of the tumour. Unresectable cholangiocarcinomas usually need treatment by biliary stenting. Urinary hormone levels (5HIAA) should be measured in patients with suspected carcinoid tumours.

■ Management

HCC may be treated by resection, orthotopic liver transplantation (OLT), local ablation, or trans-arterial chemoembolization (TACE). Resection is only feasible where there is sufficient hepatic functional reserve. Transplantion is used where the Milan criteria are met:

fit for transplantation AND

1. Single tumour < 5 cm diameter OR
2. ≤ 3 tumours (in same lobe) ≤ 3 cm diameter.

Local ablation may be performed using radiofrequency, percutaneous ethanol injection, laser or cryoablation. Ablation may be used to manage tumours up to 5 cm in diameter and give up to 50 % five-year survival in suitable patients. Only surgical resection offers a cure for cholangiocarcinoma. Resectability depends on the position of the tumour and invasion into local vascular structures. Transplantation for cholangiocarcinoma is associated with recurrence rate and is therefore not indicated. Neither HCC nor cholangiocarcinoma are sensitive to radiotherapy or chemotherapy.

■ Prognosis

Median survival after a clinical presentation of HCC is between six weeks and six months. Transplantation in carefully selected patients gives a five-year survival of 70 %. Ablation therapy may give a 50 % five-year survival. The prognosis of cholangiocarcinoma is very variable due to differences in the growth rates of the tumours. Median survival is around six months.

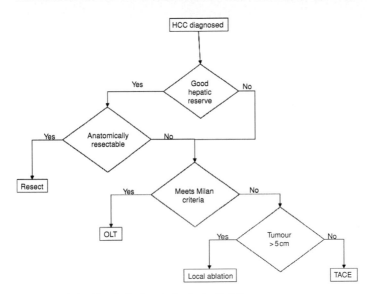

Management algorithm for treatment of patient with HCC

The spleen

ANDREW J. HEALEY AND LONG R. JIAO

■ Anatomy

Encapsulated friable organ of the left hypochondrium, forms lateral extremity of lesser sac in long axis of ribs 9, 10, 11. Weighs 150 g but atrophies with age. Visceral relations: left kidney posteriorly, stomach anteriorly and splenic flexure of colon inferiorly. Hilum contains nerves and vessels entering/leaving spleen, splenic lymph nodes and tail of pancreas. Passing to spleen are gastrosplenic ligament (containing short gastric and left gastroepiploic vessels) and lienorenal ligament (containing splenic vessels and tail of pancreas). Blood vessels: arterial-splenic artery (from coeliac axis), and venous-splenic vein (merges with superior mesenteric vein to form portal vein) (Figure 90).

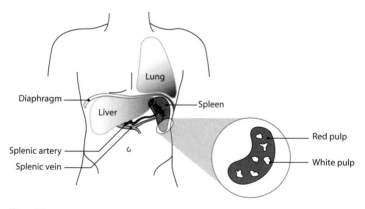

Figure 90

Hospital Surgery: Foundations in Surgical Practice, ed. Omer Aziz, Sanjay Purkayastha and Paraskevas Paraskeva. Published by Cambridge University Press. © Cambridge University Press 2009.

■ Functions

1. Filtering: spleen filters old or abnormal red cells and platelets and also abnormal white cells and cellular debris.
2. Immunological function: spleen is well adapted for removal of poorly opsonized and encapsulated pathogens and localized B-cell proliferation, differentiation and antibody synthesis.

■ Causes of splenomegaly

1. Vascular congestion: pre-hepatic (e.g. splenic or extra-hepatic portal vein thrombosis), hepatic (e.g. cirrhosis), chronic portal hypertension and post-hepatic (raised IVC pressure such as right-sided cardiac failure).
2. Infection: typhoid, chronic malaria, and viral (e.g. infectious mononucleosis).
3. Haematological disorders: haemolytic anaemia, ITP, hereditary spherocytosis, polycythaemia rubra vera and neoplasms including leukaemias, myeloproliferative disorders, Hodgkin's and non-Hodgkin's lymphoma. These can cause massive splenomegaly such that the spleen is palpable in the right iliac fossa, and the hilar notch distinguishable.
4. Immune disorders: e.g. rheumatoid disease and SLE.
5. Storage disorders: e.g. Niemann-Pick, Gaucher diseases and mucopolysaccharidoses.
6. Amyloid.

■ Indications for splenectomy

1. Trauma: CT/US can accurately characterize splenic injury in patients with blunt trauma. Non-operative support with inpatient observation for up to five days is indicated in anyone with splenic injury and haemodynamic stability, provided there is no evidence of other intra-abdominal injuries. Haemodynamic instability, bleeding > 1000 ml, transfusion of >2 units blood or other evidence of ongoing blood loss

are accepted indications in adults. Children < 14 yrs – more aggressive non-operative support justified. Splenic preservation must be considered at laparotomy if bleeding can be controlled easily, and no other intra-abdominal injuries. Children < 14 yrs – more aggressive splenic preservation attempted (for techniques see 2 below).

2. Iatrogenic: possible in any intra-abdominal procedure, especially distal oesophageal, stomach, distal pancreas or splenic flexure of colon. Injuries either direct (e.g. retractor) or indirect (from traction on splenic capsule). Splenic preservation and haemorrhage control can be attempted using suture placation, topical haemostatic agents (including absorbable mesh), electrocautery and argon beam coagulation. Splenectomy for those who require transfusion.

3. Haematological diseases: indications must be determined through close cooperation with haematologist/oncologist. Common indications: ITP (in those resistant or recurring after primary steroid treatment), hereditary spherocytosis (traditionally treated with total splenectomy but recent trials with near-total splenectomy indicate it potentially preserves immune function), thalassaemia major, autoimmune haemolytic anaemia unresponsive to medical management, and symptomatic splenomegaly. Massive splenectomy may preclude laparoscopic approach. Alternatives include open or 'hand-assisted' laparoscopic technique. Important to discuss increased operative morbidity and mortality rates and increased use of blood products postoperatively with patients before operation.

4. Others include: infection (e.g. splenic abscesses), congestion (splenic vein thrombosis or obstruction), splenic mass (cystic or neoplastic), inclusion in en-bloc resection for malignancy of adjacent organ. Distal pancreatectomy often includes splenectomy if preservation of splenic artery or vein contraindicated or technically impossible.

■ Postoperative complications

Pneumonia; thrombotic (platelet count usually increases up to 400–500×10^9/l for over a year. Thrombocytosis in excess of 1000×100/l requires antiplatelet therapy such as aspirin); wound infections; hernia formation; haemorrhage; subphrenic abscess; pancreatic pseudocyst; abscess or fistula. Loss of splenic tissue reduces capacity of body to remove immature or abnormal cells; hence target cells, siderocytes, reticulocytes and Howell-Jolly bodies often appear in postoperative blood films. Operative mortality < 1 %, except in those with myeloproliferative disorders (increased risk of postoperative haemorrhage). In trauma patients mortality is related to extent of other injuries.

■ Laparoscopic splenectomy

Feasible; increasingly common practice. Fewer severe complications. Requires greater technical care. Two approaches: anterior and lateral. Lateral suggested to enable easier dissection and mobilization, reducing operative time. However, due to the increased number of muscular layers the lateral trocars pierce, pneumoperitoneum might increase risks of abdominal wall dissection, haematoma and bleeding postoperatively. Main severe complication, rarely seen in open splenectomy, is diaphragmatic perforation (often small cautery injury of the dome enlarging under pressure of pneumoperitoneum).

■ Overwhelming post-splenectomy infection (OPSI)

All patients susceptible to fulminant bacteraemia after splenectomy. Risk greatest in young children, especially <6 yrs, because they have not yet developed extra-splenic specific immunity to encapsulated organisms. 80 % of postoperative sepsis occurs in first two years. *Streptococcus pneumoniae, Haemophilus influenzae* and meningococci are the most common pathogens. Splenectomy in children < 5 yrs should be treated by daily dose of penicillin until age 10 yrs. For non-elective splenectomy all patients should be immunized with Pneumovax (a non-viable pneumococcal vaccine). Elective cases: Pneumovax, and against *H. influenza* (HiB) and meningococcus (A and C), two or more weeks preoperatively.

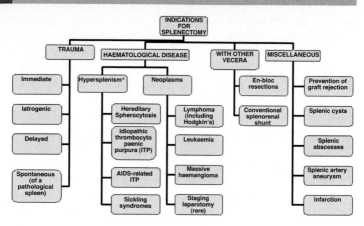

Diagram summarizing the main indications for splenectomy

Inflammatory bowel disease: Crohn's disease

RICHARD LOVEGROVE AND PARIS TEKKIS

■ Introduction

Crohn's disease (CD) is an inflammatory condition that most commonly affects the small intestine. It may, however, affect any part of the GI tract from the mouth to the anus. The colon (Crohn's colitis) or the perineum, with or without small-bowel involvement may be affected.

■ Incidence

Five new cases per 100 000 population per year in developed countries. The incidence is rising rapidly. Crohn's disease is most commonly diagnosed in 20–30 year olds, but shows a biphasic incidence, with a second peak in the sixth decade.

■ Aetiology

Unknown. Possible causes include *infective* (there are features that are similar to intestinal tuberculosis), *immunological* (there are suggestions of impaired cell-mediated immunity, and of autoantibody formation) and *diet* (possible causation of diet high in refined carbohydrates). In contrast to ulcerative colitis, smoking appears to be a risk factor.

■ Pathophysiology

Unlike ulcerative colitis, which is confined to the colon, CD can affect any part of the gastrointestinal tract. The disease is characteristically patchy in nature with normal segments of bowel between 'skip lesions'

Hospital Surgery: Foundations in Surgical Practice, ed. Omer Aziz, Sanjay Purkayastha and Paraskevas Paraskeva. Published by Cambridge University Press. © Cambridge University Press 2009.

of disease. Macroscopically there is aphthous ulceration which progresses to deep fissuring ulcers. This leads to a cobblestone appearance and tight strictures or fistulae may develop. Microscopically there is chronic inflammation of all layers of the bowel wall, with ulceration, micro-abscesses and non-caseating granulomas.

■ Symptoms and signs

The presentation of CD can vary depending on the areas affected. The most common presenting features are diarrhoea, weight loss, abdominal pain and fever. There may be steatorrhoea if the small bowel is affected, or rectal bleeding in those with Crohn's colitis. Perineal Crohn's can lead to multiple perianal abscesses and fistula formation. If strictures develop, the patient may present with bowel obstruction and may have features of malabsorption. Perforation of the bowel may occur, but this tends to be contained locally; free perforation is rare. Abscesses may form adjacent to the bowel and may discharge through fistulae to the skin, other bowel segments, bladder and vagina. Patients with Crohn's colitis are at risk of developing toxic megacolon, but this is less than is seen in ulcerative colitis (UC).

Other organs may be affected – eyes: conjunctivitis, uveitis, episcleritis; joints: arthritis/arthropathy; skin – rashes: erythema nodosum and pyoderma gangrenosum; blood: autoimmune haemolytic anaemia; liver – primary sclerosing cholangitis.

■ Important differentials

Ileocaecal CD may present with right iliac fossa pain, tenderness and fever, and should be differentiated from appendicitis. A history of an 'irritable appendix' or a family history of inflammatory bowel disease should raise the suspicion of CD; however, if indicated, the patient may need to be taken to theatre to exclude appendicitis. Colonic CD may be very difficult to differentiate from UC, but it is important to do so as to undertake restorative proctocolectomy in a patient with CD inevitably leads to failure of the ileal pouch.

■ Investigation

Blood tests may reveal raised inflammatory markers (CRP, ESR) in active disease. Iron, folate and vitamin B_{12} deficiencies are common and are a cause of anaemia. Microscopy and culture of stool specimens are required to exclude infective causes of diarrhoea.

Endoscopy allows visualization of the colon and upper GI tract and can be used to assess the extent of colonic disease as well as allowing biopsies to help differentiate from UC. Intubation of the terminal ileum allows visualization of the small-bowel and biopsy to diagnose small-bowel CD. Small-bowel follow through or video capsule endoscopy may allow further assessment of small bowel affected.

Barium studies can be used to visualize the whole of the GI tract and may show strictures, fistulae, ulcers (aphthoid, linear, collar-stud or rosethorn), cobblestoning and inflammatory pseudopolyps.

■ Treatment

The medical management of Crohn's disease aims to maintain the disease in a quiescent state. This is done through the administration of *corticosteroids* for small-bowel disease or *5-aminosalicylic acid* (5-ASA, Pentasa) or *sulphasalazine* for ileocolic and colonic disease. *Azathioprine* or *6-mercaptopurine* may be used concurrently to reduce the dose of steroids required. *Topical steroids* may be beneficial in anorectal disease. In severe attacks of Crohn's disease dietary supplements or *total parenteral nutrition* (TPN) may be required to provide nutritional support. *Monoclonal antibodies* (Infliximab) may be used to treat and prevent exacerbations.

Up to 80 % of patients with Crohn's disease will require at least one operation during the course of their disease. The aim of surgery is to

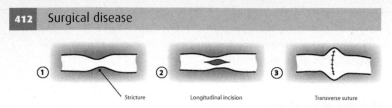

Figure 91 Strictureplasty

be as conservative as possible in order to ensure maximal bowel length and prevent short-bowel syndrome (<1 m of functioning small bowel). Strictures require either resection or a strictureplasty (Figure 91); ileo-caecal disease requires an ileocolic resection; Crohn's colitis requires colectomy and ileorectal anastomosis, or if the rectum is involved then a proctocolectomy and permanent end ileostomy. Unlike patients with UC, those with Crohn's disease can not have an ileoanal pouch. Perianal disease may be treated by laying open of fistulous tracts or passing a seton (thread) through the tract to facilitate drainage of any sepsis. More severe, intractable disease may require the creation of a colostomy or ileostomy in order to control recurrent episodes of sepsis.

Many patients with Crohn's disease require multiple operations, with the re-operation rate being 40 % by 10 years post-surgery. Some patients may, as a result of multiple resections, have too little small bowel to facilitate sufficient absorption of dietary intake. In these circumstances TPN may be required permanently, and the patient will have to learn how to administer this themselves at home.

Inflammatory bowel disease: ulcerative colitis

RICHARD LOVEGROVE AND PARIS TEKKIS

■ Introduction

Ulcerative colitis is an inflammatory condition of the large bowel that typically presents with frequent bloody stools. In acute cases presentation may be with signs of sepsis, and perforation of the colon may have occurred or be imminent.

■ Incidence

Ten new cases per 100 000 population in developed countries. Less common in Africa and Asia. Bi-modal age distribution with peak at 20–40 and a lesser peak at 60–80 years of age. Incidence is equal between the sexes.

■ Aetiology

The aetiology of ulcerative colitis remains unknown. Possible factors are genetic, as demonstrated by 15-fold increase in incidence in first-degree relatives. Other factors include infective organisms, psychosocial well-being, immunological, or defects in colonic mucus production. Smoking appears to have a protective effect.

■ Pathophysiology

The disease process usually begins in the rectum (proctitis), and spreads proximally. If the ileocaecal valve is incompetent, the terminal ileum may also be involved (backwash ileitis). Macroscopically there is diffuse inflammation with hyperaemia, pus and bleeding. Ulceration may be

Hospital Surgery: Foundations in Surgical Practice, ed. Omer Aziz, Sanjay Purkayastha and Paraskevas Paraskeva. Published by Cambridge University Press. © Cambridge University Press 2009.

evident. In long-standing cases, inflammatory polyps (pseudopolyps) may occur in large numbers. In severe fulminant (toxic) colitis, a segment of the colon, most commonly the transverse, becomes acutely dilated and the wall thins and is at risk of perforation (toxic megacolon).

Microscopically, acute and chronic inflammatory cells invade the lamina propria and crypts, and there are crypt abscesses. Goblet cell mucin becomes depleted, and the crypts are present in reduced number and atrophic. With increased duration of the disease the cells undergo dysplastic changes and there is an increase in the risk of colorectal cancer. At 20 years of disease duration, the risk is approximately 12 %.

■ Symptoms and signs

The initial presentation is usually with bloody diarrhoea, or rectal discharge which may be bloody or purulent. If the disease has been present for some time prior to presentation there may be associated signs of weight loss and malnourishment. The disease process is chronic and characterized by relapses and remissions. In the acute setting the patient will have signs of toxaemia and will be tachycardic, hypotensive and febrile. On examination there may be evidence of peritonism, but this may be masked if the patient is on high doses of steroids.

Patients with UC may have extra-intestinal manifestations, such as arthritis (15 %), spondylitis, skin lesions such as erythema nodosum and pyoderma gangrenosum, iritis and sclerosing cholangitis, which may occur in up to 70 % of patients.

■ Investigation

Blood tests may reveal anaemia, neutrophilia and raised inflammatory markers (CRP, ESR). Barium enema demonstrates a loss of haustrations, mucosal changes and the presence of pseudopolyps. The colon often appears tubular (lead-pipe appearance). Endoscopy plays an important role in disease surveillance as it allows for multiple biopsies to be taken from different colonic sites, and visualization of the response to treatment. Biopsies are important in differentiating between Crohn's disease and ulcerative colitis, and in monitoring dysplastic changes. In the acute setting a plain abdominal X-ray may demonstrate a dilated colon. If the colonic diameter is greater than 10 cm (toxic megacolon) surgical intervention is necessary to prevent perforation. An erect chest X-ray or CT scan of the abdomen may be necessary to exclude the presence of a perforation, particularly if clinical signs may be masked by steroids.

■ Treatment

The initial treatment is usually medical. Corticosteroids are the most common first-line treatment, and may be given orally, systemically or as enemas. Other agents such as 5-aminosalicylic acid (5-ASA) may be needed in slightly more resistant cases. As a last resort cyclosporine may be given. In the acute setting, large doses of hydrocortisone intravenously may be required, along with careful replacement of fluid losses. In prolonged attacks, nutritional supplementation may be required parenterally.

The surgical treatment of ulcerative colitis consists of removing the diseased bowel. In the acute setting, a total or subtotal colectomy with formation of an end ileostomy is the preferred approach. In some cases (e.g. perforation) it may be necessary to excise the rectum at this time as well, i.e. proctocolectomy. Patients generally feel much better following surgery as the cause of their toxaemia has been removed.

In the elective setting, such as for development of severe dysplasia, cancer, or frequent relapses, a restorative procedure is usually undertaken. The colon and rectum are excised, and pouch fashioned from approximately 30 cm of distal ileum. An opening at the apex of the pouch is made and this is anastomosed onto a short cuff of rectum that is left *in situ*. The patient may have a stoma, typically for eight weeks, following surgery to allow the anastomoses to heal (Figure 92). Patients generally have a good quality of life, but will find that they will need to empty their pouch 4–6 times per day.

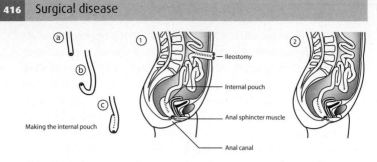

Making the internal pouch

Ileostomy

Internal pouch

Anal sphincter muscle

Anal canal

Figure 92

■ Prognosis

Most patients with UC experience recurrent episodes of acute colitis. Close surveillance is necessary to monitor for neoplastic changes, particularly after 10 years of disease duration. Patients undergoing restorative proctocolectomy (pouch procedure) have a good quality of life, but require regular follow up to monitor their pouch function and surveillance of their pouch.

Inflammatory bowel disease: infective colitis

RICHARD LOVEGROVE AND PARIS TEKKIS

Introduction: infective colitis is an inflammatory condition of the large bowel caused by the presence of pathogenic organisms, and may be primary or secondary.

Incidence: the incidence varies widely depending on the causative organism. The most common type, pseudomembranous colitis, occurs in up to 1 % of hospitalized patients, and is almost exclusively associated with antibiotic use.

■ Causative organisms

A number of different organisms have been implicated, and these include:

- *Clostridium difficile.* This organism is responsible for pseudomembranous colitis. It is associated with the use of antibiotics, particularly the macrolides. Clinically a patient who may have been steadily improving suddenly deteriorates, with tachycardia and signs of hypovolaemia. There is profuse diarrhoea which is characteristically green in colour. Blood tests show a rising white count and inflammatory markers. If dehydration is severe then renal function may become compromised. The inflammatory process causes a fibrinous pseudomembrane to develop over the colonic mucosa. Treatment is with oral metronidazole or vancomycin. Parenteral antibiotics are not effective. If treatment is delayed toxic megacolon and/or perforation may occur. Mortality is reported to be as high as 30 %.

- *Entamoeba histolytica.* This protozoal infection is most commonly seen in tropical and subtropical regions. The organism resides on

Hospital Surgery: Foundations in Surgical Practice, ed. Omer Aziz, Sanjay Purkayastha and Paraskevas Paraskeva. Published by Cambridge University Press. © Cambridge University Press 2009.

the colonic mucosa as a commensal, and as such is normally sub-clinical. The protozoa produce cysts which are passed with the stool. These are hardy, and can survive in the external environment; transmission is therefore faecal-oral. Under certain conditions, *Entamoeba* can become pathogenic. At this time the protozoa invade the mucosa and produce an amoebic colitis with ulceration and bleeding. Mild diarrhoea is common, but may become profuse in more severe cases. The infection may be complicated by colonic perforation or haematogenous spread of the protozoa to the liver where it causes abscesses. Treatment is with metronidazole and intravenous fluids if diarrhoea is severe.

- *Cytomegalovirus* (CMV). This virus belongs to the herpes family and is extremely common in the community, with 40–100 % of the population demonstrating prior exposure. CMV is excreted in a number of body fluids and is transmitted by close personal contact. In the immunocompetent CMV rarely causes clinical conditions, although a number of cases of CMV have been reported. CMV infection is most commonly seen in the immunocompromised (e.g. HIV, prolonged steroid use, post-chemotherapy or immunosuppression following organ transplantation). CMV infection of the colon causes inflammation which may mimic ischaemia histologically. Treatment is with antiviral agents such as ganciclovir. CMV colitis has a high mortality rate, being 56 % in the immunocompromised and up to 22 % in the immunocompetent.

- Other organisms such as *E. coli, Campylobacter, Yersinia enterocolitica, Salmonella, Shigella* and amoeba.

Common presentations include abdominal pain, diarrhoea (with or without the passage of blood), dehydration and sepsis. History of travel, antibiotic use and immunocompromise, and contact with others recently diagnosed with infective colitis is key to the correct diagnosis. Also it is important to remember that patients with known inflammatory bowel disease (IBD) may also contract infective colitis as well on top of their IBD.

■ Management

Early diagnosis of the pathogen is key from stool samples. However, history and thorough examination are imperative for the likely source, and to determine the severity of the presentation. Full blood count, renal function, clotting and group and save should be sent, and an erect chest and abdominal radiograph performed. A contrast-enhanced CT scan may be performed to rule out the diagnosis of ischaemic colitis and radiologically evaluate the colon.

For acutely unwell patients, aggressive resuscitation, analgesia and antibiotics (sensitive to the pathogen) are the mainstay of treatment. Large amounts of bloody diarrhoea may also necessitate blood transfusions. Severe infective colitis may lead to toxic megacolon, perforation or severe haemorrhage that warrants surgery. Patients should be optimized and often are so unwell and septic that intensive care therapy may be needed postoperatively.

In severe cases of total colitis, or if the colon has perforated and the remaining colon is severely oedematous, a *subtotal colectomy* may be performed (with or without an ileorectal anastomosis and a defunctioning ileostomy).

Patients that are stable, and where the causative organism has been identified, should be treated with the appropriate antimicrobial. For common pathogens these are:

- *C. difficile* – treat with oral vancomycin or metronidazole
- *E. coli* – typing and sensitivity is imperative to provide specific treatment
- *Salmonella* – treat with ciprofloxacin
- *Shigella* – treat with ciprofloxacin
- *Campylobacter* – treat with ciprofloxacin
- *Yersinia* – treat with ceftriaxone (severe cases)
- *Giardia* – treat with metronidazole, furazolidone, albendazole
- *Entamoeba histolytica* – treat with metronidazole.

It is important to remember that although the above antibiotics may be used to treat the named organisms, it is vital to communicate with the on-site microbiology department with regards to their therapy of choice for specific treatments.

Contact tracing is important and advice should be sought from the local public health department about which strains are reportable and what protocols should be followed during an outbreak.

Inflammatory bowel disease: non-infective colitis

OMER AZIZ AND PARASKEVAS PARASKEVA

Introduction: non-infective colitis encompasses those causes of colitis not due to pathogenic organisms. Ulcerative colitis and Crohn's colitis are considered under their relevant sections.

Aetiology and pathology: the different types of non-infective colitis will be considered below, together with their pathological features and treatment.

■ Ischaemic colitis

This is the most common form of colonic ischaemia, and presents mainly in the elderly. The classical presentation is with cramping abdominal pain followed by rectal bleeding. The bleeding is normally dark red in colour, and the attacks often settle spontaneously after a few hours. The most commonly affected area of the colon is the splenic flexure. It is in this region that the 'watershed' between the superior mesenteric and inferior mesenteric arteries exists. The marginal artery of Drummond acts as a conduit between these vessels, but may be absent or underdeveloped in 5 % of the population.

A number of precipitant causes exist, but the net effect is the same: decreased blood flow to the affected area. Atherosclerosis of the mesenteric vessels, low cardiac output states (including cardiopulmonary bypass), vasculitis and sickle cell are all common precipitants. Recurrent self-resolving attacks predispose to structuring of the affected bowel, which may necessitate resection. In the acute phase if the patient becomes shocked or develops signs of peritonism then an emergency colectomy may become necessary. If an underlying cause is identified,

Hospital Surgery: Foundations in Surgical Practice, ed. Omer Aziz, Sanjay Purkayastha and Paraskevas Paraskeva. Published by Cambridge University Press. © Cambridge University Press 2009.

then this should be treated as this may prevent or reduce the incidence of future attacks.

■ Microscopic colitis

This consists of two distinct types of colitis: collagenous and lymphocytic. In *collagenous colitis* there is an increased thickness of the subepithelial collagen and increased numbers of lymphocytes. *Lymphocytic colitis* is used to describe a colitis in which there is inflammation within the lamina propria without other histological changes. Clinically, microscopic colitis presents as chronic diarrhoea, and has an incidence of 6 per 100 000 population. Diagnosis is made on biopsies taken at the time of sigmoidoscopy or colonoscopy. Treatment is with oral budesonide and bismuth subsalicylate for collagenous colitis. There have been no controlled trials for the treatment of lymphocytic colitis. The colitis has a varying course with episodes of spontaneous remission and later relapses. Treatment: both may respond to reducing fat, caffeine and lactose in the diet, as well as 5-ASA and steroid therapy. Symptomatic diarrhoea may be treated with loperamide.

■ Indeterminate colitis

This is a chronic inflammatory condition of the colon which histologically has features of both ulcerative colitis and Crohn's colitis, and cannot be readily distinguished from either. Patients are given a diagnosis of indeterminate colitis in 10–15 % of cases of inflammatory colitis. Some patients may have features that are more favourable of diagnosis of Crohn's or UC, but nonetheless the diagnosis is not clear cut.

Treatment is as for UC and Crohn's disease and patients may need to undergo a colectomy in severe cases. Patients with indeterminate colitis may be considered for an ileal pouch, but will normally require a staged procedure with the colectomy specimen being analysed first to try and improve diagnostic accuracy.

■ Radiation colitis and proctitis

Here, inflammation and damage to the rectum, sigmoid, and left colon ensues following exposure to X-rays or other ionizing radiation as a part of radiotherapy for prostate, colonic and cervical cancer. Presentation may be acute or chronic:

Acute radiation proctitis occurs in the few weeks after completion of radiotherapy and is due to direct damage of the colonic epithelium. Presenting symptoms include diarrhoea, urgency, rectal pain and tenesmus. This is usually self-limiting, resolving after 2–3 months. Steroid enemas may help.

Chronic radiation proctitis presents anywhere from months to years following radiotherapy and is due to damage to the blood vessels which supply the colon. Symptoms include rectal bleeding, diarrhoea, pain on defaecation and rectal strictures/stenosis. Fistulae may also develop. The colon is therefore deprived of oxygen and necessary nutrients. Symptoms such as diarrhoea and painful defaecation. Treatment consists of oral opiate analgesia, stool softeners and formalin injections. Patients may require surgery for strictures of fistulae.

Colorectal disease: colorectal cancer

JAMES KINROSS AND PAUL ZIPRIN

■ Incidence

Second commonest cause of cancer deaths in both sexes after lung. 30 000 new cases per year in the UK. Increasing incidence with age, >75 yrs = 300/100 000. Increasing incidence in UK. Colon M = F, rectal M > F. More common in developed countries. Incidence increasing in less-developed nations.

■ Aetiology

1. **Family history:** if one first-degree relative, the risk is increased more than two-fold. Two first-degree relatives or one first-degree relative diagnosed < 45 yrs indicates a lifetime risk of death from colorectal cancer of 1 in 6, or 1 in 10, respectively. 5 % of colorectal-cancer patients have a **genetic syndrome**. Familial adenomatous polyposis (FAP) is an autosomal dominant mutation of the APC gene and presents with multiple colonic polyps. Hereditary non-polyposis coli (HNPCC) and Gardner's syndrome are also responsible.
2. **Inflammatory bowel disease:** ulcerative colitis for over 10 years gives an eight-fold age-related risk.
3. **Lifestyle** – increased risk with: obesity; smoking; diet – high in processed meats, low in vegetables and fibre, alcohol; reduced exercise; bile salts. Reduced risk with: folic acid, Ca^{2+}, selenium, NSAIDs (including aspirin), HRT.

Hospital Surgery: Foundations in Surgical Practice, ed. Omer Aziz, Sanjay Purkayastha and Paraskevas Paraskeva. Published by Cambridge University Press. © Cambridge University Press 2009.

■ Pathogenesis

Two-thirds of cancers develop in the colon, the rest in the rectum. Adenomatous polyps have malignant potential via adenoma-carcinoma sequence: have tubular (70 %), villous (10 %), tubulovillous (20 %) morphology. Left-sided cancers tend to be annular, stenosing and more likely to obstruct. Right-sided cancers are sessile and cause occult bleeding. 3 % of tumours synchronous, 5–10 % metanchronous. Majority are adenocarcinomas. Others: carcinoid, lymphoma, sarcoma. Cancers are graded as well, moderately or poorly differentiated.

■ Symptoms and signs

Classically right-sided lesions present with occult bleeding, weight loss and a RIF mass. Left-sided lesions present with altered bowel habit, pr bleeding or abdominal pain (obstruction/perforation). At presentation, 20 % of patients are acutely obstructed (small-bowel obstruction if ileocaecal valve involved) and 25 % have liver metastases. Also, mucus pr (rectal tumours), weight loss, loss of appetite, lethargy (anaemia), tenesmus/frequency, faecal incontinence, signs/symptoms of spread – hepatomegaly, jaundice, sacral/pelvic pain, sciatica.

■ Investigations

The aim is diagnosis, detection of complications, staging and grading. Always perform a rectal examination. Bloods: FBC for microcytic anaemia, U&E, Ca^{2+}, amylase, clotting and LFTs for liver metastases, G&S, CEA and CA19-9. CXR: for lung metastases and preoperative assessment. AXR: if possibly obstructed. Rigid sigmoidoscopy, and biopsy if non-acute. Flexible sigmoidoscopy (visible to 60 cm, detects 70 % of tumours) and colonoscopy are the gold standard (detects 90 % of adenomas and can snare/biopsy samples). CT colonography (virtual colonoscopy) if colonoscopy contraindicated. MR colonography is also now possible and emerging as a diagnostic test with good predictive indices. Double contrast barium enema may show 'apple core' lesion. Patient should have a thorax/abdomen/pelvis/staging CT scan. USS liver: can look for metastases. Contrast-enhanced CT of the abdomen/pelvis most appropriate in acute presentation, Gastrografin enema also useful. Rectal cancers: MRI or rectal endosonography scan to determine precise location and penetrance to clarify type of surgery and need for adjuvant therapy. MRI is also more useful here for assessment of mesorectal nodes and spread.

■ Treatment

All patients should be seen and diagnosed within two weeks of referral by a GP, and managed in a multidisciplinary team (MDT) setting.

Endoscopic resection may be possible for very early cancers and T1 lesions: endoscopic mucosal resections (EMR) and TEMS (transanal endoscopic microsurgery).

Surgical: 80% of cases amenable to surgery. Arrange stoma nurse review and ensure patient marked if required. Offer psychosocial support. All patients should have DVT prophylaxis (tinzaparin + TEDS) and antibiotic prophylaxis on induction. Latest evidence suggests that there is a limited benefit from bowel preparation (e.g. Kleen prep), but most surgeons request this for technical reasons, particularly for left-sided lesions if no contraindications (e.g. absolute obstruction, allergy). Ensure patient has iv access and fluids especially if elderly. If obstructed, keep NBM, aggressively fluid resuscitate ('drip and suck') before theatre. Ensure all films and endoscopy reports are available for surgery and patient has been crossmatched (2–4 units).

Laponoscopic: there is now good evidence that these procedures can be safely performed laparoscopically. The aim is curative surgery. Type of surgery dependent on location and extent of tumour in relation to blood supply and hence the draining lymph nodes.

Recurrence predicted by (1) Extent of tumour, (2) LN status (3) Circumferential resection margin (CRM) in rectal cancers.

Complications: anastomotic leak in 4–8 % of all cases (up to 15 % in rectal). Mortality from leak 6–40 %.

Emergency: patients with metastases may be stented first and then considered for palliative resection if necessary. Left-sided tumors: laparotomy +/– lavage, primary excision and anastomosis or defunctioning stoma (e.g. Hartmann's).

Treatment of metastases: 8 % of patients are potential candidates for liver resection. Options include surgical excision, radiofrequency ablation (RFA), embolization, cryotherapy, microwave therapy, laser ablation and local chemotherapy.

Chemotherapy is given as an adjuvant to surgery to Dukes' Stage C (or even aggressive Dukes' B cancers subsequent to MDT discussion): 5-FU/leucovorin (MOSAIC trial). Chemotherapy for metastatic colon cancer: irinotecan (CPT11) + 5-FU/leucovorin iv weekly for 4–6 weeks. Suitable patients should be entered into ongoing clinical trials. No benefit for Dukes' A; Dukes' B controversial and should be discussed for potentially aggressive tumours, e.g. with neurovascular invasion. Adjuvant radiotherapy can be used to treat rectal cancer preoperatively or postoperatively; usually given as a short course immediately preoperatively, but longer course in selective tumours to shrink size and facilitate curative resection. It halves the risk of local recurrence and improves five-year survival rates. The role of adjuvant radiation therapy for patients with colon cancer (above the peritoneal reflection) is not well defined.

Palliative therapy: Macmillan nursing team input is vital. Chemo/radiotherapy. Stenting: adverse effects are a 1 % mortality rate, 10 % stent migration and 10 % stent re-obstruction. Surgery: laparoscopic or open defunctioning stoma.

Future therapies: monoclonal antibodies e.g. cetuximab (erbitux), target EGF (epidermal growth factor); await COIN trial results. Bevacizumab (Avastin) is also used with chemotherapy to target VEGF (vascular endothelial growth factor); awaiting NICE review. Also antibody directed prodrug therapy (ADEPT) trial in early stage.

Prognosis: 40–50 % of patients develop liver metastases within three years of primary surgery. 20 % postoperative one month mortality rate if obstructed at presentation. Local recurrence after surgery for rectal cancer varies from less than 10 % to over 40 %.

Dukes' stage (modified)	Definition	Frequency at diagnosis (%)	five-year survival (%)
A	Confined to muscularis propria	11	85
B	Penetrating muscularis propria	35	65
C	Nodal metastases	26	40
D	Distant metastases	29	3

Colorectal disease: colonic diverticular disease

JAMES KINROSS AND PAUL ZIPRIN

Introduction: Diverticular disease is one of the commonest surgical conditions affecting the Western World, and the burden of this disease is therefore increasing with the rising numbers in the elderly population. In most patients it remains asymptomatic but its potential complications have a high morbidity and mortality rate.

■ Definition and classification

A false pulsion diverticulum. Large bowel mucosa is forced through the muscularis propria where it is pierced by the vasa recta (Figure 93). Diverticulosis implies asymptomatic disease whereas diverticulitis is symptomatic. Diverticular disease can be classified as acute or chronic and complicated or uncomplicated.

■ Incidence

Diverticulosis affects about 50 % of 60-year-olds. Increased incidence with age. F > M. It is predominantly a disease of the western World, probably related to dietary factors (but low incidence in western vegetarians).

■ Aetiology

This is predominantly an acquired disease. Commonest in the sigmoid colon. Its principle causes are thought to be a raised intraluminal

Hospital Surgery: Foundations in Surgical Practice, ed. Omer Aziz, Sanjay Purkayastha and Paraskevas Paraskeva. Published by Cambridge University Press.
© Cambridge University Press 2009.

pressure secondary to a poor diet causing bulky stools and colonic seg-
mentation: tonic and rhythmic contractions result in non-propulsive
contractions, producing isolated segments with high intraluminal pressure. A prolonged colonic transit time is also responsible.

■ Pathology

Macro: usually multiple and most frequent in sigmoid colon, right-sided
diverticula are rare, and are usually seen in young Asian populations.
Often associated with colonic structural changes e.g. elastosis of taenia
coli, muscular hypertrophy, mucosal folding. Diverticula can cause (1)
Fistulae: to bladder/vagina/small bowel/skin. (2) *Perforation:* 4/100 000
people with diverticular disease; 2000 cases/year. Most common at first
presentation. (3) *Abscess formation*: pericolic or peritonitis. (4) *Bleeding*:
it is the commonest cause of lower GI bleeds. (5) *Obstruction:* paralytic
ileus/strictures (a chronic sequelae). **Saint's triad:** diverticular disease
associated with cholelithiasis and hiatus hernia.

   Micro: histologically may show inflammation of mucosa.

■ Symptoms and signs

Spectrum of disease, only 20–30% symptomatic: (1) Pain: abdominal
findings reflect the severity and localization of disease. Patients complain of cramping abdominal pain and bloating in diverticulosis, but
localized LIF pain in diverticulitis, may be peritonitic with severe diffuse guarding +/– rebound tenderness if perforated. (2) Change in bowel
habit, usually diarrhoea but may have intermittent constipation. (3)
Fever, may be high +/– rigors if abscess or perforation. (4) Nausea and
vomiting, loss of appetite if diverticulitis. (5) Palpable inflammatory
mass or abscess. (6) pr bleed, can be torrential. (7) Signs of large-bowel
obstruction. (8) Fistulae: pneumaturia, faecaluria if colovesical, faecal
discharge from vagina if colovaginal, diarrhoea if ileocolic.

■ Investigation

Blood tests: expect raised WCC and inflammatory markers, check Hb if bleeding. U&E, amylase, G&S. **Erect CXR:** to rule out perforation/preoperative assessment. **AXR:** to rule out paralytic ileus/obstruction. **Gastrografin enema** if acute uncomplicated diverticulitis. **CT scan:** preferred if complicated. Look for pericolic disease, including intraperitoneal inflammation, perforation and abscess formation. Once acute attack settled, a **colonoscopy** (gold standard), **CT colonography** or double contrast **barium enema** (if colonoscopy contraindicated) is performed 6–8 weeks later as an outpatient to confirm diagnosis and exclude malignancy.

Hinchey classification of diverticular abscesses	
Stage I	Diverticulitis associated with pericolic abscess
Stage II	Distant abscess (retroperitoneal or pelvic)
Stage III	Purulent peritonitis
Stage IV	Faecal peritonitis

■ Treatment

Aims: relief of symptoms and prevention of complications.

Conservative: uncomplicated diverticulosis. High fibre diet (roughage, vegetables), bulk-forming laxative (e.g. Fybogel), adequate oral hydration, exercise. Advice leaflets. Antimuscarinic and antispasmodic agents e.g. hyoscine butylbromide (Buscopan). Advise about potential complications.

Medical: uncomplicated diverticulitis. Supportive therapy: bowel rest, NBM, iv fluids, analgesia and antibiotic cover (cefuroxime 1.5 g iv tds + metronidazole 500 mg iv tds or augmentin 1.2 g iv tds for *Enterococci* cover), followed by conservative measures as tolerated. Usually settles in 48 to 72 hours. An USS or CT-guided drainage for a Hinchey I and II abscess if possible. Dietary fibre supplementation also found to be beneficial. Conservative treatment results in resolution of symptoms in 70–100 % of patients. Asacol (mesalazine) may increase time to subsequent presentation.

Surgical: indications (1) Failure of medical therapy. (2) Recurrent diverticulitis (>2 attacks >40 yrs, 1 attack <40 yrs if hospitalized or immunocompromised patient). (3) Complicated diverticulitis. (4) Severe bleeding. In uncomplicated disease, bowel preparation is required so the patient must have iv access and fluids if elderly. Ensure DVT prophylaxis and prescribe antibiotics as above. Ensure that the patient is crossmatched for two units preoperatively. For sigmoid diverticulosis the operation is a sigmoid colectomy, or anterior resection with the distal anastomosis on healthy upper rectum to prevent recurrence. Most elective surgery can be done laparoscopically. Diverticulitis with free perforation is a surgical emergency: ensure that the patient is adequately resuscitated, and an early anaesthetic review is sought. Keep NBM, inform theatres, give iv antibiotics (cefuroxime and metronidazole) and consent for a potential stoma. Surgical options in complicated diverticulitis: (1) Perforation/large abscess/obstruction: laparotomy and peritoneal lavage with primary resection of the perforated or affected segment and primary anastomosis (Hinchey I and II) or a two stage procedure e.g. a Hartmann's procedure (Hinchey III and IV). (2) Large *pr* bleed requires a segmental resection if bleeding identified on angiogram, or a subtotal colectomy if not, as bleeding often right-sided. (3) Fistula: resection of diseased segment and repair of contiguous organ. Presently there is discussion about the indications for surgery in uncomplicated disease, and the guidelines are likely to be changed to a more conservative strategy. Below is a suggested algorithm.

Prognosis: the risk of recurrent symptoms following an episode of diverticulitis is 7 to 45 %. Mortality rate: 0 to 2 %, and 12–36 % for emergency operation. 27–33 % of patients have ongoing symptoms after elective bowel resection.

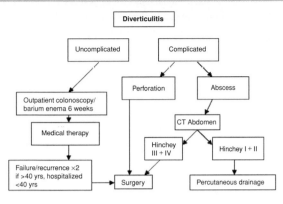

■ Complications of colonic diverticular disease

1. **Pain:** usually left iliac fossa pain as sigmoid diverticulae are the commonest, but may depend on the location of the diverticulae and may even present as for appendicitis. NB right-sided diverticulae are commoner in patients from the Far East.
2. **Bleeding:** commonly painless pr bleeding. But may also present during an attack of diverticulitis. Majority of cases are treated conservatively and resolve spontaneously and are followed up in outpatients with endoscopic evaluation; however if the patient is compromised a diagnostic/therapeutic angiogram may be indicated and followed with surgery if appropriate (see section on lower GI bleed)(Figure 93).
3. **Infection** i.e. diverticulitis: pain, fever, sepsis etc.
4. **Change in bowel habit:** intermittent diarrhoea and/or constipation. Must be evaluated with a colonoscopy or CT colonography if colon not evaluated recently, to rule out a neoplastic cause.
5. **Strictures:** inflammatory strictures may cause acute or chronic large-bowel obstruction.
6. **Perforation:** presentation as an acute abdomen. If just localized may be treated conservatively with iv antibiotics and radiologically guided percutaneous drainage. If peritonitic or systemically unwell, usually necessitates surgery: classically a Hartmann's resection for a

perforated sigmoid diverticulum; however, ideally a primary anastomosis should be considered if performed in a colorectal centre and contamination is not gross.

7. **Fistulation:**
   a. Colovesical – with the bladder
   b. Colovaginal – with the vagina (usually PMH of TAH)
   c. Colocutaneous – with the skin
   d. Colouterine – with the uterus
   e. Coloenteric – with the small bowel
   f. Colocolic – with another segment of colon.

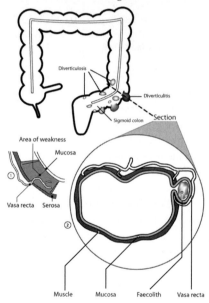

Figure 93

Fistulae should be treated as follows (SNAP):

Sepsis treated (S)

Adequate nutrition of the patient (N)

Delineate the anatomy of the fistula (A)

Carry out the relevant surgical/other procedure (P) to remove the track.

Perianal: haemorrhoids

HENRY TILLNEY AND ALEXANDER G. HERIOT

■ Introduction

Common condition resulting from engorgement of submucosal vascular beds around the anal canal. Likely to result from western diets with high fat/low fibre leading to excessive straining.

■ Definition and classification

Most commonly seen in the 3, 7 and 11 o'clock positions (with the patient in the lithotomy position). Graded into four 'degrees' (see table).

Classification of haemorrhoids	
First degree	No descent below dentate line on straining
Second degree	Prolapse on straining but reduce spontaneously
Third degree	Prolapse on straining and require manual reduction
Fourth degree	Permanently beyond dentate line, prolapsing spontaneously after reduction

■ Incidence

Estimates vary, 4.4–80 %. F > M. Prevalence increases with age to the seventh decade, when it falls. Pregnancy may predispose.

■ Aetiology

Unknown. Thought to be related to constipation/straining at stool, associated with high anal canal and intra-abdominal pressures.

Hospital Surgery: Foundations in Surgical Practice, ed. Omer Aziz, Sanjay Purkayastha and Paraskevas Paraskeva. Published by Cambridge University Press. © Cambridge University Press 2009.

■ Pathogenesis

Internal haemorrhoids derive from the superior haemorrhoidal plexus. Straining causes engorgement of the vascular cushions. Prolapse occurs as smooth muscle and connective tissue supporting the mucosa is disrupted (Figure 94).

■ Symptoms and signs

Rectal bleeding: painless/bright red. Blood mixed with stool suggests a more proximal source of bleeding.

Prolapse: sensation of a mass descending. May cause mild faecal incontinence.

Other: mucoid discharge, pruritus ani.

Not painful unless strangulated or thrombosed.

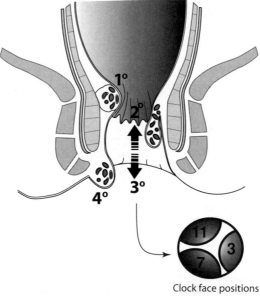

Clock face positions
of anal cushions

Figure 94

■ Investigation

History: exclude colorectal cancer (family history, change in bowel habit, blood mixed with stool).

Examination: careful digital rectal examination, rigid sigmoidoscopy and proctoscopy (confirm presence of haemorrhoids/exclude other lesions).

In atypical history/unfruitful examination, flexible endoscopy to exclude a more proximal source of bleeding is required.

■ Treatment

Over 90 % can be treated conservatively. Repeated use of 'outpatient' techniques often necessary:

1. High-fibre diet, fibre supplements, laxatives.
2. Topical hydrocortisone-based ointments.
3. Injection sclerotherapy: injection of 5 % phenol in almond oil into the submucosal space. Effective for smaller piles where prolapse is not a particular problem (see Figure 94).
4. Rubber band ligation (RBL): effective in second/third degree piles. The application of the band causes necrosis of a small area of mucosa, with the creation of an ulcer. The resulting scarring shrinks the haemorrhoid and acts to fix it back within the anal canal.
5. Infrared coagulation, laser (neodymium: YAG and CO_2).

■ Surgical options

1. Excisional haemorrhoidectomy: removal of haemorrhoids/associated skin tags. Advised for haemorrhoids non-responsive to conservative management or where prolapse is a particular problem. Techniques include 'open' (Milligan-Morgan) or 'closed' (Ferguson) or with the use of a vessel-sealing device e.g. Ligasure. Complications include bleeding, pain and sphincter damage, unhealed wound/infection.

2. Stapled haemorrhoidectomy (procedure for prolapsed haemorrhoids – PPH): anopexy with complete ring of distal rectal mucosa excised by surgical stapler, causing repositioning and fixation of haemorrhoidal tissue in anal canal.

■ Emergency presentation

Prolapse/strangulation/gangrenous.
Thrombosed.

Management: (ice, normal compression), analgesia, laxatives. Selective emergency haemorrhoidectomy if gangrenous (very rarely indicated).

Perianal: anorectal abscesses and fistula in ano

HENRY TILLNEY AND ALEXANDER G. HERIOT

■ Introduction

Anorectal abscesses and fistulae often occur together, commonly due to infection of anal glands, but can be markers of other diseases. 5 % of patients with Crohn's disease present with a perianal abscess.

■ Definition and classification

Anorectal abscess: abnormal collection of purulent material surrounded by a pyogenic membrane and granulation tissue. These may be classified by site (see Figure 95) as *intersphincteric, perianal, supralevator (pelvirectal)* and *ischiorectal*. A *horseshoe abscess* occurs if the infectious process spreads circumferentially from a space on one side to the other.

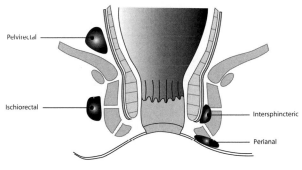

Figure 95

Hospital Surgery: Foundations in Surgical Practice, ed. Omer Aziz, Sanjay Purkayastha and Paraskevas Paraskeva. Published by Cambridge University Press. © Cambridge University Press 2009.

439

Fistula in ano: abnormal connection between two epithelialized surfaces, lined by granulation tissue. Parks' classification (see Figure 96) describes four main anatomic types named according to their relation to the external sphincter: *intersphincteric* (Type 1), *transsphincteric* (Type 2), *suprasphincteric* (Type 3) and *extrasphincteric* (Type 4).

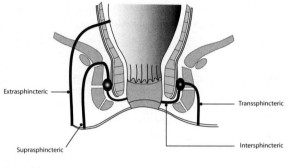

Extrasphincteric

Transsphincteric

Suprasphincteric

Intersphincteric

Figure 96

■ Incidence

Any age, increased in young adults, peak in third to fifth decades. M:F ratio 2:1.

■ Aetiology

90 % of abscesses are due to infected anal glands (*cryptoglandular theory*). Fistulae are thought to originate from the anal canal glands at the dentate line. The path of the infection determines the type of fistula produced. Associations include Crohn's disease, diabetes, neoplasia and irradiation. Prior anal surgery is also a predisposing factor.

■ Pathogenesis

Infections commonly occur in the intersphincteric plane and can extend up, down or circumferentially around the anus. If an abscess bursts both externally and within the anal canal then a fistula track is formed.

■ Symptoms and signs

Anorectal abscess: perianal pain, erythema, tenderness to palpation, systematic disturbance, fever and swelling.

Fistula in ano: persistent discharge, rectal bleeding, perianal pain, recurrent abscesses and episodes of perianal sepsis. External opening of fistula may be visible in perineum, and internal palpable on rectal examination.

■ Investigation

Examination under anaesthesia (EUA): rectal examination, proctoscopy and rigid sigmoidoscopy as well as exploration or probing of fistulous tracks. Dye or hydrogen peroxide can help to identify internal fistula openings.

■ Imaging

Endo-anal ultrasound (EAUS): sensitivity can be improved by injecting hydrogen peroxide into the external opening.

MRI: high levels of accuracy for the presence and course of abscesses and fistula tracks have been shown by MRI, which has also been shown to identify pathology missed even at surgery.

■ Treatment

Perianal abscess: incision and drainage with sufficiently wide opening to prevent healing over of the skin before the cavity has filled with granulation tissue. A *cruciate incision* is usually made and the wound probed for loculations. Avoid excessive probing due to risk of creating a fistula. Wound edges are kept open by excising the corners of the cruciate and packing the cavity.

Fistula in ano: treatment of all fistulae is based around drainage of primary infection, with identification of primary and secondary tracks.

Secondary tracks and abscess cavities are laid open. The primary fistula track is managed according to the amount of sphincter muscle caudal to the fistula (incontinence risk):

1. **Low/superficial fistulae:** involving small quantities of sphincter muscle can be definitively treated by laying open with primary fistulotomy as they carry low incontinence risk.

2. **High fistulae:** Drainage of the fistula is established with a 'drainage seton' as opposed to primary fistulotomy. This usually consists of a loosely placed braided non-absorbable suture. Secondary treatment can include a 'cutting seton' consisting of a tighter monofilament nylon suture.

3. **Complex, deep, or recurrent fistulae:** May be treated with fibrin glue, advancement flap, or in severe cases temporary colostomy.

In the management of fistula in ano, it is important to remember *Goodsall's rule* (see Figure 97), which predicts that if a line is drawn transversely across the anus, an external opening anterior to this line will have a straight radial tract, while an external opening lying posterior to this line will have a curved tract and an internal opening in the posterior midline of the anal canal. The exception to this rule is long anterior fistulae lying more than 3 cm from the anus.

Note: Also consider postoperative course of antibiotics, laxatives and GTN/Diltiazem ointments.

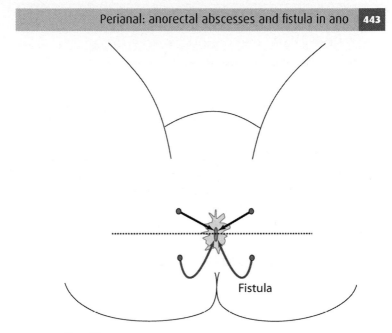

Figure 97

Perianal: pilonidal sinus and hidradenitis suppurativa

HENRY TILLNEY AND ALEXANDER G. HERIOT

■ Pilonidal sinus

INTRODUCTION

In the second World War 70 000 US servicemen were admitted to hospital due to pilonidal sinuses, staying on average 55 days. An observation of the frequency with which the condition occurred in those spending much of their time driving led to it being called 'Jeep disease'.

DEFINITION AND CLASSIFICATION

'Nest of hairs' from the Latin: pilum (hair) nidus (nest). In the natal cleft midline pits are seen, with laterally draining sinuses (see Figure 98).

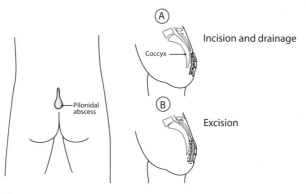

Figure 98

Hospital Surgery: Foundations in Surgical Practice, ed. Omer Aziz, Sanjay Purkayastha and Paraskevas Paraskeva. Published by Cambridge University Press. © Cambridge University Press 2009.

INCIDENCE

1 % in males and 0.1 % in females, but proportionately more females undergo surgery (M:F 4:1). Rare before puberty or after age 40. Incidence is highest in Caucasians and least in Africans and Asians. As an observation, pilonidal sinuses often occur in more hirsute populations.

PATHOGENESIS

Congenital: 'pit theory' (discredited).

Acquired: infection in a natal cleft hair follicle extends into the subcutaneous fat, forming an abscess which drains laterally. Follicle persists as a remnant in the midline which communicates with the abscess through which loose natal cleft hairs are forced, collecting inside.

Squamous carcinoma has been reported in long-standing pilonidal sinuses but the incidence is extremely low.

SYMPTOMS AND SIGNS

Acute: 50 % present first with an acute pilonidal abscess.

Chronic: sinus in the natal cleft with, or without, a prior history of an abscess. Symptoms: pain and/or discharge of pus from a midline or lateral pit.

Examination: single/multiple midline pits in natal cleft. Local tenderness/discharge.

INVESTIGATION

Exclude diabetes. Consider spinal abnormalities in atypical presentations.

TREATMENT AND PROGNOSIS

Asymptomatic pits: no acute management is required although elective excision is recommended. Advise hair removal.

Acute abscess: drain with laterally placed incisions.

Chronic sinus: although conservative management with shaving of natal cleft, extraction of hairs, brushing of the pits and injection of phenol has been described, results are poor. Surgical treatment is the mainstay and consists of:

- *Midline incision with curettage of sinus and packing:* requires daily dressing and has long healing time as wound heals by secondary intention.

- *Excision of sinus with primary closure:* has a high rate of wound breakdown.

- *Lateral incision with excision of sinus cavity (Bascom/Karydakis repair)*: The incision is usually to the left of the midline, to improve healing rates.

- *Plastics procedures (Limberg flap):* may be used for complex disease/unhealed wounds. For example Z-plasties and rotational flaps.

Patients should be advised that all techniques involving primary closure heal quicker but have a higher risk of recurrence.

■ Hidradenitis suppurativa

INTRODUCTION

This is a chronic, indolent, relapsing, suppurative disease occurring in apocrine follicles. It can result in subcutaneous induration, sinus, and fistula formation. Affects skin bearing apocrine glands, most commonly the axilla, groin and perineum.

INCIDENCE

Most common in the third decade of life. Prevalence in industrialized countries 0.3–4 %. More common in white and black populations and is rarely observed in Asians.

PATHOGENESIS

Keratin comedones → Occlusion of the apocrine ducts → Superimposed inflammation and infection → Abscess formation → Chronic infection and spread → Induration and sinus and fistula formation.

SYMPTOMS AND SIGNS

Initial presentation involves solitary, painful nodules that persist for weeks or months. Subcutaneous extension results in indurated plaques, seen as linear bands in the axilla and groin. Bilateral and multiple site involvement are common. Eventually pustules form and rupture, exuding purulent material. Subsequent healing and fibrosis occur and the process begins again. Chronic sinuses ultimately form and discharge serous, purulent, or bloodstained fluid intermittently.

INVESTIGATION

Exclude diabetes. Microbiology and culture may guide antibiotic treatment. Often shows coagulase-negative staphylococci, *E. coli, Streptococcus milleri*, and the anaerobic *Bacteroides* species. CT scanning may be used to plan surgery in extensive cases.

TREATMENT

Acute disease
- Lifestyle changes – weight loss and good hygiene.
- Antibiotics – two week course of erythromycin and metronidazole, minocycline, or clindamycin.
- Steroids – intralesional injection of early nodules with 5–10 mg triamcinolone diluted with water.

Chronic disease

- Long-term erythromycin and tetracycline to treat chronic infection.
- Steroids may reduce inflammation.
- Retinoids have been shown to be effective but are teratogenic.
- Surgery – may involve incision and drainage, block dissection, or total wide excision and healing with secondary intention or flaps and grafts.

Perianal: anal fissure

HENRY TILLNEY AND ALEXANDER G. HERIOT

■ Introduction

Anal fissures are painful linear tears or ulcers found in the lower anal canal, usually in the posterior midline.

■ Definition and classification

Longitudinal tears occur in the anoderm between the dentate line and anal verge (Figure 99). They may be acute or chronic (>1 month). 80 % are in the posterior midline (six o'clock with the patient in the lithotomy position) and 20 % are anterior (more common in women). In 5 % both anterior and posterior fissures co-exist. Anal fissures that are away from the midline should prompt suspicion of unusual pathology.

■ Incidence

M.F = 1:1, more common in young adults. Occasionally occur in children and rare in the elderly.

■ Aetiology

Primary fissures result from shearing forces on the anoderm, often associated with the passage of hard stool. *Secondary fissures* may be caused by malignancy, inflammatory bowel disease, venereal infection, trauma, tuberculosis and chemotherapy.

Hospital Surgery: Foundations in Surgical Practice, ed. Omer Aziz, Sanjay Purkayastha and Paraskevas Paraskeva. Published by Cambridge University Press. © Cambridge University Press 2009.

■ Pathogenesis

Pain results in spasm of the internal sphincter, reducing blood flow to the anoderm, inhibiting healing. A vicious circle of painful defaecation, constipation, hard stool, and exacerbation of fissure ensues.

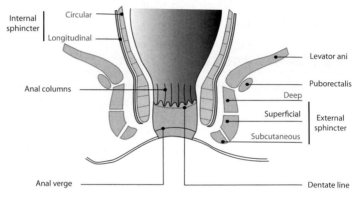

Internal sphincter — Circular

Longitudinal

Anal columns

Anal verge

Levator ani

Puborectalis

Deep

Superficial — External sphincter

Subcutaneous

Dentate line

Figure 99

■ Symptoms and signs

Pain on defaecation and for up to two hours after, which is often burning in nature.

Bright red rectal bleeding often on the toilet paper.

■ Examination

Should consist of digital rectal examination. Proctoscopy and rigid sigmoidoscopy are required but may not be possible at presentation because of severe pain. In this case, treatment should be initiated and patient re-examined at four to six weeks. Failure to improve warrants formal examination under general anaesthesia. On proctoscopy the fissure can be seen as a tear or narrow ulcer most often at six o'clock with the patient in the lithotomy position. The fissure may be associated with an external tag or '*sentinel pile*' distal to it. Exposed internal sphincter fibres imply chronicity.

■ Investigation

Diagnosis is clinical, with empirical treatment initiated even if the fissure is not visualized. *Atypical features* or a *failure to heal* warrant examination under anaesthesia, proctoscopy and biopsy of the fissure edge, and rigid sigmoidoscopy.

■ Treatment

- *Dietary and lifestyle advice* to maintain a high-fibre diet with soft stools. Spicy foods may aggravate the fissure.
- *Faecal softeners* and bulk laxatives may be used.
- *Topical treatments:* 0.2–0.4 % glyceryl trinitrate (GTN) or 2 % diltiazem ointment (side effects include headaches) to relax the sphincter. 40 % heal using topical treatments.
- *Botulinum toxin* can be injected into the sphincter to perform a 'chemical sphincterotomy', the effect of which lasts approximately three months.
- *Surgery* is reserved for patients who fail medical therapy. This involves a *limited lateral internal anal sphincterotomy* with a controlled division of the muscle to the height of the proximal extent of the fissure created (Figure 100). This results in a healing rate of up to 95 %. The practice of anal stretching (*Lord procedure*) for the management of anal fissures is discredited due to the potential for uncontrolled damage to the internal sphincter. *Anorectal advancement flap procedures* may be used to manage resistant fissure.

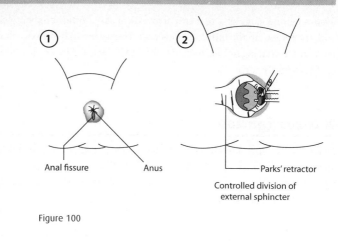

Figure 100

■ Prognosis

Up to 95 % of anal fissures heal with the management described. Consider other diagnoses if non-healing fissure is present, including Crohn's disease, anal carcinoma and tuberculosis.

Chronic limb ischaemia

RAVUL JINDAL AND MICHAEL JENKINS

■ Definition

Chronic limb ischaemia occurs as a result of slow and progressive occlusion of large arteries, mainly due to atherosclerosis. Upper and lower-limb blood supplies are shown in the Figures 101 and 102.

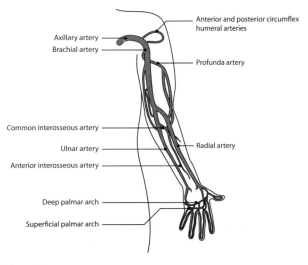

Figure 101

Hospital Surgery: Foundations in Surgical Practice, ed. Omer Aziz, Sanjay Purkayastha and Paraskevas Paraskeva. Published by Cambridge University Press. © Cambridge University Press 2009.

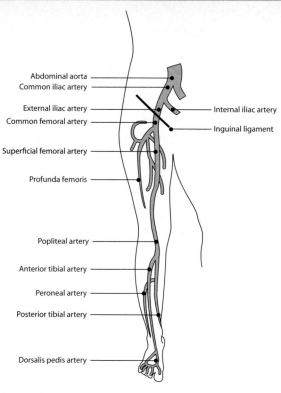

Abdominal aorta	
Common iliac artery	
External iliac artery	Internal iliac artery
Common femoral artery	Inguinal ligament
Superficial femoral artery	
Profunda femoris	
Popliteal artery	
Anterior tibial artery	
Peroneal artery	
Posterior tibial artery	
Dorsalis pedis artery	

Figure 102

■ Incidence

The incidence of peripheral artery disease is 17 % between the ages of 55 and 70 years. Without treatment, 10–15 % of the patients with intermittent claudication improve over 5 years, and 60–70 % do not progress over the same period. The 10–15 % with worsening symptoms can be treated with intervention. The overall survival for patients with intermittent claudication is only 72 % at 5 years and 50 % at 10 years; this is mainly due to coronary artery disease.

■ Aetiology

Atherosclerosis is the most frequent cause of occlusive disease of the major branches of the aorta. Although its aetiology remains unclear, its incidence and progression are clearly accelerated by the presence of diabetes mellitus, hypertension, hyperlipidaemia and smoking.

Another cause is thromboangiitis obliterans or Buerger's disease, which usually affects young male smokers. It is a chronic inflammatory process that involves the entire neurovascular bundle and is also associated with venous thrombosis. It usually involves distal vessels of the hand and feet and therefore surgical reconstruction is usually difficult.

Vasculitis involves the small arteries and arterioles, and treatment depends on recognition and treatment of the underlying disease process. Trauma is usually associated with acute ischaemia but rarely it is missed during the first presentation and can present later with chronic ischaemia.

Cystic adventitial disease and popliteal entrapment syndrome are rare causes affecting young healthy patients and surgical treatment is associated with good outcome.

■ Pathogenesis

Atherosclerosis is a disease affecting the intima and involves inner media. It is a generalized disease but with a segmental distribution mainly at arterial bifurcations and in areas of posterior fixation and acute angulations. Plaque is a deposit of fatty material on the inner lining of an arterial wall and is a characteristic of atherosclerosis.

■ Symptoms

Patients present with claudication, a term applied to cramp-like pain felt in muscle groups when blood flow becomes inadequate to meet the metabolic requirements during exercise. Pain is reproducible on walking for the same distance and is relieved by rest. Claudication in the buttock and thigh usually indicates proximal aortoiliac disease and calf pain signifies superficial femoral artery disease. When the blood flow is so poor that it is not able to meet the metabolic requirements at rest, continuous pain is felt in the foot and toes, called 'rest pain'. Rest pain is characterized by an unremitting burning pain at night, which is relieved by hanging the legs over the side of the bed to allow gravity to aid flow. It signifies critical limb ischaemia and the involved limb may subsequently develop gangrene and tissue loss.

■ Signs

Physical signs include absent pulses below the occlusion and a thrill or bruit at the site of a stenosis. Pallor of the skin especially with elevation of the leg, and rubor on dependency (Buerger's sign) is due to cutaneous reactive vasodilation in response to chronic ischaemia and usually signifies severe foot ischaemia. Signs of chronic ischaemia are also evident on epidermal structures in the form of thin shiny skin, loss of hair and brittle nails and punched-out ulcers on the foot.

Measurement of ankle brachial pressure index (ABPI) gives an objective evidence of limb ischaemia. This is the measure of systolic pressure at the ankle (dorsalis pedis/posterior tibial arteries) divided by brachial pressure, to give a ratio or index. A normal ABPI is around 1.0, falling to 0.7 in claudication and <0.5 in critical ischaemia. Note that the ABPI may be >1 or falsely raised in diabetics due to vessel calcification.

■ Investigations

Routine blood investigations are performed to check for FBC (anaemia, infection), CRP, ESR (arteritis), electrolytes, renal function, lipid levels, clotting and group and save if planning for further investigations or treatment. Non-invasive investigations (duplex scans and MRA (magnetic resonance angiography)) are improving rapidly, but at present most surgeons rely on angiography to look at vessels below the knee prior to reconstruction. Care must be taken with all contrast investigations in patients with impaired renal function.

■ Treatment

INDICATIONS

Indications for treatment include patients with disabling or life-style limiting claudication, rest pain, ulceration or gangrene.

CONSERVATIVE

More than 75 % of the patients with intermittent claudication remain stable or even improve without intervention. All patients should stop smoking, require control of hypertension and blood sugar, statin and antiplatelet treatment. Supervised exercise has been shown to be equivalent to angioplasty in some studies.

ENDOLUMINAL

Percutaneous transluminal (PTA) or subintimal angioplasty has gained widespread acceptance for the treatment of the occlusive peripheral arterial disease in selected groups. PTA is usually more successful in short lesions <10 cm and the results in long occlusion and multiple long stenoses are limited.

It has advantages of reduced cost, morbidity, good initial success rates and ease of reapplication but with lower long-term patency rates as compared with surgery. The patency rate varies depending on site of PTA (aortic 93–100 %, iliac 65–75 %, femoropopliteal 50–60 % at four years, tibioperoneal around 60 % at one year).

Complication rates vary from 5 to 10 % with a mortality rate of 0.2 % (mainly due to myocardial infarction or vessel rupture). Acute thrombosis and distal embolization resulting in limb loss occur in 0.2 % of cases.

PTA can cause acute limb ischaemia requiring urgent surgery in around 2 % of cases.

SURGERY

Reconstruction: surgical options include endarterectomy or surgical bypass. Autogenous vein is the preferred vascular conduit for bypass as the patency rates are superior to the prosthetic conduits available. Long saphenous vein is preferred and can be used either *in situ* with destruction of vein valves, or reversed. If there is no good quality vein then prosthetic (PTFE or Dacron) can be used and a vein boot at the lower end improves the patency of the graft. Vein bypass has an up to 90 % one-year and 75 % 5-year patency rate for the femoropopliteal segment, but the patency rate deteriorates for distal bypass to crural vessels.

Amputation: this is mandatory for non-viable tissue. It is also used in the face of intractable pain without a reconstructive option.

Abdominal aortic aneurysms

RAVUL JINDAL AND MICHAEL JENKINS

■ Introduction

Prevalence of abdominal aortic aneurysm (AAA) is 3% in those
>50 years. The frequency increases steadily in men >55 yrs, reaching
a peak of 5.9% at 80–85 yrs. In women, the peak is 4.5% at age > 90
years. Male: female ratio is 4:1. Abdominal aortic aneurysms are 3–7
times more common than thoracic aneurysms. Other aneurysms co-
existing with abdominal are iliac (20–30%) and femoropopliteal (15%).
Popliteal aneurysms are a marker of AAA. AAAs are present in 8% of
patients with unilateral and in 50% with bilateral popliteal aneurysms.
Cigarette smoking is associated with an increased incidence of AAA, 8:1
as compared with non-smokers. Popliteal aneurysms are the most common peripheral arterial aneurysms. Atherosclerotic in 95%, M:F 30:1,
sixth to seventh decade, bilateral in 50%. Rare causes are entrapment
syndrome or trauma.

■ Definition

An aneurysm is a permanent localized dilation of an artery with an
increase in diameter of greater than 50% (1.5 times) its normal diameter. Ectasia refers to dilation of an artery that does not reach the above
threshold.

■ Classification

True (contains all components of the arterial wall – intima, media
and adventitia) or *false* (only adventitia). *Congenital* or *acquired*
(atherosclerosis, trauma, infection, or medial cystic necrosis). *Saccular*

Hospital Surgery: Foundations in Surgical Practice, ed. Omer Aziz, Sanjay
Purkayastha and Paraskevas Paraskeva. Published by Cambridge University Press.
© Cambridge University Press 2009.

(arising from one part of the arterial wall) or *fusiform* (generalized dilation of the arterial wall) (Figures 103 and 104). The aneurysms can also be divided into: aneurysms of the aortoiliac area, peripheral aneurysms and splanchnic aneurysms. They may present electively or in an emergency.

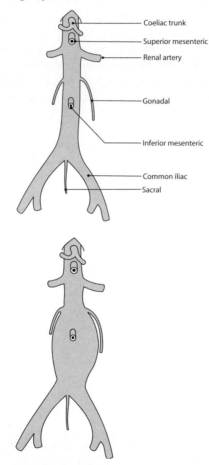

Coeliac trunk

Superior mesenteric

Renal artery

Gonadal

Inferior mesenteric

Common iliac

Sacral

Figure 103 Fusiform aneurysm

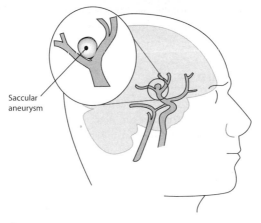

Saccular
aneurysm

Figure 104 Berry aneurysm

■ Aetiology

The current evidence suggests that atherosclerosis (and particularly hypertension) is the major aetiological factor for aneurysm formation. Other uncommon causes are cystic medial necrosis, dissection, infection (mycotic) and connective-tissue disorders (Ehlers-Danlos and Marfan's syndrome). Only about 25 % are associated with occlusive disease. There appears to be genetic susceptibility to aortic aneurysm formation. Around 20–30 % have a first-degree relative with the same condition.

■ Symptoms and signs

Approximately 70–75 % of infrarenal AAAs are asymptomatic when first detected. Tender aneurysms make up around 13 % of cases. Physical examination alone can miss 33 % of AAAs. Abdominal aortic aneurysm can rupture, occlude, throw off emboli and rarely compress surrounding structures (duodenum, inferior venae cava, ureter or nerves). Popliteal artery aneurysms are usually asymptomatic or present with distal embolization, occlude, rupture (rare 5 %), or with local compressive symptoms–venous obstruction or nerve involvement resulting in pain.

■ Investigations

Plain abdominal or lateral spine radiograph may reveal an aneurysm if the wall is calcified. CT or US can detect aneurysms and are useful in depicting size, relation to surrounding structures and in showing anomalies. MRI can also be used as it avoids radiation exposure. Angiogram may not show the presence of an aneurysm as it only shows the lumen which may be of normal calibre regardless of the aneurysm size.

■ Risk of rupture

Large aneurysms expand faster compared to smaller ones. Size of the aneurysm is the most important risk factor for rupture. *The yearly risk of rupture for AAA is < 1 % for 4–5.4 cm, 5 % for 5.5–5.9 cm, 10 % for 6 cm and around 20 % for 7 cm aneurysms.* Average rate of aneurysmal enlargement is 0.5 cm/year (see Leaking AAA Chapter).

■ Indications for aneurysm repair

Size is the main indication for repair. Evidence would suggest this is >5.5 cm for AAA and >2–2.5 cm for femoropopliteal. Mycotic and saccular aneurysms are dangerous regardless of size. Ruptured aneurysms require emergency repair to prevent imminent death (see Leaking AAA Chapter).

■ Treatment

Operative mortality in elective patients varies from 1 to 5 % for repair of infrarenal AAAs. Age > 80 years and renal failure carry a worse prognosis. Mainstay of the treatment remains open surgery, but this is changing.

The aorta may be approached intraperitoneally or retroperitoneally and replaced with a Dacron (or PTFE) tube or bifurcated graft depending on iliac involvement.

Endovascular repair (EVAR) involves inserting a covered stent graft from the femoral arteries and deploying it just distal to the renal arteries. An adequate proximal neck and iliac 'landing zone' is necessary and about 40–60 % of AAAs are suitable with current technology.

Published trials suggest the perioperative risk is less than the open surgery (1.7 vs. 4.7 % mortality), but the long-term durability is unclear. Patients require long-term follow-up imaging to identify potential complications: endoleak (blood leak back into the sac), continued sac expansion or graft failure (migration or stent fracture). EVAR is therefore currently reserved for older or high-risk patients.

■ Complications of surgery

Mortality (elective repair AAA 1–5 %, ruptured AAA 70–90 %), myocardial infarction (fatal 4 %, non-fatal 16 %), haemorrhage, renal failure, bowel or ureteric injury, colonic ischaemia, paraplegia, lower-limb ischaemia or trash foot, graft infection and aortoduodenal fistula.

■ Prognosis

About 50 % of patients with a ruptured aneurysm die before reaching hospital. Another 25 % arrive at the hospital alive but die before an operation can be performed. Only 10 % of the patients with free intraperitoneal rupture survive, but up to 80 % of patients survive if a small-contained leak is present.

Diabetic foot

RAVUL JINDAL AND MICHAEL JENKINS

■ Introduction

About 27 % of people > 55 yrs of age have peripheral arterial disease (PAD). Diabetics are 2–4 times more likely to have PAD. Around 15 % develop PAD after 10 years of diabetes and 45 % after 20 years. Diabetic foot accounts for the highest number of non-traumatic lower extremity amputations.

■ Definition

A neuroischaemic condition leading to soft tissue loss +/– infection over pressure-bearing areas.

■ Incidence

84 % of patients with a 20-year history of diabetes have vascular disease and 75 % die of vascular disease or its complications; primarily IHD and stroke. Gangrene occurs 50 times more commonly in diabetic males and 70 times more commonly in female diabetic patients as compared with non-diabetic patients.

■ Pathogenesis

Arterial occlusive disease in diabetics is a different pattern compared with atherosclerosis in non-diabetics. It mainly affects the distal popliteal segment, the tibial and metatarsal vessels with sparing of inflow and peroneal artery. Microscopically: thickening of the intima, increased thickness of the basement membrane, patchy distribution – diabetic microangiopathy.

Hospital Surgery: Foundations in Surgical Practice, ed. Omer Aziz, Sanjay Purkayastha and Paraskevas Paraskeva. Published by Cambridge University Press. © Cambridge University Press 2009.

Neuropathy: segmental demyelination of both sensory and motor nerves (defect in metabolism of Schwann cells) causing delayed nerve conduction. Distal nerves are affected more than proximal. Initial night cramps and paraesthesia progress to loss of vibratory sense and perception of light touch and pain and finally deep tendon reflexes are lost.

Motor dysfunction results in malfunction of the intrinsic muscles of the foot leading to distortion of foot architecture. It consists of extensor subluxation of the toes, plantar prominences of metatarsal heads and imbalance in action of flexors and extensors. The metatarsal arch then collapses. In its extreme form, the mid foot deteriorates leading to the so-called *Charcot's foot.*

Infection: As a result of neuropathy, minor soft-tissue injuries are common. Infection spreads faster because of impaired defence function, reduced blood supply and neuropathy. Usually polymicrobial and therefore a synergistic effect. Both gram positive and negative and aerobic and anaerobic pathogens are involved.

Osteomyelitis: may be present in absence of severe clinical signs of sepsis. The signs of osteomyelitis can be confused with Charcot's joint which has signs of chronic inflammation.

■ Symptoms

Neuropathic symptoms (numbness, tingling and burning, often worse at night) and ischaemic symptoms (rest pain, gangrene or foot ulceration).

■ Signs

Examine for neuropathy (decreased sensation in stocking distribution (especially vibration), monofilament test, and postural hypotension). Muscle atrophy along with varied signs of joint abnormalities. Examine arterial system (absent pulses). Thickened nails (slow growth at the nailbed), loss of hair growth and chronic fungal infections. Other signs of ischaemia noted are decreased capillary refill, dependent rubor (chronic vasodilation) and elevation pallor.

Doppler pressure measurements – may be falsely elevated due to non-compression of calcified vessels (ABPI may be >1). All signs are more marked in IDDM patients. Toe vessels are not affected therefore toe pressures are more reliable. If toe pressures are <30 mmHg, the chance of a local amputation healing is poor.

On the foot itself, a wide spectrum of clinical signs may be present. Cellulites, blisters (infection up to dermis), sinus (chronic deep infection with discharging fluid to the skin), chronic sub-clinical osteomyelitis, gangrene – dry or wet (infected).

Ulcer examination: neuropathic ulcers are punched out, painless in an area of callous with signs of superadded infection; involved areas are pressure sites such as sole of foot at head of metatarsal. Arterial ulcers affect the dorsal foot or the toes distally; necrotic ulcers usually painful (unless associated with neuropathy).

Bony examination may show bony deformity as outlined above.

■ Investigation

Bloods (glucose, anaemia, high white cell count and CRP); blood cultures, wound swabs, foot X-ray shows gas in soft tissues or osteomyelitis (osteopaenia focally and destruction of cortical or medullary bone). MRI shows low signal intensity on T1-weighted images and high signal intensity on T2-weighted images. Angiography is mandatory prior to arterial reconstruction.

Microbiology is crucial to plan treatment and the ideal specimen for culture is aspirated pus or necrotic tissue. Bone is difficult to culture, as organisms lie deep in the cancellous bone. Both aerobic and anaerobic cultures should be used.

■ Treatment

Antibiotics to cover polymicrobial flora including anaerobes. First line of drugs should be started (augmentin and flucloxacillin) and change antibiotics according to the swab results.

Surgery is indicated for infection (debridement or amputation), severe ischaemia in the form of gangrene or rest pain (revascularization – radiological or arterial bypass surgery). Important principles include saving as much of the foot as possible, revascularize if indicated before amputation, infection control, leave wound open if residual infection or any doubt of flap viability with delayed skin grafts or secondary healing for open wounds.

During an amputation the cartilagenous surface of the metatarsal head should be removed as it is avascular. When the hallux is amputated the sesamoid bones should be removed as they may also be infected. If pus is present in the plantar surface a longitudinal incision along the midline of the foot can drain the infection and save the functional status of the foot. If infection is around the malleolus level the foot is rarely salvageable.

■ Prevention

Education for patient to examine their feet regularly (often compounded by poor eyesight). Appropriate comfortable, well fitting shoes (with weight-distributing cradles) are essential and barefoot walking should be avoided. Regular chiropody to take care of foot lesions.

■ Prognosis

Aggressive and early surgical care offers the best chance of avoiding major amputation. Patients with critical limb ischaemia have a high mortality rate (40 % die within two years) and morbidity. Use of newer anti-diabetic agents (e.g. glitazones), islet cell transplantation, tissue-engineered skin for foot ulcers and angiogenic growth factors (medical bypass) in patients with unreconstructible vascular disease.

Carotid disease

RAVUL JINDAL AND MICHAEL JENKINS

■ Introduction

The earliest link reported between carotid disease and stroke was credited to Savory in 1856. In 1954 Eastcott reported the first carotid artery reconstruction to prevent stroke at St. Mary's Hospital in London. Main diseases affecting carotid artery are occlusive, dissection, aneurysms, trauma and inflammatory.

■ Definition

There are three clinical presentations of carotid occlusive disease.

1. Asymptomatic: patients with no history of cerebral symptoms
2. Transient ischaemic attacks (TIA): temporary neurological deficits <24 hours with complete recovery. Crescendo TIA suggests repeated frequent embolization with complete recovery in between. The average reported rate of risk of stroke ranges from 5 % within the first 2 days and 20 % within the first month to 10.5 % within 90 days. The benefit from intervention is greatest for patients undergoing surgery within two weeks of their last ischaemic event.
3. Stroke: permanent neurological deficit – defect ranging from minimal with good recovery to massive causing death.

■ Pathogenesis

Up to 30 % of cerebral events are caused by embolization from atherosclerotic lesions at the carotid bifurcation, or low-flow related

Hospital Surgery: Foundations in Surgical Practice, ed. Omer Aziz, Sanjay Purkayastha and Paraskevas Paraskeva. Published by Cambridge University Press. © Cambridge University Press 2009.

ischaemic events. Other causes include embolization from the aortic arch, intracerebral bleeds and tumours.

■ Symptoms and signs

Presentation is usually in the form of discrete motor or sensory dysfunction contralateral to the side of the ischaemic event. Since the left hemisphere is dominant in 95 % of the population, an ischaemic event affecting the left hemisphere may also cause receptive or expressive aphasia. It can also present as transient visual loss (*amaurosis fugax*) in the ipsilateral eye. Patients typically describe a curtain drawn over the eye, or field defect.

A bruit suggests turbulent flow at the carotid bifurcation but this is unreliable in estimating the presence or degree of stenosis.

■ Investigations

Initial evaluation is by duplex scanning to assess the stenosis of the internal carotid artery and also to assess the nature of the plaque. CT scan of the brain will reveal the presence and size of infarcts and exclude other intracranial pathologies. MRI of the brain is more sensitive in identifying infarctions earlier than CT. Imaging of the arch and extracranial carotid tree is only necessary to plan for the placement of a carotid stent.

Carotid angiography is rarely indicated, only if conflicting information is obtained from duplex and MRI or CT or if non-invasive study is unsatisfactory, or if the clinical picture is unexplained by non-invasive imaging.

■ Trials

SYMPTOMATIC PATIENTS

Both NASCET (North American symptomatic carotid endarterectomy trial) and ECST (European carotid surgery trial) showed that patients with high-grade carotid stenosis (70–99 %) benefit from surgery over medical treatment in reducing risk of fatal and non-fatal strokes.

ASYMPTOMATIC PATIENTS

Both ACAS (asymptomatic carotid atherosclerosis study) and ACST (asymptomatic carotid surgery trial) showed that patients with >70 % carotid stenosis who are <75 years of age (and with a life expectancy of >5 years) benefit from surgery over medical treatment by reducing the risk of stroke from 12 to 6 % over the following five years.

■ Treatment

CAROTID ENDARTERECTOMY (CEA)

CEA is performed either under general or regional anaesthesia. Regional anaesthesia has the advantage of allowing assessment of conscious level and hence brain perfusion, and maintaining the autoregulatory mechanisms controlling cerebral blood flow. When the carotid artery is clamped, it is therefore easier to safely judge cerebral blood flow and the requirement for needing to use a shunt is reduced.

This involves dissection of the common, external and internal carotid artery. After clamping, an arteriotomy is made. An intimectomy plane is established between the atherosclerotic plaque and part of the media, attempting to leave circular medial fibres attached to adventitia. While the carotid is clamped, the majority of patients have enough collateral blood supply to the brain (especially under local anaesthetic). A number, however, require the insertion of a shunt to allow blood flow proximal to the common carotid clamp to distal to the internal clamp. Literature supports patch closure after endarterectomy of the carotid artery, especially in female patients, and in patients who have small internal carotid artery or who continue to smoke, as it reduces risk of recurrent carotid stenosis and early acute occlusion.

Postoperatively patients are monitored for blood pressure and continued on antiplatelet agents. Complications include <5 % combined morbidity and mortality in symptomatic patients and <3 % in asymptomatic patients. These are stroke, cranial nerve injury, haematoma, numbness, hypotension or hypertension and headache.

CAROTID ARTERY STENTING (CAS)

This is an evolving alternative treatment to carotid endarterectomy. There have been a number of trials to date, but much of the data is flawed. A new trial (ICSS) is currently recruiting. At present, CAS is reserved for patients with symptomatic high-grade stenosis in a high-risk surgical group (recurrent stenosis, post-radiation, previous neck surgery or high lesions). Patients with common carotid artery (CCA) origin stenosis, tortuous brachiocephalic or CCA making sheath placement difficult are probably managed better surgically.

The technique involves transfemoral access and like any other transluminal angioplasty, the stenosis is crossed and a balloon-mounted stent is deployed. To prevent micro-emboli causing cerebral damage, a distal protection filter is placed in the internal carotid prior to ballooning.

■ Other carotid diseases

1. *Aneurysms:* causes include atherosclerosis, trauma, mycotic, congenital and dissection. Presentation includes distal embolization, thrombosis, rupture or pressure on the surrounding structures. Treatment involves open repair or stenting in selected cases.
2. *Dissection:* secondary to atherosclerosis, fibro muscular dysplasia, cystic medial necrosis, or trauma. Presentation includes the sudden onset of a temporal headache or cervical pain associated with a neurological or visual deficit or Horner's syndrome.
3. *Takayasu's arteritis:* non-specific arteritis resulting in constriction or occlusion and occasional aneurysm formation. Two phases: acute

and occlusive stage. These are not usually amenable to endarterectomy and require bypass surgery.

4. *Radiation injury:* causes accelerated atherosclerosis years after radiation therapy.

5. *Carotid body tumour:* are paragangliomas located at carotid bifurcation, 95 % being benign. Present as painless mass and diagnosis is made on CT scan or angiogram. Treatment is by surgical resection with or without repair of the carotid artery.

Raynaud's syndrome

RAVUL JINDAL AND MICHAEL JENKINS

■ Introduction

In 1862 Maurice Raynaud described an episodic digital ischaemia due to vasospasm of the small arteries and arterioles of the extremities, precipitated by cold or emotion. It consists of intense pallor (vasoconstriction), cyanosis (spasm relaxation with a trickle of blood flow causing rapid desaturation) and rubor (increased blood flow into dilated capillaries), with full recovery in 15–45 minutes. The fingers remain normal in between the episodes.

The term 'Raynaud's phenomenon' is used when the cause is unknown, and if underlying cause is identifiable, it is known as Raynaud's disease. However, the syndrome is better classified into spastic and obstructive type depending on the causative factor.

■ Incidence

The prevalence varies with climate and probably ethnic origin. In cooler countries (UK, Scandinavian) the prevalence varies from 20 to 25 %. It affects all age groups but mainly young women. Around 40–80 % of Raynaud's patients have associated disease, scleroderma being the most common.

■ Pathogenesis

Two types: obstructive and spastic.

Obstructive arterial disease causes a decrease in resting digital arterial pressure and, in these patients, even normal vasoconstrictive response to cold or emotion is sufficient to cause symptoms. Spastic type has

Hospital Surgery: Foundations in Surgical Practice, ed. Omer Aziz, Sanjay Purkayastha and Paraskevas Paraskeva. Published by Cambridge University Press. © Cambridge University Press 2009.

normal resting digital pressure and symptoms are caused due to an increased intensity of cold-induced arterial spasm. Both $\alpha2$ adrenoceptors and presynaptic β receptors are implicated in its causation.

Raynaud's disease can be associated with autoimmune diseases (SLE, RA, Sjögren's syndrome, mixed connective-tissue disorders, scleroderma), haematological diseases (mixed cryoglobulinaemia, monoclonal gammopathies, leukaemia, cold agglutinins, thrombocytosis), trauma, vibrating tools, arteriosclerosis, frostbite, Buerger's disease, hypothyroidism, thoracic outlet obstruction, and drugs. Autoimmune vasculitis can cause digital and palmar arterial occlusion and use of vibrating tools causes digital artery obstruction due to repeated shear stress.

■ Symptoms

Obstructive disease: usually involves one or several fingers, male = female distribution, usually >40 years of age. It can cause fingertip ulceration. Symptoms are usually coldness, numbness or mild discomfort. Significant pain is usually absent. Most episodes are induced by cold; however, the cold threshold varies from patient to patient.

Spastic disease: involves young female patients. Both hands are affected equally, thumb being frequently spared. It is usually not associated with finger ulceration. Only 10 % have primary lower extremity involvement.

■ Diagnosis

The physical examination is frequently normal and the diagnosis relies on history and non-invasive tests. History of symptoms, occlusive vascular disease, drugs, trauma or frostbite, malignancy, connective-tissue disorders (arthralgia, dysphagia, skin tightening, xerophthalmia or xerostomia). Look for associated autoimmune disease and also evaluate for peripheral pulses and assess hands for sclerodactyly, telangiectasias, calcinosis and fingertip ulcerations. Carpal tunnel syndrome is associated in around 15 % of patients with Raynaud's disease.

■ Investigations

The *digital photoplethysmography* provides qualitative information on the character of the arterial waveform. Normal digital blood pressure is within 30 mmHg of brachial pressure. Patients with obstructive Raynaud's syndrome (RS) have blunted waveforms, whereas patients with vasospastic RS have either normal waveforms or a peaked pulse. The peaked pulse pattern reflects increased vasospastic arterial resistance.

A *cold challenge test* is used to verify cold sensitivities. A liquid-perfused cuff is placed on the proximal phalanx of the target finger. The cuff is inflated to suprasystolic pressure for five minutes while it is perfused with cold water. The pressure at which blood flow is detected on deflation of the cuff is recorded. A control finger on the same hand is tested at room temperature and the result is expressed as percentage drop in finger systolic pressure with cooling. Digital blood pressure response to five minutes of digital occlusive hypothermia has proved to be 87 % specific and 90 % sensitive in diagnosing Raynaud's syndrome but it does not differentiate between obstructive and spastic causes.

X-ray hand for calcinosis or tuft resorption, full blood count, ESR, RF (rheumatoid factor), and antinuclear antibodies to detect autoimmune disease. If there is a sudden onset of symptoms, digital ischaemia should also be evaluated for hypercoagulable states. Duplex scanning or angiography is required in patients with digital ulceration to detect proximal arterial lesions. Echocardiogram helps to rule out a cardiac source of emboli.

■ Treatment

Warm clothes, cessation of smoking, electrically heated mittens are the cornerstones of the treatment. Avoid drugs such as ergot alkaloids or β blockers. More than 90 % will respond to conservative treatment and even patients with obstructive symptoms and ulceration may have a healing rate of 80–85 % with conservative measures.

DRUGS

- Nifedipine: 10–20 mg/8 hr po or extended release nifedipine (30 mg every night) is used. Patients with spastic disease are more likely to respond than those with an obstructive disease pattern. It is indicated in patients with severe symptoms and ulceration. There is 70 % subjective benefit but 10–20 % of patients have side-effects (headache, ankle swelling, pruritis, severe fatigue).
- Second-line drugs include an α blocker (phenoxybenzamine hydrochloride) or losartan (angiotensin II receptor blocker).
- Iloprost (0.5 nanogram/kg/min iv) (stable analogue of PGI2) may salvage digits with ulcers or near gangrene; but the effect is short lived (approximately 3–4 months), relapse is common and the best results are in patients with systemic sclerosis.

Sympathectomy may also help in severe disease (good results noted only in lower limbs and associated with relief in 90 % of patients). Temperature biofeedback, TENS (transcutaneous electrical nerve stimulation) and acupuncture have been used with limited success. Surgery may be required to correct any proximal arterial obstruction. Reconstruction of the palmar arch and direct microvascular bypass of occluded segments of palmar and digital arteries have been performed in selected patients with limited success.

■ Prognosis

It is a relatively benign condition. Patients with associated arterial disease or positive serology are more likely to develop finger ulceration or ischaemia in the future. Patients without a diagnosable connective-tissue disorder on presentation have a 2–6 % chance of progressing to one if serology is negative, and a 30–75 % chance if serology is positive on presentation. Fingertip amputations are rarely required to aid healing.

Varicose veins

RAVUL JINDAL AND MICHAEL JENKINS

■ Incidence

More than 50 % of men and two-thirds of women have physically identifiable disease. The appearance of varicose veins in childhood is rare
although adolescents have incompetent valves. European data indicate
that up to 1.5 % of adults will suffer a venous stasis ulcer at some point
in their lives. Annual healthcare cost in the UK for venous ulceration is
estimated at £290 million.

■ Definition

Varicose veins are abnormal tortuous, dilated, elongated superficial
veins. These are most commonly found in the long (LSV) and short
saphenous vein (SSV) distribution. Spider veins are dilated smaller cutaneous venules (Figure 105).

■ Classification: CEAP (clinical, etiological, anatomical, pathological)

Clinical: 0 – no signs of venous disease, 1 – reticular veins, 2 – varicose
  veins, 3 – oedema, 4 – skin changes (lipodermatosclerosis), 5 – skin
  changes with healed ulceration, 6 – active ulceration

Aetiological: congenital, primary (no cause), secondary (deep vein
  thrombosis, traumatic, etc.)

Anatomical: superficial, perforator or deep; location (long or short
  saphenous)

Pathological: reflux, obstruction, both.

Hospital Surgery: Foundations in Surgical Practice, ed. Omer Aziz, Sanjay
Purkayastha and Paraskevas Paraskeva. Published by Cambridge University Press.
© Cambridge University Press 2009.

■ Aetiology

The risk factors for varicose vein include prolonged standing, hereditary, female sex, parity and history of phlebitis. Venous ulcers on the other hand have different risk factors and include old age, obesity, hypertension, trauma, history of venous thrombosis, and low socioeconomic status.

■ Symptoms

Symptoms range from cosmetic to intractable pain. A burning sensation over the varicose veins is caused by local pressure on cutaneous sensory nerves. In early stages, it causes mild swelling, heaviness and easy fatigability. Dull pain and aching usually starts in the afternoon after long standing and is relieved with leg elevation. Itching is a manifestation of local cutaneous stasis and precedes the onset of dermatitis. The skin and subcutaneous tissue are normal. The magnitude of the symptoms is not related to the length or diameter of the varicose veins.

Later, with chronic venous insufficiency (CVI), moderate to severe swelling occurs with large varicosities, pigmentation and induration (lipodermatosclerosis). With continued damage, ulceration occurs.

■ Complications

Ulceration, bleeding, thrombophlebitis.

■ Pathogenesis

The main theories suggested for primary varicose veins are a defect in elastin and collagen in the venous wall, anatomical difference in location of superficial veins in legs, intrinsic incompetence of the valve system, acquired valve damage (monocytic infiltration), and venous hypertension (hydrostatic pressure, dynamic hypertension from muscle compartment). Female hormones (progesterone) are associated with venous dilation and thus more symptoms occur in the second phase of the menstrual cycle and during pregnancy. Capillary permeability leads to transcapillary leakage of osmotically active particles, especially fibrinogen, which in turn leads to fibrin deposition and skin damage. Raised intra-abdominal pressure (tumours and fetus) can also predispose to varicose veins.

■ Investigations

Duplex scanning is the single most useful test for venous disease. It gives information as to reflux at junctions, perforator vein status and patency of the deep veins. Use of venography and plethysmography is rarely needed. Confirm competence of the deep venous system.

■ Treatment

Indications include symptoms (pain, fatigue, heaviness), recurrent thrombophlebitis, bleeding, skin changes and complications (ulceration).

NON-OPERATIVE TREATMENT

Compression therapy remains the mainstay of treatment. It is highly effective in controlling symptoms of varicose veins and promotes healing of venous ulcers. It works by decreasing the effects of venous hypertension on the skin and subcutaneous tissue. It improves skin microcirculation and thus promotes healing of ulcers. Compression stockings are adequate for varicose veins, but four-layer bandaging is necessary to heal ulceration.

SCLEROTHERAPY

Venules < 1 mm can be treated with 0.2 % sodium tetradecyl or hypertonic saline injection used as a sclerosing agent. Similarly,

1–3 mm venules can be treated with 0.5 % sclerosant. It is also used in patients with recurrent, isolated or residual varicosities. Main side-effects include anaphylaxis, allergy, thrombophlebitis, pigmentation and cutaneous necrosis.

SURGERY

The veins are marked with a permanent marker with the patient standing. Valvular incompetence at saphenofemoral and saphenopopliteal junction causing truncal varicosities requires ligation of the junction and stripping of the veins. Saphenofemoral junction (SFJ) is ligated after dealing with all tributaries of LSV. Stripping of the LSV is done to knee level to avoid saphenous nerve injury. Multiple stab avulsions are performed for varicosities. Postoperative pressure dressings are applied and patient can usually go home the same day as surgery.

Complications include venous thrombosis, bruising, paraesthesia, infection and recurrence (10–20 %). Redo surgery for residual or recurrent varicose veins can be complex. Veins are marked using duplex scan. Redo groin exploration greatly increases the risk of complications – seroma or lymphatic leak and wound infection.

■ New methods

A number of less-invasive treatment methods have recently found favour. Radiofrequency ablation and laser both involve an energy source causing collagen contraction to occlude the LSV without destroying the venous wall integrity. The catheter is inserted at knee level under duplex guidance, positioned to the SFJ and then slowly withdrawn. Foam sclerotherapy works in a similar way to any sclerosing agent, but can expand to fill a large area of the superficial venous system. The long-term results of all these treatments are yet to be determined.

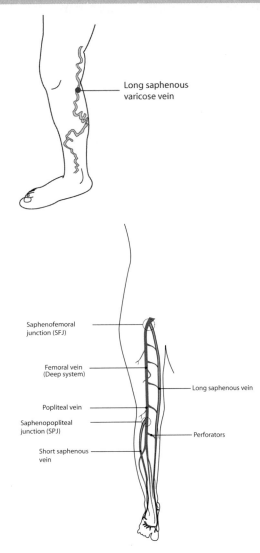

Figure 105

General aspects of breast disease

PARASKEVAS PARASKEVA

■ History

The history from the patient is essential in helping you to establish the causes of disease and assessing whether there is an increased risk of malignancy. The history should be taken in a private place and it should be done with sympathy, as most breast patients are very anxious. This should cover:

Age of the patient: this is very important. Remember, cancers are uncommon below the age of thirty.

Lump: always ask about: the length of time it has been present. Its relation to the menstrual cycle. Exact location (note which breast). Does its size vary? Is it getting larger?

Pain: is the lump painful? Is this cyclical?

Nipple discharge: ascertain colour, quantity, pattern, frequency.

Skin changes of the breast/nipple.

Shape of breast: ask if she has noticed any nipple retraction, breast distortion.

Metastatic related symptoms: e.g. back pain, shortness of breath, jaundice.

Previous breast disease, and whether this was investigated/treated.

Family history: this is extremely important, and many clinics offer family counselling and screening.

Other risk factors for breast cancer (see Breast cancer Chapter).

Genetics of breast cancer: 5–10 % of breast cancers are inherited in a dominant fashion. They are of an early onset and are associated with other tumours e.g. bowel, ovarian. The following genes have been

Hospital Surgery: Foundations in Surgical Practice, ed. Omer Aziz, Sanjay Purkayastha and Paraskevas Paraskeva. Published by Cambridge University Press. © Cambridge University Press 2009.

isolated: BRCA1 (chromosome 17q21), BRCA2 (chromosome 13q24), P53 gene on chromosome 17p (associated with Li-Fraumeni syndrome).

Medication: HRT, OCP.

Gynaecological/obstetric history: all these symptoms should be related to the woman's normal cycle. An obstetric history should also be taken e.g. parity, age when she had first child, did she breast feed or not? When was her last period?

■ Examination

This should occur in appropriate surroundings and with a chaperone (even if the examiner is female). Make sure you explain what you are going to do, and that your hands are clean and warm.

1. Undress the patient to the waist.
2. Sit the patient up on a couch facing you at 45 degrees.
3. Ask patient to raise her arms – look for:
   - Asymmetry
   - Scars
   - Fungating lesion
   - Nipple discharge/inversion
   - Peau d'orange (skin tethering)
   - Eczema around the nipple (it may be Paget's disease)
   - Erythema/oedema (and lymphoedema of the arms).
4. Ask the patient if she has a lump and if so to point to it.
5. Ask the patient to raise her arms above her head. Also ask her to put hands on waist and push inwards. Took for tethering of breast lesions.
6. Start to palpate the normal breast first using the flat of the hand in a systematic way, either in a concentric circle or in quadrants (Figure 106). Do not forget to palpate the axillary tail. If a lump is found, treat it as any other lump.
7. Fixity – test the skin mobility and ask the patient to press on her hips to fix pectoralis. Is the lump fixed to the muscle?
8. Ask the patient to produce any nipple discharge.

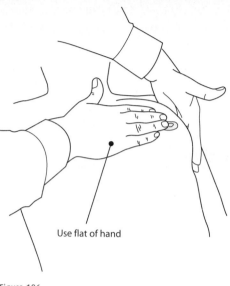

Use flat of hand

Figure 106

9. Examine the axilla – look for lymphadenopathy.
10. Palpate cervical and supraclavicular regions for lymphadenopathy.
11. Palpate the liver – if hepatomegaly think metastases.
12. Percuss spine for pain from metastasis.
13. Always cover the patient when you have finished.
14. Finally, encourage regular self examination.

■ Investigations

The following investigations may be used:

USS   This is most useful in the under forty age group as the density of the glandular tissue reduces the sensitivity of mammography. It can, however, be used to accurately guide FNA in older women.

Mammography This is used in screening programmes. Oblique and craniocaudal views are used and it is particularly useful in dense or bilateral tumours. It has a false negative rate of 10 %. Mammography is not useful in women with very small breasts and those under the age of 35 as their breast tissue is too dense.

MRI MRI scanning is increasingly being used for investigation of the breast and can be used in an interventional manner to guide surgery.

FNAC This procedure involves adequate localization of the lump (through palpation or USS), the use of local anaesthetic and a green (18G) needle. Continual aspiration is used as the needle is inserted and about 10 passes through the lump or cyst are required. The resulting aspirate is then sent for cytology, and in good hands this can have about 95 % sensitivity.

Core biopsy Histological information regarding a suspicious breast lump can be obtained via a core (Tru-Cut) biopsy needle which comes in manual and spring-loaded varieties; this is a procedure that can be done under local anaesthetic. Tissue can be examined also for receptor status (Figure 107).

If a breast cancer is diagnosed it must be managed in an MDT setting (see Multidisciplinary team chapter).

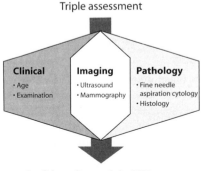

Figure 107 Triple assessment: the mainstay of evaluating breast disease

Benign breast disease

PARASKEVAS PARASKEVA

■ Congenital abnormalities

Congenital absence of the breast – complete absence of both the breast and nipple (amastia). Breast hypoplasia is more common and some degree of asymmetry can be seen in many women.

Accessory nipples – caused by failure of the regression of the primitive milk line, present in 1 % of people; can be excised if problematic.

Accessory breast – polymastia.

■ Developmental disorders

Excessive breast enlargement – minor degrees of enlargement can occur in infancy related to maternal oestrogens.

Male breast enlargement occurs in 30 % of boys at puberty. Usually reverses spontaneously.

Gynaecomastia can occur in juveniles with hormonal abnormalities or hormone-secreting tumours. Other causes: hypogonadism, liver disease, hormone-secreting tumours and drugs e.g. spironolactone, cimetidine, isoniazid, omeprazole, finasteride, marijuana, thyroxine and digoxin.

■ Disorders of cyclical change

Benign mammary dysplasia – this usually affects pre-menopausal women and is characterized by pre-menstrual breast nodularity and pain commonly in the upper outer quadrant. If there is concern that a nodule may be malignant then a mammogram and a FNAC (fine needle aspiration and cytology) should be performed. This is an aberration of

Hospital Surgery: Foundations in Surgical Practice, ed. Omer Aziz, Sanjay Purkayastha and Paraskevas Paraskeva. Published by Cambridge University Press. © Cambridge University Press 2009.

normal development and involution (ANDI) and includes the following conditions:

1. Fibrosis
2. Adenosis – multiplication of acini
3. Cyst formation – macro or microcysts
4. Epitheliosis – hyperplasia of epithelium
5. Papillomatosis – papillomatous overgrowth within the ducts.

Management – usually reassurance, analgesia, a well-fitting bra and evening primrose oil may help. Occasionally drugs such as danazol, tamoxifen or bromocriptine may be used. In very rare circumstances a mastectomy may be considered for symptomatic treatment.

Cystic disease – cysts occur commonly in women who are approaching the menopause and aspiration should be attempted. A green brown fluid is usually obtained in which case the patient can be reassured. Persistence of a mass or blood-stained fluid needs FNAC and an ultrasound scan.

Fibroadenomas – these are developmental masses rather than true neoplasms. They occur between the ages of 15 and 40 and account for about 20 % of discrete breast masses. They are firm, smooth, mobile and they can be multiple (and are thus sometimes referred to as 'the breast mouse'). The size and consistency of the lesion may change with the menstrual cycle. Peri-canalicular fibroadenomas tend to be small and hard while intra-canalicular ones are large and soft.

Management – fibroadenomas can be observed as they may regress, but if there is any doubt in the diagnosis FNAC is advised and then excision. Occasionally fibroadenomas are giant in size (>5 cm) and malignant change occurs in 0.001 %. These are usually excised.

■ Infective disorders

Mastitis neonatorum occurs in neonates on the third or fourth day of life, and usually disappears by the third week. This is because of the maternal prolactin affecting the neonates' breast tissue.

Lactational breast abscess – common in the first month after delivery, usually following a cracked nipple caused by infection with *S. aureus*. This can be treated with antibiotics in the early stages, but if there is fluctuance then incision and drainage with a biopsy is indicated.

Non-lactating infections of the breast can also occur and are caused by *S. aureus* (most common), streptococci, and more rarely tuberculosis, syphilis and actinomycosis. Bacterial mastitis is usually acute and is the most common cause of mastitis. This requires cultures to be taken, bed rest, analgesia and appropriate antibiotic cover.

■ Inflammatory disorders

Periductal mastitis affects young women and can present as mastalgia, nipple discharge and nipple retraction. Treatment consists of adequate analgesia and antibiotics. This is important because it can progress to abscesses or fistulae.

Duct ectasia – duct dilation with a cheesy or blood-stained discharge.

Fat necrosis – occurs after trauma; fibrosis and calcification results in a mass that may simulate carcinoma.

Mondor's disease – thrombophlebitis in the region of the internal thoracic vein. Treatment includes rest, ice packs, and NSAIDs.

■ Benign neoplasms

Duct papillomas – commonly present with blood-stained nipple discharge. These usually present in women between 35 and 50 years old and they are more likely to be unilateral. Treatment is with microdochectomy or duct excision.

Lipoma – as per lipomata on other parts of the body.

■ Others

1. Non-cyclical breast pain
2. Haematoma

3. Amyloid
4. Silicone granuloma
5. Galactocoele
6. Sebaceous cysts
7. Eczema of the nipple – need biopsy to exclude Paget's disease.

Breast cancer

PARASKEVAS PARASKEVA

Incidence: affects 1 in 12 women in the UK.

There are 20 000 new patients per year in the UK. The incidence is rising but the mortality is falling, however there are still about 15 000 deaths from this cancer per year.

Age: it is very rare under the age of 30, incidence increases with age.

Geography: disease of developed countries.

Aetiology/risk factors:

1. Early menarche, late menopause
2. First child over 30 years
3. Family history in first-degree relatives
4. Previous breast cancer
5. Radiation exposure
6. Exogenous hormones
7. High intake of saturated fats, alcohol.

■ Pathology

Tumour type:

1. **Non-invasive ductal carcinoma *in situ* (CIS)** – this is a premalignant condition that can be seen as microcalcification on mammography. This can be unifocal (indicating a localized removal or lumpectomy) or widespread (which may require a mastectomy).
2. **Non-invasive lobular CIS.**

Hospital Surgery: Foundations in Surgical Practice, ed. Omer Aziz, Sanjay Purkayastha and Paraskevas Paraskeva. Published by Cambridge University Press. © Cambridge University Press 2009.

3. **Invasive ductal** – this is the most common. The lump feels hard ('scirrhous').
4. **Invasive lobular.**
5. **Medullary** – 5 % of breast cancers. The tumour is soft, and it tends to affect younger patients.
6. **Colloid/mucinous** – occur in the elderly. May mimic a benign mass on mammogram.
7. **Papillary.**
8. **Paget's** – this is a superficial presentation of an underlying cancer and it appears as an eczema-like condition of the nipple. Importantly this persists, therefore all eczema of the nipple lasting >2 weeks should be biopsied.

■ Staging of cancer

This is either using the TNM classification or a clinical staging process (Figure 108):

Tis (no tumour palpable). CIS/Paget's
T1 <2 cm. No skin fixation
T2 2–5 cm. Skin distortion
T3 5–10 cm. Ulceration + pectoral fixation
T4 >10 cm. Chest wall extension, skin involved.

N0 No nodes
N1 Ipsilateral mobile nodes
N2 Ipsilateral fixed nodes
N3 Internal mammary nodes.

M0 No mets
M1 Mets in liver, lung, bone.

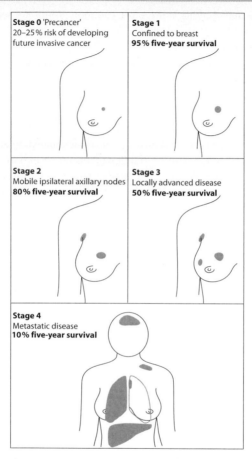

Figure 108

■ Clinical features

The main features to grasp from the history and examination have already been eluded to, however, here are the most important signs and symptoms to look out for:

1. Firm irregular painless lump usually in the upper outer quadrant
2. Nipple discharge
3. Nipple retraction
4. Axillary lymph nodes
5. Paget's disease
6. Peau d'orange
7. Signs of metastases
8. Asymptomatic following screening.

These begin with the *triple assessment*, but then progress to more invasive procedures and will also include the staging procedures mentioned before.

1. Blood tests (as mentioned already)
2. Ultrasound
3. Mammogram – oblique, craniocaudal
4. FNAC
5. Tru-Cut biopsy
6. Excision biopsy
7. Wire-guided biopsy
8. Bone scan
9. CT
10. Breast MRI.

■ Treatment

This is an individual process taking into account the age of the patient and their respective fitness to undergo surgery, their wishes regarding the treatment options available and the clinical stage of the tumour.

Principles of surgical approach:

Local tumour control
Staging the axilla

■ Treatment of early breast cancer

1. SURGICAL

Before surgery it is important to involve the breast counselling nurse and to ensure that the tumour is marked on the correct breast. The goal of surgery is to gain local control.

There are two basic treatment options; these both have the same survival rates:

A. Wide local excision (WLE) + radiotherapy (DXT)

(1 cm excision margin is required.)

B. Mastectomy

Mastectomy is useful where radiotherapy is not possible, in those tumours that are particularly large (>3.5–4 cm) and in central tumours. It also has a lower rate of recurrence compared to WLE. However, there are obvious cosmetic and psychological implications to having a breast removed compared to simply having a lump excised.

Nodal status is important in invasive carcinomas, to stage the disease and also to clear it. Therefore at the time of surgery, the following are practiced:

i. **Axillary sampling** = removal of the lower axillary nodes, which if involved, will then need clearance or radiotherapy.
ii. **Axillary clearance** = removal of contents below the level of the axillary vein. This can be done to varying levels (most commonly level 1, about eight lymph nodes):
   - Level 1 = below pectoralis minor
   - Level 2 = behind pectoralis minor
   - Level 3 = above pectoralis minor.

iii. **Sentinal node mapping,** which is now coming into fashion as this allows visualization of draining lymph nodes (LNs). The sentinal node is the first node that a section of the breast drains to, and therefore if this can be removed and proven to be clear on frozen section then there is little point in further dissecting other nodes as they are also likely to be clear. This procedure is therefore done at the time of surgery and involves the injection of a radioisotope which collects in the LNs. This can then be detected with the aid of a probe and the sentinel node easily localized.

Complications of mastectomy

1. Wound infection
2. Haematoma
3. Seroma
4. Frozen shoulder
5. Intercostal brachial nerve numbness
6. Lymphoedema – this can be reduced with stockings or by raising the arm.

Reconstructive surgery should be offered to the patient either at the same sitting or as a delayed procedure. Possible options include:

1. Implants – Silastic or saline inflatable
2. Latissimus dorsi flap
3. TRAM flap (transfer of rectus abdominis myocutaneous) flap
4. Nipple tattoo.

But, not everyone is suitable for plastic surgery and there are complications. It obviously requires further surgery and therefore results in more trauma, and it may not even be possible to attain perfect symmetry. Also immediate reconstruction may interfere with postoperative radiotherapy and the scarring may make detection of recurrence more difficult.

2. SYSTEMIC TREATMENT

This can be:

■ Adjuvant
■ Neoadjuvant (primary).

A. Radiotherapy

This can be used in three circumstances:

  i. Breast and chest wall
 ii. Axilla
iii. Palliation (e.g. for bony tenderness).

B. Chemotherapy

There are no hard and fast rules as to when this should be used, and many patients receiving chemotherapy are invariably part of a trial. However, this treatment can be used in the following circumstances:

  i. Recurrent disease
 ii. <70 years old with >1 +ve axillary node
iii. Very large tumours.

Chemotherapy is usually offered to pre-menopausal women, but it can also be offered to post-menopausals.

Monotherapy is used but combination therapy is also indicated e.g. CMF (cyclophosphamide, methotrexate, 5-FU). Neoadjuvant chemotherapy is offered to women with large or inflammatory tumours in an attempt to shrink them down to make them more amenable to surgery.

C. Endocrine therapy

Tamoxifen is a partial agonist at oestrogen receptors (ER) and therefore it tends to have its best effect in ER +ve females. However, up to 15 % of ER –ve females also respond. (Most well-differentiated and lobular tumours are ER +ve, while few metastases are ER +ve.)

Newer drugs affecting the aromatase enzyme include Arimidex (anastrozole).

The thyroid gland

JAMES ARBUCKLE AND BILL FLEMING

■ General principles

Thyroid gland disease is usually benign. Thyroid cancer is rare and the majority of patients have an excellent prognosis if treated correctly at first presentation. Presented below are the principles of the Endocrine Surgery Unit at the Hammersmith Hospital:

1. Make the diagnosis: *history, examination, investigations*
2. Make the patient safe: *if toxic, airway problem etc.*
3. Localize the lesion: *if solitary*
4. Does the patient need an operation: *if so, which operation?*
5. Replace the deficit following operation.

■ History

- Most have lump in neck – ask duration, how did patient notice lump, any change since first noticed, any other similar lumps.
- Hyperthyroid symptoms – irritability, weight loss, heat intolerance, vomiting, diarrhoea, tachycardia, irregular periods, tremor.
- Hypothyroid symptoms – weight gain, cold intolerance, mental changes (depression, myxoedema madness), constipation, irregular periods, deafness, decreased libido, hair loss, coarse dry skin, carpal tunnel syndrome.
- Past history – thyroid disease, surgery in the neck, surgery of adrenals or pancreas; radiation to neck.
- Family history – thyroid cancer, MEN syndrome.

Hospital Surgery: Foundations in Surgical Practice, ed. Omer Aziz, Sanjay Purkayastha and Paraskevas Paraskeva. Published by Cambridge University Press. © Cambridge University Press 2009.

■ Examination

(Diagram of thyroid anatomy, see Figure 109.)

Inspection   Obvious goitre
              Previous scars, check for previous radiation
              Signs of toxicity.
Palpation   Diffuse or nodular goitre
              Single or multiple nodules
              Tracheal deviation
              Retrosternal extension
              Lymphadenopathy.

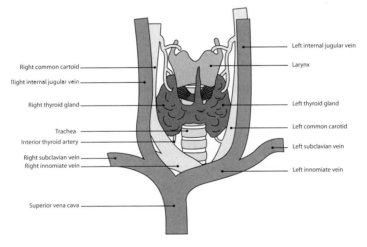

Right common cartoid
Right internal jugular vein
Right thyroid gland
Trachea
Interior thyroid artery
Right subclavian vein
Right innomiate vein
Superior vena cava

Left internal jugular vein
Larynx
Left thyroid gland
Left common carotid
Left subclavian vein
Left innomiate vein

Figure 109

■ Investigations

Blood tests: thyroid function tests. Calcium and phosphate. PTH and vitamin D. Thyroid autoantibodies if thyroiditis suspected. Calcitonin and CEA if medullary carcinoma suspected.

Imaging: ultrasound. Isotope scan – only in toxic patients to differentiate toxic nodule from Graves' disease. CT neck and mediastinum – if retrosternal extension. MRI – useful if malignant lymphadenopathy.

Cytology FNA +/– ultrasound guidance: result may be benign, malignant or non-diagnostic and highly dependent on quality of cytologist:

- Colloid nodules and inflammatory thyroid disease (Hashimoto's thyroiditis, TB), straightforward diagnosis
- Papillary, medullary, anaplastic carcinoma and lymphoma, relatively straightforward diagnosis
- Follicular carcinoma, near impossible diagnosis on FNA.

■ Informed consent

Warn patient of risks associated with general anaesthetic (GA), wound infection, scar (hypertrophic, keloid), bleeding necessitating return to theatre – NB airway obstruction.

Recurrent laryngeal nerve damage (more common in redo surgery, neck dissection and extensive carcinoma): temporary – hoarse voice for days/weeks; permanent – 1/1000.

Thyroxine replacement – always after total thyroidectomy; in 30 % of patients after hemithyroidectomy.

Parathyroid injury – requiring calcium and vitamin D supplements (may be temporary or permanent depending on extent of surgery).

■ Goitre

Definition: goitre means enlarged thyroid gland – may affect one lobe or entire gland.

Goitres may be physiological (puberty, pregnancy) or pathological: benign or malignant.

BENIGN CAUSES OF GOITRE

Reduced dietary iodine intake ('Derbyshire neck', mountainous areas)
Multinodular goitre

Thyroid cyst
Thyroid adenoma
Thyroiditis.

MALIGNANT CAUSES OF GOITRE

See section on thyroid cancer.

WHO CRITERIA TO DESCRIBE GOITRE

Grade 0   Goitre not visible or palpable, even with neck extended
Grade 1a   Goitre palpable
Grade 1b   Goitre palpable, and visible when neck extended
Grade 2   Goitre visible with neck in normal position
Grade 3   Large goitre visible from distance.

TREATMENT

There is no effective medical treatment for multinodular goitre.

The operation for benign goitre is total thyroidectomy. A subtotal thyroidectomy is rarely performed due to the 15 % risk of recurrence.

INDICATIONS FOR SURGERY

Cosmetic appearance (patient request)
Pressure symptoms (dysphagia, dyspnoea – particularly on lying flat, suddenly waking up at night)
Concern about malignancy
Retrosternal extension
Thyrotoxicosis (usually recommend radioiodine).

■ Thyroid cancer

Less than 1 % of all cancers – in the UK 1200 new cases diagnosed per year.

■ 90 % thyroid cancers are well differentiated papillary, follicular or Hurthle cell (variant of follicular) tumours.

- 10 % poorly differentiated, such as anaplastic or medullary tumours and lymphoma.
- 25 % of thyroid nodules in children are malignant.

PREDISPOSING FACTORS

1. Follicular cancer more prevalent in iodine deficient areas (check for slightly elevated TSH).
2. Ionizing radiation:
   - initiator of papillary cancer, especially if age < 10 years
   - exposure over age of 20 years does not increase risk
   - radiotherapy to treat head and neck childhood conditions increases risk, but risk falls with time from exposure.
3. Hashimoto's thyroiditis – predisposes to lymphoma.

CLINICAL FEATURES OF MALIGNANCY

Hoarseness, dysphagia
Painless, fixed, hard thyroid mass
Isolated lymph node enlargement.

WELL-DIFFERENTIATED CANCERS (90 %)

Papillary cancer

Arises from follicular cells
F:M 3:1, aged 30–50 years
Lymph node metastasis
Treatment: total thyroidectomy and radioiodine (micropapillary cancers < 1 cm do not need radioiodine); neck dissection for involved nodes
Excellent prognosis.

Follicular cancer

Arises from follicular cells
More common in women – peaks later in life than papillary

Bloodborne metastasis to lung, bone, brain

Two types: minimally invasive and widely invasive

Treatment: total thyroidectomy and radioiodine

Excellent prognosis.

Hurthle cell tumour

Variant of follicular cancer and often difficult to determine malignancy

Does **not** take up radioiodine

Treatment: total thyroidectomy and radioiodine (to ablate remaining thyroid).

POORLY DIFFERENTIATED CANCERS (10 %)

Medullary cancer

Originates in parafollicular cells or C cells and secretes calcitonin

80 % sporadic – solitary thyroid nodules and involved lymph nodes

Familial forms:

- MEN associated (MEN2a or MEN2b) or non-MEN form
- all patients should be screened for ret proto-oncogene mutations

Treatment: total thyroidectomy and routine lymph node dissection (central compartment and jugular nodes); radioiodine of no use due to C cell origin

Children carrying genetic abnormality require prophylactic thyroidectomy by three years if MEN2a , and by one year if MEN2b (may differ according to local endocrine surgical unit policy)

Overall good prognosis (85 % at 10 years).

Anaplastic cancer

Almost always p53 mutation – enhances transformed phenotype

Usually lethal within months

Occurs in elderly, presenting as a rapidly enlarging mass, invading local structures

Treatment: surgery to debulk +/– tracheostomy. External beam radiotherapy and chemotherapy (doxorubicin) may palliate for short time.

Lymphoma

Hashimoto's thyroiditis increases the risk 70 fold

Most are intermediate to high grade, but important to distinguish low grade MALTomas which rarely disseminate

Stage with total body scan and bone marrow biopsy

Treatment: external beam radiotherapy and chemotherapy (radiotherapy only for MALTomas); no role for thyroidectomy or radioiodine.

Parathyroid

NEIL WALKER

■ Introduction

Overt **primary hyperparathyroidism (PHPT)** is defined as a hypercalcaemic state due to excessive parathyroid hormone (PTH) secretion from one or more parathyroid glands. Cardinal features include a persistent **hypercalcaemia** (elevated serum calcium) and **hypercalciuria** with an elevated (or inappropriately normal) PTH concentration (Figure 110).

■ Incidence

Primary hyperparathyroidism has an overall incidence of 25 per 100 000 of the UK population. In women over the age of 45 it may affect 1 in 500. Over 1 % of post-menopausal women have raised serum calcium.

■ Aetiology

Primary hyperparathyroidism occurs due to benign pathology in the vast majority of cases (85 % caused by a single adenoma). Hyperplasia accounts for 14 % of cases, and accounts for hereditary conditions such as MEN1 or MEN2. Parathyroid carcinoma is rare (<1 %).

■ Symptoms and signs

Most patients diagnosed are asymptomatic or have mild disease. It is always worth enquiring about symptoms related to end organ damage such as: **'stones'** – loin pain from renal stones; **'bones'** – bone pains, arthralgia, low-impact fractures suggestive of osteoporosis;

Hospital Surgery: Foundations in Surgical Practice, ed. Omer Aziz, Sanjay Purkayastha and Paraskevas Paraskeva. Published by Cambridge University Press. © Cambridge University Press 2009.

'groans' – peptic ulcer disease, pancreatitis; 'psychic overtones' – fatigue, reduced intellectual capability and depression.

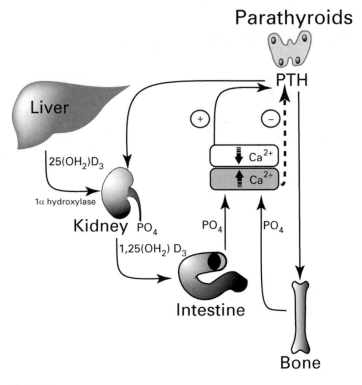

Figure 110

■ Investigations

Ca^{2+}, albumin, phosphate, alkaline phosphatase, PTH, U&E, 24 hr urinary calcium. Once the diagnosis is confirmed bone density DEXA scans and renal ultrasound should be considered to assess end organ damage. Urinary collections are used to help differentiate familial hypocalciuric hypercalcaemia which has a low urine calcium excretion. The abnormal gland is often localized using a combination of ultrasound and technetium-99m sestamibi scanning. If used in combination the success rate is extremely high. This localization is important preoperatively.

■ Medical treatment of hypercalcaemic crisis

- Rehydration with normal saline
- Correct hypokalaemia and hypomagnesaemia
- Furosemide-induced forced diuresis
- Bisphosphonates (pamidronate) may inhibit bone resorption
- Urgent referral to endocrinologist for further advice. Steroids may be used and dialysis can be used to lower serum calcium rapidly.

■ Indications for surgery

Parathyroidectomy is the treatment of choice in symptomatic primary hyperparathyroidism. However as the majority of patients diagnosed are asymptomatic, the subject of surgical resection has become controversial. Indications from surgery from the National Institute of Health in the USA include:

- <50 years of age
- Patient cannot participate in appropriate follow-up
- Serum calcium level >1.0 mg/dl above the normal range
- Urinary calcium > 400 mg/24 hours
- 30 % decrease in renal function
- complications of PHPT, including nephrocalcinosis, osteoporosis (*T*-score < 2.5 standard deviation (SD) at the lumbar spine, hip, or wrist)
- a severe psychoneurologic disorder.

PARATHYROIDECTOMY PROCEDURE

Traditionally involves a collar incision, bilateral exploration of the neck, identification of all four parathyroid glands, and removal of the diseased gland or glands. Patients with accurately and reliably localized single gland parathyroid disease may be treated with a minimal access approach. Minimally invasive parathyroidectomy can often be done in less than 20 minutes, with a local anaesthetic cervical block and sedation or laryngeal mask airway. This can now be done as a day case procedure.

PROGNOSIS

PHPT remains a relatively common disorder of calcium metabolism that is readily cured by a low-risk operation in 95 to 98 % of patients when performed by a qualified surgeon. Follow-up of patients with PHPT treated with surgery has shown a 10–12 % increase in bone mineral density at the lumbar spine and hip, that is sustained over 10 years with no documented recurrence of renal stones over the same period.

Follow-up: patients with mild asymptomatic primary hyperparathyroid without surgical indications should have follow-up which includes annual measurement of calcium, PTH, creatinine and bone mineral density at distal radius.

■ Complications of surgery

- ■ Transient hypocalcaemia. The dominant parathyroid may have suppressed the remaining normal glands resulting in temporary hypocalcaemia following surgery. Disruption of vascular supply may lead to hypoparathyroidism.
- ■ The main feature of hypocalcaemia is neuromuscular irritability. This can be mild with tingling and numbness in the peripheries, but it can become severe with tetany, laryngospasm and seizures. Bedside tests include:

    Trousseau's sign: inflate a blood pressure cuff to 10 mmHg above the systolic pressure for 3 min. Monitor for carpo-pedal spasm which is a positive sign.

Chvostek's sign: tap the facial nerve anterior to the tragus of the ear. Monitor for facial contractions which is a positive sign. (Note this sign is not specific for hypocalcaemia and may be present in healthy adults).

■ Hypomagnesaemia (arrhythmias)– check the Mg and correct if needed.

■ Treatment of hypocalcaemia

Symptomatic hypocalcaemia requires **urgent treatment:**

■ 10 ml of 10 % calcium gluconate iv diluted with 100 ml sodium chloride 0.9 % and infuse over 10 minutes. This can be repeated up to three times to control symptoms.
■ To maintain plasma calcium infuse 100 ml of 10 % calcium gluconate added to 1 l sodium chloride 0.9 % via a volumetric pump over 24 hr.
■ Titrate to maintain serum calcium in the low normal range.
■ When the patient's calcium is stable start on oral calcium treatment.
■ If the patient has underlying heart disease they should be placed on a monitor.
■ Continue to monitor the calcium on a six hourly basis.

Adrenal pathology

NEIL WALKER

■ Introduction

Located on the superior/medial aspect of both kidneys, the adrenal glands are triangular shaped and measure approximately 1.5 cm in height and 7 cm in length. The inner part, the *adrenal medulla*, secretes adrenaline and noradrenaline while the outer part, the *adrenal cortex*, secretes cortisol, aldosterone, and sex-hormone precursors (Dehydroepiandrosterone (DHEA) and its S isomer) (see Figure 111).

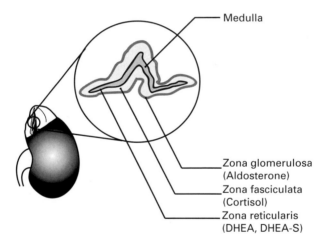

Medulla

Zona glomerulosa
(Aldosterone)
Zona fasciculata
(Cortisol)
Zona reticularis
(DHEA, DHEA-S)

Figure 111

Hospital Surgery: Foundations in Surgical Practice, ed. Omer Aziz, Sanjay Purkayastha and Paraskevas Paraskeva. Published by Cambridge University Press. © Cambridge University Press 2009.

Although the majority of adrenal tumours are benign and non-functioning, up to 20 % can be functioning. Rarely these tumours are malignant.

There are a number of pathological conditions which benefit from adrenal surgery and each will be looked at in turn.

■ Cushing's syndrome (secondary to a cortisol-secreting adenoma)

INCIDENCE

Approximately 15 % of all cases of Cushing's syndrome are secondary to cortisol-secreting adrenal adenomas (10 % are benign and 5 % malignant).

SYMPTOMS AND SIGNS

Characteristic clinical features include weight gain (especially of the face and trunk), hypertension, proximal muscle weakness, fragile skin, abdominal purple striae, facial acne and a plethoric complexion. Symptoms include mood disturbances, low libido, easy bruising and menstrual irregularities.

COMPLICATIONS

Diabetes mellitus, osteoporosis and cardiovascular disease secondary to hypertension.

INVESTIGATIONS

Initial screening tests can help to demonstrate excess cortisol production but these do not distinguish the exact cause. The excess cortisol could be secondary to excess pituitary ACTH production, ectopic ACTH production or excess cortisol secretion from an adrenal tumour.

- *24 hr urinary free cortisol collections* – although these are relatively sensitive they lack specificity.
- *Overnight dexamethasone suppression test* – 1 mg of dexamethasone is administered at 23.00 hours. At 9 a.m. the next morning the cortisol reading should suppress to less than 50 nmol/l. Failure to suppress is suggestive of Cushing's syndrome.

Patients with any abnormal screening tests should be referred to an endocrinologist who will carry out further inpatient tests to confirm the diagnosis. This will include *midnight cortisol measurements* and a *low-dose dexamethasone suppression test*. To ascertain the underlying cause measurement of ACTH is required. A low reading (<5 pg/ml) suggests an ACTH-independent origin, therefore, an adrenal tumour. The diagnosis can be difficult to secure and an experienced endocrinologist's opinion is crucial.

RADIOLOGY

After biochemical confirmation *CT scanning* of the adrenal glands is required. This will be helpful in identifying whether there is a solitary cortisol-producing tumour or the rare diagnosis of nodular adrenocortical hyperplasia. It also provides information as to whether the tumour has any malignant features.

TREATMENT

Unilateral adrenalectomy is the treatment of choice for adenomas. Pre-treatment with drugs to suppress steroid production may take place using metyrapone or ketonazole.

PROGNOSIS

Cortisol-secreting adenomas which are fully resected have a good prognosis. Special care must be taken in the postoperative period as these patients are often at higher risk of infections and wound breakdown. With unilateral adrenalectomy the contralateral adrenal is likely to be suppressed and steroid cover is required. Adrenal carcinoma has a very poor prognosis and is discussed in more detail later.

■ Phaeochromocytoma

INTRODUCTION

These tumours arise from chromaffin cells, and secrete catecholamines and their metabolites. The majority arise in the adrenal medulla, however very rarely they can be extra-adrenal (Paragangliomas).

INCIDENCE

Rare tumours occurring in 0.1–0.3 % of hypertensive individuals. Peak incidence is in the third to fifth decades of life. 10 % are bilateral, 10 % familial, 10 % extra-adrenal and 10 % malignant. Bilateral tumours are more common in familial syndromes including multiple endocrine neoplasia 2a and 2b, von Hippel-Lindau disease, and neurofibromatosis.

SYMPTOMS AND SIGNS

Hypertension may be sustained or paroxysmal. Other symptoms include headaches, palpitations, tachycardia, anxiety and sweating.

COMPLICATIONS

Cardiac dysrhythmias. Persistent hypertension leads to end organ damage including nephropathy, retinopathy and cardiac dysfunction. Rarely hypertensive encephalopathy.

INVESTIGATIONS

- *24 hr urinary collections* in acid bottles for free catecholamines and metabolites. At least two should be performed. Tricyclic antidepressants need to be stopped.

■ *Plasma catecholamines/metanephrines* are available in some centres and can be a useful diagnostic tool.

RADIOLOGY

Imaging gives information on the localization and extent of the tumours. Initial studies include a *chest X-ray* and an *abdominal CT/MRI scan*. *I-131 meta-iodobenzylguanidine (MIBG)* scans are useful as a localization agent. MIBG has a sensitivity of 80 % but very high specificity.

TREATMENT

Surgical resection is the treatment of choice. Prior to this the patients need to be adequately α blocked, usually with phenoxybenzamine. When a significant postural drop is obtained, β blockade is then initiated. An experienced anaesthetist is essential. During theatre hypertension is managed with drugs such as nitroprusside.

PROGNOSIS

If the primary tumour is benign then survival is that of the normal age-matched population. Metastatic disease has an overall survival of less than 50 %.

■ Conn's syndrome

Caused by small adenomas of the adrenal cortex secreting aldosterone. They are nearly always benign. Aldosterone acts on the distal nephron causing sodium retention with potassium and hydrogen ion loss. This leads to hypertension, alkalosis and hypokalaemia.

INCIDENCE

They are the cause of hypertension in approximately 3–4 % of patients. Peak incidence occurs in the third to sixth decades of life. Twice as common in women.

SIGNS AND SYMPTOMS

The hypertension can be severe and resistant to conventional treatment. Hypokalaemia is usually asymptomatic but can lead to fatigue and muscle weakness. Rarely, it causes nephrogenic diabetes insipidus which presents as polyuria or nocturia.

COMPLICATIONS

Persistent hypertension leads to end organ damage including nephropathy, retinopathy and cardiac dysfunction.

INVESTIGATIONS

- *Biochemistry* results typically show hypernatraemia, hypokalaemia and a metabolic alkalosis. Serum potassium can be normal in up to 40 % of cases.
- *Screening tests* include measurement of plasma renin and aldosterone. Plasma renin is suppressed due to the excess aldosterone. Aldosterone:renin ratios can be calculated. A high ratio is suggestive of primary hyperaldosteronism. When an abnormal ratio has been identified the diagnosis needs to be confirmed by further measurements of renin/aldosterone under more stringent conditions e.g. overnight recumbancy. The potassium level should be normalized and certain antihypertensives withdrawn prior to testing as these can interfere with the results. α blockers can be used.

These tests confirm primary hyperaldosteronism, but further tests are required to confirm the diagnosis of a Conn's adenoma. Imaging is crucial to help differentiate between an adenoma and bilateral adrenal hyperplasia.

RADIOLOGY

CT or MRI scanning is used for localization. If accurate diagnosis is difficult *adrenal vein sampling* or *radiolabelled iodocholesterol scanning* may be required.

Multiple endocrine neoplasia (MEN)

MATHEW ROLLIN AND BILL FLEMING

A group of genetically-based syndromes consisting of benign or malignant diseases of several endocrine glands, occurring either synchronously or spaced over many years. Also known as multiple endocrine *adenopathy (MEA)*, with reference to the fact that not all manifestations are necessarily neoplastic.

■ Definition and classification

MEN1	Parathyroid hyperplasia/adenoma	95 % occurs of cases
(Wermer's)	Pituitary adenoma	70 % of cases
	Pancreatic tumours	50 % of cases
	Gastrinoma	
	Insulinoma (single or multiple)	
	Glucagonoma (rare)	
	VIPoma (rare)	
	Non-functioning adrenal adenoma	40 % of cases
	Thyroid adenoma (single or multiple)	20 % of cases
MEN2a	Medullary thyroid carcinoma	95 % of cases
(Sipple)	Phaeochromocytoma	95 % of cases
	Parathyroid hyperplasia	60 % of cases
MEN2b	*(Occasionally also known as MEN3)*	
	Medullary thyroid carcinoma	95 % of cases

Hospital Surgery: Foundations in Surgical Practice, ed. Omer Aziz, Sanjay Purkayastha and Paraskevas Paraskeva. Published by Cambridge University Press. © Cambridge University Press 2009.

Phaeochromocytoma   70 % of cases

Characteristic habitus:

   Multiple mucosal neuromas (lips, cheeks, tongue, eyelids)

   Ganglioneuromas of GI tract

   Marfanoid appearance

   Delayed puberty

   Predisposition to SUFE (slipped upper femoral epiphysis)

(NB there is **no** parathyroid disease in MEN2b)

■ Incidence

Most commonly presents in third to fifth decades. No geographical or sex distribution.

Onset of MEN-related tumours occurs at a younger age than the same tumours caused by sporadic mutations. Incidence of bilaterality and multicentricity is also greater in MEN-related tumours than sporadically-mutated counterparts.

MEN accounts for one in five cases of medullary thyroid carcinoma – so should be considered in every such patient.

■ Aetiology

Genetic: familial inheritance (autosomal dominant) or new mutation.

■ Pathogenesis

Both MEN1 and MEN2 are caused by mutations in tumour suppressor genes. The MEN1 gene has been localized to chromosome 11. Its product, 'menin', controls the activation of transcription factors. MEN2 is caused by mutations in the ret proto-oncogene, on chromosome 10.

These mutations are not commonly found in relation to sporadic single endocrine tumours.

■ Symptoms and signs

Symptoms of hypercalcaemia are non-specific (lethargy, polydipsia, vague bone pain), so MEN syndromes often present due to urinary tract stones, symptoms of pituitary tumour (visual disturbance, acromegaly), symptoms of pancreatic tumour (recurrent hypoglycaemic attacks), symptoms of phaeochromocytoma (paroxysmal severe hypertension), or with lumps in the neck.

■ Investigation

Primary hyperparathyroidism:	Raised calcium + inappropriately high PTH
	USS or nuclear medicine scanning
Medullary thyroid carcinoma:	Significantly raised calcitonin
	USS or CT to look for local invasion and nodes
Pituitary adenoma:	Full pituitary hormone screen
	Visual field testing
	Head CT or MRI imaging
Pancreatic tumours:	Raised hormone levels appropriate to history
	Abdominal CT or MRI
Phaeochromocytoma:	Raised plasma and urinary catecholamines (24 hr urine sample, 9 a.m. bloods)
	Abdominal CT or MRI.

When diagnosis is established, first and second-degree relatives must be screened: tests include plasma calcitonin, PTH, and urinary catecholamines. If these are suggestive, then irrefutable diagnosis can be obtained by using PCR to detect genetic mutation.

■ Treatment

Surgical excision of tumours and their local nodes. Long-term surveillance is required, as recurrent or related tumours may develop many years after initial treatment.

Relatives testing positive for genetic mutations should be counselled and if calcitonin is normal, prophylactic surgery offered, enabling pre-emptive cure before neoplasia has developed. If calcitonin is already raised then treatment should be along the standard lines for medullary thyroid carcinoma. Total thyroidectomy is recommended for all susceptible children by the age of three years.

■ Prognosis

Dependent on disease state at presentation. With early surgery and good long-term surveillance, potentially excellent.

Obstructive urological symptoms

ERIK MAYER, ED ROWE AND JUSTIN VALE

■ Introduction

Obstructive urinary symptoms result from mechanical obstruction to the flow of urine at time of micturition. The level of obstruction can be anywhere from the bladder neck to the external urethral meatus. The term **bladder outflow obstruction (BOO)** is often used to describe the constellation of symptoms that results. Sometimes urologists will elect to use the term **'lower urinary tract symptoms' (LUTS)** if the patient's symptoms are both obstructive and storage (irritative) in nature.

■ Definition and classification

- **Obstructive symptoms** include: hesitancy, straining, decreased force of urination, intermittent stream, prolonged micturition, post-micturition dribbling and a sensation of incomplete bladder emptying.
- **Objective measurements** include use of basic urodynamic flow studies and completion of validated symptom score e.g. I-PSS (international prostate symptom score).
- **It is important to distinguish these from storage symptoms**, which include frequency, nocturia, urgency and dysuria. Although storage symptoms may result from bladder outlet obstruction, their presence should prompt investigation for a more sinister cause, e.g. carcinoma in situ of the bladder.

Hospital Surgery: Foundations in Surgical Practice, ed. Omer Aziz, Sanjay Purkayastha and Paraskevas Paraskeva. Published by Cambridge University Press. © Cambridge University Press 2009.

■ Incidence

Obstructive urinary symptoms are far more common in men by virtue of benign prostatic hyperplasia (BPH). Incidence and therefore prevalence is difficult to determine, as there is no standardized definition for BPH. Histologically this is not found in males under 30 years old but is found in 88 % of 90-year-old men.

■ Aetiology

The most common causes include:

- **BPH**
- **Urethral strictures.**

Other causes include:

- Bladder neck hypertrophy
- Marked prostatitis
- Urethral calculi
- Urethral meatal stenosis
- Phimosis
- Neurogenic detrusor/sphincter dysfunction.

Prostatic carcinomas, which form in the prostatic peripheral zone, are unlikely to cause significant obstructive symptoms in isolation.

In women, causes of BOO include:

- Idiopathic urethral narrowing
- Urethral strictures
- Atrophic urethritis
- Various forms of pelvic prolapse.

■ Pathogenesis

BPH is characterized histologically by nodular glandular hyperplasia and hyperplasia of the intervening fibromuscular stroma in the peri-urethral component of the prostate.

Any insult to the urethral epithelium that results in healing by formation of scar tissue will lead to a **stricture**; common examples include urinary instrumentation, infective urethritis (typically gonorrhoea), and external trauma.

■ Symptoms

A **full history** must be taken including symptoms suggestive of UTIs/STDs and previous urological procedures. It is important to be aware of pre-existing neurological conditions.

Drug history may be relevant: many antidepressants have antimuscarinic side-effects and reduce bladder contractility.

■ Signs

Examine the prepuce and external urethral meatus and formally assess the prostatic lateral lobes on **digital rectal examination** (DRE). It is important to remember that the impalpable prostatic middle lobe influences the degree of BOO more than lateral lobes. In women urethral lesions, atrophic changes and pelvic prolapse should be excluded. Symptoms are subjective and can often go unnoticed for long periods with an insidious onset; correlation with the objective degree of BOO is therefore poor.

■ Investigation

Blood tests: FBC (raised WCC in UTI), U&E (look for obstructive uropathy). **Urine** should be sent for MC&S and cytology if there are storage symptoms or a patient is 'high-risk' for bladder cancer. An **ultrasound urodynamogram** will assess for hydronephrosis in the presence of high pressure BOO. Assessment of the distended bladder will indicate moderate to severe trabeculation with or without diverticula. Any degree of post-micturition residual volume will be recorded. Although not as accurate as **transrectal ultrasound**, an estimate of prostatic size and any significant indentation of an enlarged middle lobe can be made. The patient will be asked to void into a **uroflowmeter**; voided volumes, maximum and average flow rates and flow patterns will be quantified. More formal **videourodynamics** may be required in the assessment of neurogenic pathologies. A **flexible cystoscopy** performed under local anaesthetic can provide additional diagnostic information prior to instigation of treatment. An **ascending urethrogram** may be necessary to provide anatomical information on urethral strictures.

■ Treatment

Non-surgical treatments: α antagonists (tamsulosin, doxazosin, alfuzosin), which relax smooth muscle fibres at the level of the bladder neck and prostate. 5-α reductase inhibitors (dutasteride, finasteride) will reduce prostatic volume by approximately 30 % after a four-month period and may therefore be useful adjunctive treatment in BPH.

Surgical: bladder neck hypertrophy can be managed surgically by *endoscopic resection* or *incision* of the bladder neck. Patients with BPH who fail medical management or present with significant urinary retention may be suitable for *transurethral resection of the prostate (TURP)*. Smaller glands may only need a *transurethral incision to open up the prostatic urethra (TUIP)*, and occasionally very large glands require *open retropubic (Millins) prostatectomy*. In patients not suitable for surgery, prostatic stents, *clean intermittent self-catheterization (CISC)*, or long-term *indwelling catheterization* may be suitable alternatives. Urethral strictures can be managed according to their site, extent and severity. Options include urethral dilation, optical urethrotomy and urethroplasty. CISC is often necessary following any definitive treatment, to reduce the risk of early recurrence. Meatal stenosis can be treated with recurrent dilations or more definitive meatotomy/meatoplasty.

■ Prognosis

BPH is a progressive disease. Treatment with 5-α reductase inhibitors can reduce the incidence of acute urinary retention and the requirement for prostatectomy. α antagonists increase the rate of successful trial without catheter following an episode of urinary retention. Urethral strictures frequently recur: the best long-term results are seen with complete excision of the area of fibrosis and reconstruction (urethroplasty).

Testicular lumps and swellings

ERIK MAYER, ED ROWE AND JUSTIN VALE

The important diagnoses to make in the setting of acute testicular pain are **testicular torsion** or **testicular rupture** when there has been preceding trauma. Prompt surgical intervention is required for a satisfactory outcome.

There are multiple other scrotal pathologies which may mimic the above and thus cause diagnostic dilemma for the surgeon including (Figure 112):

- Hydrocoele
- Epididymal cyst/spermatocoele
- Testicular torsion (see Testicular pain Chapter)
- Torsion of the appendix testis (see Testicular pain chapter)
- Testicular tumour
- Epididymitis/epididymo-orchitis
- Varicocoele
- Inguinal hernia.

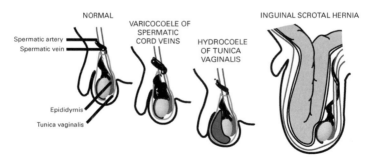

Figure 112

Hospital Surgery: Foundations in Surgical Practice, ed. Omer Aziz, Sanjay Purkayastha and Paraskevas Paraskeva. Published by Cambridge University Press.
© Cambridge University Press 2009.

■ Definitions

Hydrocoele – an abnormal accumulation of excessive serous fluid between the visceral and parietal layers of the tunica vaginalis. Four types are described (Figure 113):

- Congenital
- Infantile
- Vaginal (most common type, can either be primary or secondary)
- Hydrocoele of the cord.

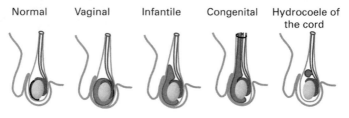

| Normal | Vaginal | Infantile | Congenital | Hydrocoele of the cord |

Figure 113

Epididymal cyst/spermatocoele – when the fluid contained within an epididymal cyst is turbid from the presence of spermatozoa, it is known as a spermatocoele.

Testicular tumour – testicular tumours can be benign or malignant and primary or secondary.

Epididymitis/epididymo-orchitis – Epididymitis is inflammation, pain and swelling of the epididymis. It may be acute or chronic (occurring for >6 weeks). Although initially the testicle may be tender, resulting from the surrounding inflammation, it is unlikely to be directly involved.

Varicocoele – an abnormal collection of dilated and tortuous veins of the pampiniform plexus of the spermatic cord.

■ Incidence

Hydrocoele is the most common benign scrotal mass and occurs in an estimated 1 % of adult males. **Epididymal cysts** are also common with

spermatocoeles accounting for 10 % of all epididymal cysts. **Testicular cancer** only accounts for 1 % of all cancers, but is the most common cancer in men 15–35 years old. A second peak in incidence occurs in late adulthood (>60 years old). Teratoma typically occurs in the third and seminoma in the fourth decades of life. **Varicocoeles** are present in 15 % of adult males and 30 % of subfertile males. 90 % are left sided.

■ Aetiology

Hydrocoele: the serous layers of the tunica vaginalis are likened to the pleural and peritoneal linings and are thus subject to the same changes. *Primary vaginal hydrocoeles* result from failure of the normal reabsorption patterns and are common in heart failure, hypoalbuminaemia, and lymphatic disturbances. *Secondary hydrocoeles* result from excessive production of serous fluid and occur with infection, tumours and torsion. *Congenital, infantile* and *encysted cord hydrocoeles* all result from total or partial abnormal occlusion of the processus vaginalis.

Epididymal cyst/spermatocoele: *epididymal cysts* result from focal epididymal degeneration whereas *spermatocoeles* represent retention cysts of the epididymis.

Testicular tumours: testicular cancer likely results from genetic and environmental factors. A known risk factor is *cryptorchidism*, which confers a 3–14 fold relative risk of developing testicular cancer in the affected testicle. *Orchidopexy* does not affect cancer risk but delivers the testicle into a position that can more easily be monitored. Other postulated risk factors include trauma, hormonal imbalances and testicular atrophy.

Epididymitis/orchitis: in children results from infection by *gram negative bacilli* often with an underlying structural defect of the urethral tract. In males up to 35 *Chlamydia trachomatis* and *Neiserria gonorrhoea* become the commonest causative organisms, and it is thus associated with urethritis. In men older than 35 years, coliforms, especially *Escherichia coli*, are usually isolated. Factors such as urethral strictures, incomplete bladder emptying, prostatitis and urinary instrumentation are additional precipitants.

Varicocoele: abnormalities in the venous drainage of the testicle likely explain the aetiology of varicocoeles, supported by the predominance of left-sided varicocoeles and the differing venous drainage from right to left. Higher left-sided venous pressures, incompetent venous valves and collateral venous anastomosis have all been postulated.

■ Pathogenesis

Testicular tumours: *germ cell tumours* e.g. seminoma, teratoma, account for 90–95 % of all primary malignant testicular tumours. *Non-germ cell tumours* are less common and include Leydig and Sertoli cell tumours. *Secondary testicular tumours* can result from lymphoma, leukaemia or granulomatous infections. *Retroperitoneal lymph node involvement* can occur with cancer restricted to the testicular parenchyma. Any involvement of epididymis or cord may result in iliac or inguinal lymph node spread.

Epididymitis/epididymo-orchitis: epididymitis is thought to result from an ascending infection from the bladder, prostate and/or urethra. Infected urine can enter the ejaculatory ducts at the level of the verumontanum and ascend via the vas deferens. There may be a causal relationship between exertion, e.g. lifting, and straining to pass urine, which further exacerbates urinary reflux into the ejaculatory ducts.

Varicocoele: this is an area of much debate, but an increasing incidence during adolescence raises the possibility of changes that occur around the time of puberty.

■ Symptoms and signs

Hydrocoeles are invariably painless accumulations of fluid and are often ignored, particularly in the elderly, until they become very large (>300 ml). There is a diffuse non-tender swelling, fluctuant in two planes, in the affected hemiscrotum. One can get above the swelling and the testicle will not be palpable separately if the hydrocoele is tense. If lax, palpation of the testicle may still be possible posterior to the fluid sac. A hydrocoele is brilliantly transilluminable. Congenital hydrocoeles associated with a patent processus vaginalis will often appear during ambulatory activity and disappear overnight.

Epididymal cyst/spermatocoeles are smooth spherical swellings often found in the head of the epididymis. They are therefore separate from the testicle and located posterior or posterosuperiorly to it. Epididymal cysts are transilluminable, whereas some spermatocoeles may not be.

Testicular tumours usually present with the finding of a testicular lump on self-examination. Typically there is no associated pain, but in 10 % of men pain can be the presenting factor. Often an episode of trauma draws attention to a pre-existing lump. In 10 % of cases, patients present with symptoms of metastatic disease. Examination will reveal a solid lump, which is not separate from the testicle. It does not transilluminate. There may be an associated secondary hydrocoele. Systems review should aim to identify evidence of metastases, such as supraclavicular or retroperitoneal lymphadenopathy.

Epididymitis/epididymo-orchitis presents with a gradual onset of pain and swelling to the affected hemiscrotum. The pain may radiate to the lower abdomen as in testicular torsion. There may be episodes of fevers and/or symptoms of urinary tract infection or a urethritis. In the early stages the epididymis will be distinguishable as a warm, swollen, tender mass posterior to the testicle. Late in the disease process the testicle may not be distinguishable and may also be tender. On DRE there may be prostatic tenderness associated with concurrent prostatitis.

Varicocoeles result in an aching pain tending to be worse after long periods of standing. The patient may also describe variability of the degree of swelling from morning to night. On examination a swelling is felt posterior to the testicle, which is separable. It is likened to a 'bag of worms'. The swelling is exacerbated by standing and manoeuvres which increase intra-abdominal pressure. Beware the left-sided varico-coele that does not disappear on lying the patient down; it may indicate obstruction at the level of the renal vein (Figure 114).

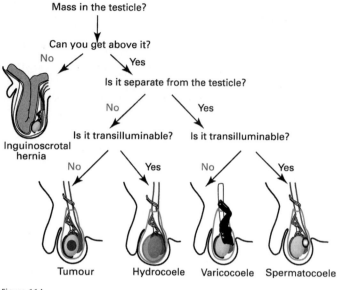

Figure 114

■ Investigation

For scrotal pathology, **ultrasound** is the best first-line investigation. It will confirm diagnoses made clinically and also exclude testicular tumours if palpation is not possible with tense hydrocoeles. Ultrasound, even with Doppler flow studies, should not be relied on in confirming or excluding a testicular torsion, where the need for surgical exploration remains a clinical decision. Investigations for epididymitis should additionally include **urine MC&S** and **urethral swabs** if urethritis is suspected. With the diagnosis of a testicular tumour a **chest/abdomen/pelvis CT scan** should be arranged. Serum **tumour markers** (AFP, LDH and β-HCG) also need to be requested. Facilities for sperm storage should be available if required. All patients should be investigated appropriately as part of any preoperative optimization.

■ Treatment

Hydrocoele: surgical excision of the hydrocoele only becomes necessary if there is associated pain, or its size impinges upon daily activities or cosmesis. In patients with significant co-morbidities, simple aspiration may be all that is required to provide temporary relief. No intervention should be embarked upon until an underlying testicular tumour has been excluded.

Testicular tumours: surgical management is by means of radical orchidectomy performed via an inguinal incision. This should be performed promptly as germ cell tumours have a doubling time of 10–30 days. All patients should be offered a prosthesis. Simultaneous biopsy of the contralateral testicle should be considered. Adjuvant treatment will depend on tumour type, grade and staging investigations. Possibilities include surveillance, radiotherapy, chemotherapy or retroperitoneal lymph node dissection, alone or in combination. Treatments available for a primary tumour will dictate the management of its secondary deposits within the testicle.

Epididymal cyst/spermatocoele: treatment is by surgical excision if they become symptomatic or a nuisance to the patient. As they probably arise from the rete testis, excision may be contraindicated if fertility is to be preserved.

Epididymitis/epididymo-orchitis: antibiotic selection is guided by likely causative pathogens according to the age of the patient. A quinolone is usually a good first-line agent without knowing the causative pathogen. It is important that culture specimens are obtained prior to initiating treatment.

Varicocoele: mild and moderately symptomatic varicocoeles can be managed conservatively with advice on the use of scrotal supports. Surgical treatment options include transvenous embolization or vein ligation at varying levels performed open or laparoscopically.

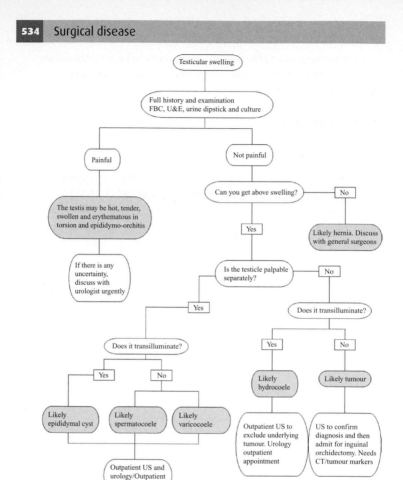

Management algorithm for patient with testicular swelling

■ Prognosis

Hydrocoele: reaccumulation of fluid is inevitable with aspiration alone and will therefore need to be repeated at risk of introduction of infection.

Testicular tumours: prognosis, like treatment, will depend on tumour type, grade and staging investigations. It is however one of the most curable solid neoplasms with five-year survival greater than 95 % even in the presence of metastases.

Varicocoele: the estimated failure rate of varicocoele surgery is 0–10 % and results from the extensive collateral network of the pampiniform plexus.

Haematuria

ED ROWE, ERIK MAYER AND JUSTIN VALE

■ Introduction

Haematuria is alarming for the patient and can be a sign of serious underlying pathology. Painless macroscopic haematuria is indicative of cancer in the urinary tract until proven otherwise after full and thorough investigation.

■ Definition and classification

The presence of blood in the urine is described as microscopic (the presence of ≥ 3 red blood cells per high power field on microscopic evaluation of urinary sediment from two of three samples), or macroscopic (frank) haematuria, and is further categorized as either painful or painless.

■ Incidence (prevalence)

The estimated prevalence of asymptomatic microscopic haematuria is between 0.19 to 16.1 %. It is reportedly higher in older screened populations (10 to 21 %). Macroscopic haematuria is less common (prevalence 2.5 %), but the chances of significant underlying pathology are up to five times greater.

■ Aetiology

Tumours of the urinary tract (renal cell carcinoma, transitional cell carcinoma) are the commonest cause. Also infection (pyelonephritis, cystitis, prostatitis); trauma, including iatrogenic injury to the kidney,

Hospital Surgery: Foundations in Surgical Practice, ed. Omer Aziz, Sanjay Purkayastha and Paraskevas Paraskeva. Published by Cambridge University Press. © Cambridge University Press 2009.

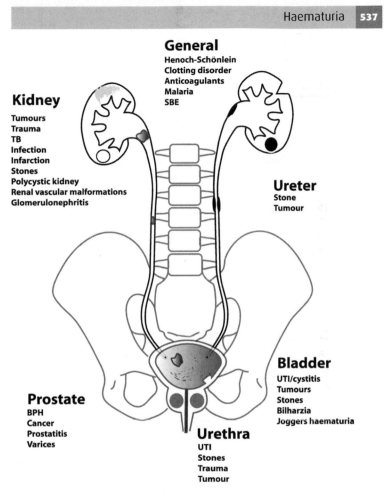

General
Henoch-Schönlein
Clotting disorder
Anticoagulants
Malaria
SBE

Kidney
Tumours
Trauma
TB
Infection
Infarction
Stones
Polycystic kidney
Renal vascular malformations
Glomerulonephritis

Ureter
Stone
Tumour

Bladder
UTI/cystitis
Tumours
Stones
Bilharzia
Joggers haematuria

Prostate
BPH
Cancer
Prostatitis
Varices

Urethra
UTI
Stones
Trauma
Tumour

Figure 115 SBE: Subacute bacterial endocarditis

ureter, bladder, and urethra; stones including staghorn calculi, ureteric calculi (see Renal colic Chapter) and bladder stones. Other causes include glomerulonephritis, papillary necrosis, Berger's disease, renal infarct, polycystic disease, bleeding diathesis and warfarin. The risk of significant underlying pathology increases with age (>40 years) and if the haematuria is macroscopic (see Figure 115).

■ Symptoms and signs

The patient may complain of macroscopic haematuria, or be found to have microscopic haematuria on urinalysis (e.g. Multistix). The timing of the blood in the urinary stream may indicate its source. Initial haematuria is suggestive of a bleed from the distal urinary tract such as the anterior urethra, while terminal haematuria usually arises from the prostatic urethra or bladder trigone. Total haematuria is suggestive of pathology above the bladder neck. The association of pain may help alert the clinician to the aetiology. A history of smoking and chemical/dye exposure (benzenes and aromatic amines) increase the risk of a neoplasm. There may be a history of urinary tract infection, irritative voiding symptoms or pelvic irradiation. On examination, the patient may be shocked and/or septic. A mass in the loin in conjunction with pain and haematuria may be part of the classic triad found in renal cell carcinoma.

Note that urine may be discoloured by conditions such porphyria, foods such as beetroot and some drugs (e.g. rifampicin). A negative test using urine dip sticks will exclude the presence of blood in the urine, but false positives are obtained with haemoglobinuria and myoglobinuria. Therefore, the presence of red blood cells on urine microscopy is most accurate (≥3 RBCs per high power field) provided the sample is examined fresh (if there is a delay to microscopy the red blood cells will lyse).

■ Investigation

FBC, U&E, clotting, group and save. Renal ultrasound, IVU, flexible cystoscopy, urine cytology and culture.

■ Treatment

Analgesia, and treat shock/sepsis if necessary. The passage of macroscopic haematuria with clots requires the insertion of a three-way irrigation catheter and bladder washout. Definitive treatment will depend on the underlying cause.

■ Prognosis

Typically a cause for bleeding is found in up to 40 % of those with macroscopic haematuria. Pathology is identified in up to 11 % of those with microscopic haematuria depending on the population.

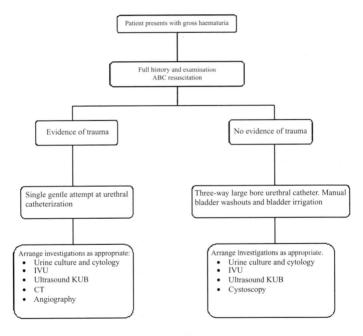

Management algorithm: haematuria

Brain tumours

ANDREAS DEMETRIADES AND JOAN GRIEVE

■ Introduction

2 % of all cancer deaths are due to brain tumours and 20 % of paediatric neoplasms are in the CNS. Overall they account for 10 % of all malignancies. Although it is difficult to generalize about all brain tumours, there are some common themes.

■ Classification

May be according to *cell origin* (see table) or *histological grading* by the World Health Organization (WHO):

■ *Grade I*: benign – growth is slow, cells are similar to normal cells and rarely spread into adjacent tissue; total excision can be curative.
■ *Grade II*: growth is slow but local spread possible. The tumour may 'transform' into higher grade.
■ *Grade III*: malignant – growth is quick, cells are pleomorphic with higher nuclear-to-cell ratio. Local spread likely.
■ *Grade IV*: highly malignant – aggressive growth with high mitotic rate.

■ Incidence

15–20 per 100 000 (primary and metastatic); 35 000 new cases per annum (USA).

20–30 % of patients with systemic cancer will have brain metastases. Gliomas 7 per 100 000; meningiomas 1.2 per 100 000. Meningiomas and pituitary adenomas slightly commoner in women. 3.6 per 100 000 children per annum have a primary brain tumour, the second commonest

Hospital Surgery: Foundations in Surgical Practice, ed. Omer Aziz, Sanjay Purkayastha and Paraskevas Paraskeva. Published by Cambridge University Press. © Cambridge University Press 2009.

cause of paediatric cancer after leukaemia, and the most prevalent solid tumour in children.

■ Aetiology

Unknown in most cases. *Developmental abnormality*: teratoma, dermoid, epidermoid, craniopharyngioma, chordoma, hamartoma, angioma, ganglioneuromas. *Hereditary*: haemangioblastoma in von Hippel-Lindau disease; meningiomas and acoustic neuromas in neurofibromatosis; astrocytomas in tuberous sclerosis. *Immunosuppression*: lymphoma. *Radiation*: meningioma, sarcoma, glioblastoma.

■ Symptoms

Benign slow growing tumours may reach large size without causing significant symptoms. Onset of symptoms is normally gradual, but acute deterioration may result from intratumoural bleeding or obstructive hydrocephalus. *Headache* (54 %): classically early morning and exacerbated by cough or straining; often associated with nausea, vomiting and drowsiness; due to raised intracranial pressure; beware change in pattern or new onset in adults. *Seizures* (26 %): may be focal or generalized; a tumour must be excluded in adults first presenting with seizures. *Focal symptoms* (68 %) include weakness, ataxia, visual disturbance, dysphasia or dysarthria.

■ Signs

Focal neurological deficit that may localize as follows:

- Bitemporal hemianopia in pituitary adenomas
- Anosmia in frontal tumours
- Homonymous hemianopia in occipital tumours
- Ataxia, incoordination, nystagmus with cerebellar tumours
- Unilateral deafness with involvement of the facial, vestibular and cochlear nerves in cerebello-pontine angle tumours.

False localizing signs include diplopia from sixth nerve palsy and may occur with raised ICP. *Papilloedema* suggests long-standing raised ICP (>1 week).

■ Investigation

Skull X-rays generally not useful but can demonstrate hyperostosis associated with meningiomas, enlarged sella with pituitary tumours, lytic lesions (metastases). *CT* is 80–90 % accurate. *MRI* gives clearer anatomical definition and differentiates between tumour (T1) and oedema effect (T2). Pre- and post-contrast T1 images show blood-brain-barrier breakdown. *Angiography* helps illustrate the vascular supply of tumours, especially at the skull base, and may allow selective preoperative embolization. *MR spectroscopy* and *PET* are still experimental.

Tissue type	Tumour	
Neuroepithelial	**Gliomas**	Astrocytoma, oligodendroglioma, ependymoma,glioblastoma multiforme (GBM),choroid plexus papilloma/carcinoma
	Embryonal/ neuronal tumours	Medulloblastoma, ganglioglioma, gangliocytoma,primitive neuroectodermal tumour (PNET)
	Pineal tumours	Germ cell tumour, germinoma, pineoblastoma,pineocytoma
	Nerve sheath tumours	Schwannoma, neurofibroma, nerve sheath tumour
Meninges	Meningiomas, meningeal sarcomas	
Adenohypophysis	Pituitary adenoma/carcinoma	
Teratoid and other	Teratoma, dermoid, epidermoid, craniopharyngioma, chordoma, lymphoma, colloid cyst	
Blood vessel origin	Haemangioblastoma, glomus jugulare	
Metastatic	Breast, lung, kidney, skin (melanoma), colon	

■ Management

Dexamethasone (4 mg qds) with gastric protection. Can help with symptomatic control and reduce surrounding oedema. Indications for *surgery* include: histological diagnosis, cure, tumour debulking (volume reduction) to treat raised ICP, and local delivery of chemotherapeutic agents (e.g. carmustine). The type of operation depends on likely histological cell type, tumour location and the patient's age and functional status. Surgery ranges from biopsy (open or stereotactic) through to craniotomy and debulking and full resection. *Radiotherapy* may be whole brain (fractionated) or stereotactic (radiosurgery) using gamma knife, linac (linear accelerator) or Bragg peak. With regards to *chemotherapy*, new trials are in progress and this is an ever-evolving area.

■ Prognosis

Surgical procedures: mortality for craniotomy and stereotactic biopsy is similar (1 %) but morbidity doubles with the former (10 % vs. 5 %). *Postoperative complications:* seizures, stroke, intratumoural haemorrhage, subdural or extradural haematoma, tumour bed swelling, systemic complications. Age: <45 have four times higher expected survival than >65 year olds with same grade tumour. But, the leading cause of death in oncology patients younger than 35 years old. *Performance status:* Karnofsky performance score of 100 is better prognostically than <65. *Histological prognosis is as follows:*

WHO GRADE

- Patients with high grade tumours (III and IV) have far lower expected survival than those with low grade (I and II).
- WHO Grade I tumours: complete resection can be curative.

CELL TYPE

- Glioma: median survival rates with GBM are 1.5–3 months (no treatment) vs. 3–4 months (surgery) vs. 9–10 months (surgery + RTX (radiotherapy)) vs. 9 months (biopsy + radiotherapy) vs. 9–11 months (surgery + radiotherapy + chemotherapy).
- Metastases: complete resection of all intra-cranial metastases can improve symptom-free survival.

Hydrocephalus

ANDREAS DEMETRIADES AND JOAN GRIEVE

■ Definition

Hydrocephalus (HC) is a hydrodynamic disorder of CSF due to a disturbance of formation, flow or absorption of CSF that leads to an increase in volume occupied by this fluid within CNS. (Note: increased CSF volume also observed in cerebral atrophy but this is not due to a hydrodynamic disorder, but a passive filling of the increased vacant space; hence the old term *'hydrocephalus ex vacuo'*.)

■ Classification

Functional:

1. *Obstructive* or *non-communicating*: block is proximal to arachnoid granulations with an obstruction of CSF flow in the ventricular system or its outlets to the subarachnoid space.
2. *Communicating*: full communication exists between the ventricles and subarachnoid space with CSF circulation blocked at level of arachnoid granulations. Causes: decreased CSF absorption, venous drainage insufficiency, or CSF overproduction (rare).

Alternative classifications:

1. *Acute* (over days) / *subacute* (weeks) / *chronic* (months or years).
2. *Congenital* or *acquired*.
3. *Arrested HC*: stabilization of known ventricular enlargement after compensation. These patients are prone to decompensation, e.g. with a minor head injury.

Hospital Surgery: Foundations in Surgical Practice, ed. Omer Aziz, Sanjay Purkayastha and Paraskevas Paraskeva. Published by Cambridge University Press. © Cambridge University Press 2009.

4. *Normal pressure hydrocephalus (NPH):* a triad of dementia, abnormal gait, and urinary incontinence, in the absence of papilloedema and in the presence of normal CSF pressures on lumbar puncture.

Incidence: 3/1000 live births with congenital HC. Incidence of acquired HC unknown, but about 100 000 V-P (ventriculo-peritoneal) shunts performed in developed countries per annum.

Gender: M:F=1:1. In *NPH M>F*. X-linked HC in Bickers-Adams syndrome.

Age: bi-modal age curve with peaks in infancy and adulthood (40 %).

■ Aetiology

Congenital: Sylvian aqueduct stenosis (10 %); Dandy-Walker malformation (2–4 %); Arnold-Chiari malformation (ACM) Types I and II; congenital toxoplasmosis; foramen of Monro agenesis; Bickers-Adams syndrome (7 % males – aqueduct stenosis, mental retardation, thumb deformity).

Acquired:

1. *Infectious*: most common cause of communicating HC. Caused by meningitis (bacterial or viral), cysticercosis, toxoplasmosis, cryptococcus.
2. *Post-haemorrhagic*: subarachnoid haemorrhage (in up to 30 %), intraventricular haemorrhage, trauma.
3. *Space occupying lesion (SOL):* non-neoplastic (abscess, haematoma, vascular malformation). Neoplastic (colloid cyst, astrocytoma, medulloblastoma, ependymoma, giant cell astrocytoma, choroid plexus papilloma, craniopharyngioma, pituitary adenoma, hypothalamic or optic nerve glioma, hamartoma, metastases).
4. *Postoperative.*
5. *Increased venous sinus pressure* (in craniosysnostosis, achondroplasia, venous thrombosis).
6. *Iatrogenic*, e.g. hypervitaminosis A.
7. *Idiopathic.*

■ Pathophysiology

Normal CSF production is 0.3–0.35 ml/min, produced by the choroid plexus (Figure 116). Total adult CSF volume is 150 ml. Normal CSF route:

1. Choroid plexus
2. Lateral ventricle
3. Interventricular foramen of Monro
4. Third ventricle
5. Sylvian aqueduct
6. Fourth ventricle
7. Two lateral foramina of Luschka and midline foramen of Magendie
8. Subarachnoid space
9. Arachnoid granulations
10. Dural sinus
11. Venous drainage.

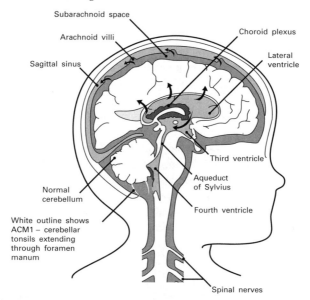

Figure 116

When production exceeds absorption, ICP rises. This causes a drop in CSF production. Temporal and frontal horns of lateral ventricles dilate first.

■ Symptoms and signs

These depend on age, aetiology, location of obstruction, duration and speed of onset.

Infants	Children	Adults	NPH
Irritability	Reduced mental capacity	Cognitive decline	Gait disturbance (may precede other symptoms by months)
Reduced activity	Morning headaches	Morning headaches	Dementia
Poor feeding	Vomiting	Nausea and vomiting	Urinary incontinence
Vomiting	Blurred vision	Blurred vision	Parkinsonism
Lethargy	Double vision Neck pain (tonsillar herniation) Stunted growth (third ventricle dilation and pituitary pressure) Gait disturbance Lethargy	Double vision Neck pain Incontinence Lethargy	Aggressive behaviour

Signs			
Infants	Children	Adults	NPH
Head circumference > 98th percentile	Papilloedema or optic atrophy	Papilloedema or optic atrophy	Normal strength
Suture diastasis	Unsteady gait	Truncal and limb ataxia	Ataxia with short steps like Parkinsonism, inability to tandem walk *(cont.)*

Infants	Children	Adults	NPH
Dilated scalp veins	Large head, despite closed sutures	Large head (if since childhood)	Hyperreflexia, including Babinski
Tense fontanelle	Unilateral or bilateral sixth nerve palsy	Unilateral or bilateral sixth nerve palsy	Sucking and grasping reflexes in late stages
Sunset eyes	Upward gaze failure, Parinaud's syndrome (pressure on tectal plate)	Failure of upward gaze	
Hypertonicity or spasticity	Macewen's sign (crackpot sound on head percussion)	Spasticity	

■ Investigations

In preparation for operative shunting: blood tests: general tests (FBC, U&E, LFTs, CRP, glucose, clotting, G&S). Infection screen and inflammatory markers when infection suspected as the cause of hydrocephalus.

In cases of suspected shunt malfunction: exclude other causes of symptoms, particularly in children (WBC, ESR, CRP, blood cultures, CXR, urine dipstick and MSU, stool culture). Exclude infection as a cause of shunt blockage (CSF gram stain and culture; NB not in cases of obstructive hydrocephalus unless obtained direct from shunt proximal reservoir).

Imaging: *CT* for ventricular size, differentiation between communicating and non-communicating HC, presence of obstructive lesion. Comparison with previous imaging useful. *MRI* for Chiari malformation or tumours. *USS* through anterior fontanelle in infants for IVH or subependymal haemorrhage. *Shunt series of radiographs* (lateral skull, CXR, AXR) may show disconnection.

LP (lumbar puncture) should only be done after a CT: Opening pressure should normally be <18 cm H_2O. In marginal cases, CSF pressure monitoring may be used to assess likelihood of need or response to shunting.

■ Treatment

Conservative treatment is not effective long term. Acetazolamide decreases CSF secretion by choroid plexus in infants.

Repeated LP in HC after intraventricular haemorrhage may allow resolution, but only indicated in communicating HC.

Surgery is the mainstay of treatment with the following options:

1. *CSF shunting*: from the ventricles into most commonly the peritoneum (Figure 117), but also pleura. From lumbar canal to peritoneum in communicating HC (complications include over drainage, under drainage, blockage, infection).

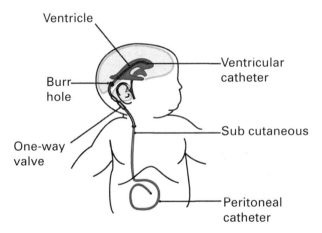

Ventricle

Burr hole

One-way valve

Ventricular catheter

Sub cutaneous

Peritoneal catheter

Figure 117

2. *Endoscopic third ventriculostomy* is being increasingly used in obstructive HC and obviates the need for shunting.
3. *Direct surgical removal of obstructive SOL.*
4. *Emergency treatment* in rapid onset HC: ventricular tap (infants); external ventricular drainage; lumbar puncture (post-haemorrhagic or meningitic HC); shunting.

■ Prognosis

Long-term outcome relates to cause of HC. 50 % of infants with IVH need lifelong shunting compared to 20 % of children after excision of posterior fossa tumour. Shunt malfunction rate in first year in paediatric population is 17 %. In NPH response is better if gait disturbance was the first symptom.

Spinal cord injury

ANDREAS DEMETRIADES AND JOAN GRIEVE

Spinal cord injury (SCI) involves an insult to the spinal cord with resultant disturbance in motor, sensory or autonomic function which may be temporary or permanent.

■ Important definitions

Paresis: partial loss of power; weakness.

Plegia: total loss of power; paralysis.

Myelopathy: caused by damage to the spinal cord, which ends at L1.

Radiculopathy: damage/compression to nerve roots with symptoms in the distribution of the root.

Tetraplegia or quadriplegia: injury involving all four limbs.

Monoplegia: of one limb.

Paraplegia: bilateral lower-limb involvement.

Neurogenic shock: triad of hypotension, hypothermia and bradycardia due to interruption of sympathetic nervous system input (T1–L3) with unopposed vagal input. Note: hypovolaemic shock causes *tachy*cardia.

Spinal shock: a transient physiological reflex with depression of spinal cord function associated with loss of all motor and sensory function, including reflexes and anal tone, below the level of injury. Catecholamine release will lead to a transient hypertension, followed by hypotension and accompanied by flaccid paralysis, double incontinence and priapism. Duration may be hours to days until function returns to the reflex arcs below the injury level.

Hospital Surgery: Foundations in Surgical Practice, ed. Omer Aziz, Sanjay Purkayastha and Paraskevas Paraskeva. Published by Cambridge University Press. © Cambridge University Press 2009.

■ Classification

ASIA (American Spinal Injury Association) impairment scale: A (complete motor and sensory loss including S4–5); B (incomplete: sensory but no motor function preserved below injury); C (incomplete: motor function preserved below injury with power < 3); D (incomplete: motor function preserved below injury with power ≥ 3); E (normal). An incomplete lesion may progress to a complete lesion and vice versa. The clinical level of injury may worsen due to developing oedema and ischaemia.

  MRC (Medical Research Council) grading of motor strength: 5 normal power; 4 power against resistance but reduced; 3 antigravity power; 2 movement with gravity eliminated; 1 flicker of movement; 0 no movement.

■ Incidence

Traumatic SCI is commoner in the under forties with >50 % of injuries occurring in the 16–30 age group; non-traumatic SCI is more common in the over forties. Traumatic SCI affects 30–60 new cases per million population per annum; the prevalence is estimated at 800 cases per million population in the US. M:F ratio is 4:1. Commonest levels of injury are C4, C5, and C6. SCIWORA (spinal cord injury without radiological abnormality) is commoner in children.

■ Aetiology

Trauma: road traffic accidents (45 %), falls, violence (blunt or penetrating injuries), sports e.g. diving.

Tumours: direct involvement of neural structures or compressive from neighbouring bone (primary or secondary; intramedullary or extramedullary; intradural or extradural).

Degenerative: (cervical spondylosis, disk prolapse, canal stenosis).

Inflammatory: (e.g. rheumatoid arthritis).

Infective: (e.g. vertebral osteomyelitis or intraspinal abscess; *Staphylococcus, Streptococcus, E. coli*, TB).

Vascular (haemorrhagic or ischaemic).

■ History

It is important to acertain: (1) Mechanism of injury, (2) Length of symptoms, (3) Rapidity of symptom progression, and (4) Co-morbidity including medication.

■ Examination and assessment

- In traumatic SCI, immobilize neck in neutral position with hard collar, sandbags and tape. Four-person lift for transfer.
- Assessment should start with a primary survey according to ATLS protocol. Consider a spinal injury in all head injuries, trauma, falls.
- Remember: airway *and C-spine control*. Intubation if necessary in the neutral neck position (fibre-optic). Careful suction, as oropharyngeal stimulation will cause bradyarrhythmia.
- Assessment of breathing in SCI is essential: pallor, cyanosis, respiratory rate, chest wall expansion, abdominal wall movement, increased accessory muscle use, agitation from poor oxygenation. Check saturations and arterial blood gases.
- Respiratory compromise caused by a high cervical SCI may be made worse by associated decreased central respiratory drive (head injury, drugs or alcohol).
- Differentiate between haemorrhagic and neurogenic shock. Hypotension or shock with an injury below T6 is haemorrhagic until proven otherwise. Haemorrhagic shock with an injury above T6 may be falsely attributed as neurogenic due to the associated sympathetic disturbance preventing tachycardia and vasoconstriction. If haemorrhagic, treat shock and cause appropriately. If neurogenic, start fluid resuscitation with isotonic crystalloid, aiming at SBP 100 mmHg and a pulse of 60–100. Atropine for bradycardia.
- Log roll all patients.
- As part of the secondary survey do a full neurological examination, considering a concurrent head injury.
- Assess motor and sensory function according to myotomes and dermatomes (Figure 118). Distinguish between a complete and

incomplete SCI; important prognostically. The only preservation in an incomplete SCI might be sacral sparing – remember to assess the perineum.

- Deep tendon reflexes.
- Ileus is common – insert a nasogastric tube to prevent aspiration pneumonia.
- Catheterize and monitor urine output.
- Prevent pressure-sores.

RED FLAGS suggesting a serious spinal condition		
History	Presenting complaint	Examination
Cancer	Predilection for haemorrhage	Anal sphincter weakness
Unexplained weight loss	New onset back pain in older patient	Perineal/perianal sensory loss
Fever, recent infection	Pain when supine or at night	Major motor weakness in legs
Immunosuppression	Major trauma	Fever
Intravenous drug abuse	Minor trauma in elderly	Pulsatile abdominal mass
Metabolic bone disorder	Saddle anaesthesia	Raised inflammatory markers
Young or advanced age	Recent bladder or bowel dysfunction	Neurologic deficit not attributable to a monoradiculopathy
	Bilateral radiculopathy Severe or progressive motor and sensory deficit	

■ Investigation

FBC, U&E, LFTs, clotting, CRP (ESR if suspecting infection or abscess); bone profile and PSA (if suspecting malignancy). Electrophoresis of serum and urine for light chains for multiple myeloma.

■ Imaging

Standard radiographs: C-spine AP, lateral and odontoid peg views. The C7-T1 junction must be adequately visualized. If not, Swimmer's view or CT is recommended. Thoracic spine AP and lateral views with special attention at T-L junction. Dynamic flexion/extension views for ligamentous injury in the absence of C-spine fracture. Three normal view C-spine X-rays and dynamic flexion/extension views has >99 % negative predictive value. In bullet penetrating injuries X-rays are most useful as CT may have a lot of artefact, while MRI may be impossible due to foreign body metallic content.

CT scan with coronal and sagittal 3D reconstructions indicated if X-rays inadequate or suspicious of an abnormality.

MRI scan is the investigation of choice for spinal cord lesions, ligamentous injuries and non-bony lesions like haematoma, tumour, abscess, disk prolapse, oedema and contusion.

■ Management

- Treatment of associated life-threatening injuries.
- *Steroids in traumatic SCI* is controversial. Check local policy. The NASCIS studies recommend that methylprednisolone is given within 3 hours of traumatic SCI for 24 hours (30 mg/kg bolus over 15 minutes and an infusion of methylprednisolone at 5.4 mg/kg/hr for 23 hours beginning 45 minutes after the bolus) or for 48 hours if given between 3–8 hours of injury.
- Careful monitoring. Beware of a delayed deterioration in ventilation from cord ischaemia or oedema particularly with mid to high cervical injuries.
- After stabilization and imaging, discuss with neurosurgery/ orthopaedics.

■ Prognosis

In traumatic SCI 10–20 % will not make it to hospital and 3 % will die in hospital. Death is mainly from pneumonia, cardiorespiratory disease or septicaemia. Complete SCI has <5 % chance of recovery. In incomplete SCI there is a 50 % chance that the patient will walk if some sensory function is preserved. Five-year survival in quadriplegics is >90 % with 90 % returning home and regaining independence (Figure 119).

Table summarizing spinal neural tracts

Position in cord	Tract haem	Direction	Spinal arterial supply	Decussation	Associated deficit
Posterior	Dorsal columns	Ascending	Posterior	Medulla	Ipsilateral vibration, proprioception, light touch
Lateral	Lateral (pyramidal) corticospinal	Descending	Anterior	Medulla	Ipsilateral weakness
Lateral	Lateral spinothalamic	Ascending	Anterior	Within 3 segments of origin	Contralateral loss of pain and temperature
Anterior	Anterior corticospinal	Descending	Anterior	Within same segment	Contralateral weakness
Anterior	Anterior spinothalamic	Ascending	Anterior	Within 3 segments of origin	Contralateral light touch

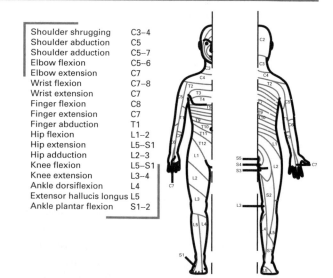

Shoulder shrugging	C3–4
Shoulder abduction	C5
Shoulder adduction	C5–7
Elbow flexion	C5–6
Elbow extension	C7
Wrist flexion	C7–8
Wrist extension	C7
Finger flexion	C8
Finger extension	C7
Finger abduction	T1
Hip flexion	L1–2
Hip extension	L5–S1
Hip adduction	L2–3
Knee flexion	L5–S1
Knee extension	L3–4
Ankle dorsiflexion	L4
Extensor hallucis longus	L5
Ankle plantar flexion	S1–2

Figure 118 Key myotomes and key dermatomes

Central cord syndrome	Associated with cervical injuries, giving greater upper limb motor weakness than in the lower limbs. Distal weakness is more than proximal. Variable sensory loss but pain and temperature more commonly affected than vibration and proprioception. Upper limb dysaesthesia and sacral sparing common.	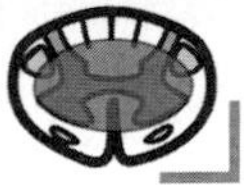
Anterior cord syndrome	Variable motor weakness and pain/temperature sensory loss, with preservation of vibration and proprioception.	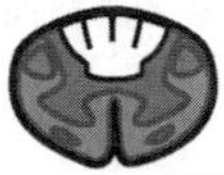
Brown-Sequard syndrome	Greater ipsilateral weakness and proprioceptive loss, with contralateral loss of pain and temperature, due to a hemisection of the cord.	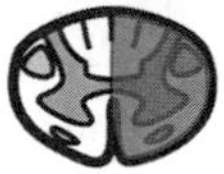
Conus medullaris syndrome	An injury to the sacral elements of the spinal canal with or without lumbar nerve root injury, causing areflexic bladder, bowel and lower limbs. Variable motor and sensory loss in the legs.	N/A
Cauda equina syndrome	Often from a central lumbosacral disc herniation. Damage to the lumbosacral nerve roots in the spinal canal leading to an areflexic bladder and/or bowel with variable lower limb motor and sensory loss. As this is a nerve root injury and not a true SCI, the affected limbs have no reflexes.	N/A
Spinal cord concussion	Transient neurological deficit that fully recovers without structural damage.	N/A

Figure 119

Superficial swellings and skin lesions

OMER AZIZ

■ Approach to examining a lump

INSPECTION – assess the following:

- **Site**
- **Size** (width, length and depth)
- **Shape** (e.g. spherical)
- **Surface** (irregular vs. smooth)
- **Skin changes** (including discolouration, ulceration and tethering)
- **Scars** (indicating previous surgery).

PALPATION

- **Edge** (well-defined vs. diffuse)
- **Consistency** (soft, firm, hard)
- **Fluctuance** (if two areas on the opposite end of a lump bulge when a third area is compressed). This is best elicited by placing thumb and index finger either side of lump and compressing it with the index finger of the other hand)
- **Compressability** (if the lump disappears and then reforms)
- **Reducibility** (a characteristic of hernia)
- **Cough impulse** (a key characteristic of hernia)
- **Pulsatility** (implies that the lump lies adjacent to an artery). If it is **expansile** (can be felt by placing a hand either side of the lump), this suggests the presence of an aneurysm
- **Layer of origin** (e.g. skin, fat, muscle, bone)

Hospital Surgery: Foundations in Surgical Practice, ed. Omer Aziz, Sanjay Purkayastha and Paraskevas Paraskeva. Published by Cambridge University Press. © Cambridge University Press 2009.

- **Tethering**
- **Fixity** (whether it is attached to a deeper structure. Fixity to muscle can be demonstrated by contracting the underlying muscle and seeing the effect this has on its mobility)
- **Regional lymph nodes**.

AUSCULTATION

- **Bruits**
- **Bowel sounds**.

OTHER

- **Transillumination** (transmission of light through the swelling suggests a fluid content).

■ Approach to examining an ulcer

INSPECTION – assess the following:

- **Site** (e.g. venous ulcers commonly found in the gaiter area around the medial malleolus; neuropathic ulcers on pressure-bearing points of foot; ischaemic ulcers are found peripherally and also on pressure points)
- **Size** (width, length and depth)
- **Shape**
- **Depth** (superficial, full thickness, soft tissues and tendons, bone)
- **Edge** (see Figure 120)

    Punched out – rapid skin death such as in neuropathic, vascular and syphilitic ulcers

    Everted – edge of ulcer grows rapidly onto the skin surface such as in squamous cell carcinomas

    Undermined – commonly occur with infections such as TB

    Sloping – commonly with venous ulcers that are healing

    Rolled – indicates a slow growing ulcer edge as with basal cell carcinoma

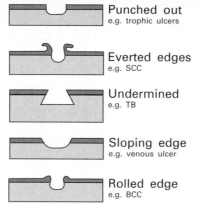

Punched out
e.g. trophic ulcers

Everted edges
e.g. SCC

Undermined
e.g. TB

Sloping edge
e.g. venous ulcer

Rolled edge
e.g. BCC

Figure 120

- **Base** (healthy, sloughed, necrotic, pale/avascular)
- **Surrounding tissues**.

PALPATION

- **Temperature**
- **Capillary refill**
- **Peripheral pulses**.

OTHER

- **Peripheral vascular examination**
- **Neurological examination**.

■ Benign lesions

Lipoma – a benign slow-growing fatty tissue tumour that may be found on almost any part of the body. Usually soft and relatively moveable, they consist of fat cells that have clustered and become distended. Generally painless and not noticed until they reach a certain size. Malignant transformation is rare. Dercum's disease is afamilial lipomatosis syndrome.

Freckle – normal number of melanocytes in normal position producing excess melanin.

Lentigo – increased number of melanocytes in normal position producing excess melanin.

Pigmented naevus (mole) – increased number of melanocytes in abnormal position producing excess melanin. May have varying degrees of dysplasia (mild/moderate/severe).

Sebaceous cyst – (trichilemmal cyst) is more correctly called an epidermal cyst. This is a subcutaneous cyst with a lining resembling the uppermost part (infundibulum) of a hair follicle. The cyst contains *sebum*, a fatty, white, semi-solid material produced by sebaceous glands in the epidermis. These are commonly found on the scalp but may occur on any hair-bearing skin. May possess a punctum or overlying opening onto the skin, and may also become infected.

Neurofibroma – a benign nerve sheath tumour with both ectodermal and mesodermal components. Often present as multiple painless lumps. Occur in neurofibromatosis (Von Recklinghausen's disease).

Pyogenic granuloma – raised, shiny, well-defined nodule arising from skin. Neither pyogenic nor a granuloma, this is an overgrowth of granulation tissue. Commonly gingival in pregnant women (lips and gums), and found on hands and face where trauma may precipitate them.

Dermatofibroma – a round, brownish to purple growth commonly found on the legs and arms. Benign neoplasm of dermal fibroblasts.

Dermoid cyst – a teratoma containing developmentally mature skin, with hair follicles and sweat glands. May also contain fat, bone, nails, teeth and cartilage. May be congenital (*inclusion dermoids* occur at sites of fusion of skin dermatomes such as lateral and medial eyebrow, midline of nose and midline of neck) or acquired (*implantation dermoids* occur in areas with repeated trauma, such as fingers).

Haemangioma – an abnormal proliferation of vascular networks. Represents a type of *hamartoma* (increased number of normal cells in their normal location). Examples include *strawberry naevus, spider naevi* and *port wine stain.*

Papilloma – a benign epithelial tumour involving overgrowth of all layers of skin.

Seborrhoeic keratosis – resemble flattened or raised warty lesions, ranging from pink or yellow through brown and black.

Warts – 'cauliflower'-like skin lesions commonly found on hands or feet. Caused by human papillomavirus (HPV) infection and contagious on contact.

Hypertrophic scars – excessive fibrous tissue response during healing resulting in a more prominent scar. The fibrosis is confined to the scar and is not progressive.

Keloid scars – excessive fibrous tissue response during healing that extends beyond the wound and into normal tissues, continuing to grow for long periods after the wound has healed. More common with pigmented skin, a family history, and in patients with previous keloid scars.

■ Premalignant skin lesions

Solar keratosis – 'squamous cell carcinoma in situ'. Precancerous skin lesion found on sun-exposed parts of the body. Often start off as small reddish-brown patches ranging in size from a few millimetres to a few centimetres in diameter. Rapidly growing.

Bowen's disease – 'carcinoma in situ'. A gradually enlarging, well demarcated erythematous plaque with an irregular border and surface crusting.

Keratoacanthoma – overgrowth of hair follicle cells with a central keratin plug. Also known as adenoma sebaceum and found on sun-exposed regions of the body. A premalignant condition predisposing to squamous cell carcinoma.

■ Malignant skin lesions

Basal cell carcinoma – a common type of slow-growing skin cancer.

Incidence – most common skin cancer, seen in lighter-skinned people, more common with increasing age and male sex (M:F = 2:1).

Aetiology – acquired: sunlight, X-rays, immunosuppression; congenital: BC naevus syndrome.

Clinical presentation – pearly raised lesions with rolled edges and over-lying fine blood vessels. May have central ulceration and occur most commonly on the face (90 % above a line joining the angle of the mouth to external auditory meatus).

Treatment – excision has excellent results. If large may have radiotherapy.

Prognosis – rarely metastasizes and spreads by local growth and infiltration ('rodent ulcer').

Squamous cell carcinoma – common invasive skin cancer that metastasizes.

Incidence – increases with age and more common in men. Mainly on sun-exposed areas of the body (face and hands).

Aetiology – sunlight, X-Rays, tar/soot exposure, immunosuppressants, chronic ulcers undergoing malignant transformation (Marjolin's ulcer), Bowen's disease, solar keratosis.

Clinical presentation – typically an ulcer with raised everted edge and a central scab.

Treatment – wide surgical excision +/– radiotherapy. Nodal spread may be treated with block dissection +/– radiotherapy.

Prognosis – higher local recurrence rate than basal cell carcinoma (BCC). Metastasizes in 5 %.

Malignant melanoma – a highly invasive malignant tumour of melanocytes with high potential for metastatic spread.

Incidence – 1/10 000 in UK, 4/10 000 in Australia. More common in fair-skinned people, but do occur in people with dark skin.

Aetiology – sunlight exposure, sun-bed use (UVA and UVB). May have familial inheritance.

Types – superficial spreading, nodular, lentigo maligna and acral lentiginous.

Clinical presentation – may occur de novo or in pre-existing moles. Signs to look out for include: (1) Rapid change in size, (2) Bleeding,

(3) Itching, (4) Pain, (5) Ulceration, (6) Change in pigmentation, (7) Presence of nodules, (8) Lymph node spread.

Treatment – surgical excision +/– reconstructive surgery. Lymph node dissection and radiotherapy. Isolated limb perfusion. Need specialist referral and must be discussed at MDT meeting.

Prognosis – Clark level and Breslow thickness determine prognosis. AJCC/UICC system is used for staging.

The cancer multidisciplinary team

TESS CANN AND SUSAN CLEATOR

■ The origins of the site-specific cancer multidisciplinary team

- In 1991 the UK Department of Health consultative document '*The Health of the Nation*' concluded that cancer accounted for 25 % of all deaths, and that death and ill health from cancer should be reduced.

- In 1995 the *Calman-Hine report* took this further, setting out that 'all patients should have access to a uniformly high quality of care . . . wherever they may live.' This was the origin of the term 'post-code lottery' in relation to cancer care.

- In 1997 the NICE Clinical Outcomes Guidelines (COG) for colorectal cancer suggested that there were 'significant variations both in process and outcomes of colorectal cancer care across the country' recommending that treatment of cancers should be carried out by 'a coordinated team with particular interest and expertise in this field'.

- In 2000, the NHS Cancer Plan was published, stating that 'every patient diagnosed with cancer will benefit from pre-planned care' and that this care should be 'delivered by specialist teams in line with evidence on best practice'.

The cancer multidisciplinary team aims to bring together cancer diagnosticians and those involved in cancer treatment and patient support to discuss the diagnostics and all aspects of care of each cancer patient.

Hospital Surgery: Foundations in Surgical Practice, ed. Omer Aziz, Sanjay Purkayastha and Paraskevas Paraskeva. Published by Cambridge University Press. © Cambridge University Press 2009.

Specific responsibilities of the multidisciplinary team (MDT) are to:

- Agree appropriate membership and ensure attendance.
- Develop systems that collect and present all the relevant information needed for decision making.
- Ensure that the care of every cancer patient is discussed at MDT meetings.
- Record the decisions that are made.
- Disseminate that decision to relevant individuals and departments.
- Ensure a rapid referral process between members of the MDT.
- Ensure all patients' needs are addressed, i.e. nutrition, palliative care.
- Capture information for audit and research and improve recruitment into clinical trials.
- Aid compliance with National Cancer Wait targets.

As cancer MDTs have developed, they have gone on to:

- Agree evidence-based protocols for care delivery.
- Use MDTs to discuss more complex cases that fall outside protocols.
- Monitor outcomes information and use this to further refine care.
- Redesign roles and care pathways.

■ Members of the cancer multidisciplinary team

Membership is divided into core and extended members, led by a lead clinician from any medical specialty. An example of membership of a colorectal MDT is highlighted below. Each member also has specific cover.

Core team members	Extended team members
Lead surgeon	Representatives from other tumour site MDTs (e.g. liver, lung)
Oncologist	MRI radiologist
Gastroenterologist/endoscopist	Research trials coordinator
Radiologist	Dietician
Histopathologist	Clinical geneticist
Colorectal nurse	Benefits advisor
Stoma care nurse	Social worker
MDT coordinator	
Palliative care team	

■ Recommendations for setting up MDT meeting

- A dedicated MDT facility with projection system to display histopathological slides and imaging, ideally with a workstation to download scans in-house and from referring trusts.
- Robust systems to ensure collection and presentation of all relevant information prior to the meeting, to minimize multiple discussions and ensure effective decision making.
- Adequate preparation so the meeting runs efficiently and promotes good attendance.

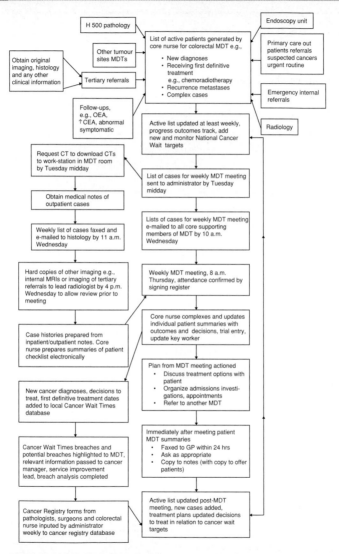

An overview of the organization and process supporting a cancer MDT: example, colorectal

Tumour types

EMMA J. ALEXANDER AND SUSAN CLEATOR

Tumours can be classified as *benign* or *malignant*. Benign tumours are slow growing, retain normal cell morphology and do not invade tissue or metastasize. They tend not to cause damage to neighbouring structures unless compressive in nature, secondary to being large, or in a critical site e.g. brain, spinal cord. The cardinal characteristics of malignant tumours are their ability to invade and metastasize.

If a malignant tumour remains localized, surgery is the mainstay of curative treatment. Radiotherapy and chemotherapy can be added to reduce the risk of recurrence. If a tumour has metastasized, treatment typically consists of chemotherapy and radiotherapy and, except in the case of highly treatment-sensitive cancers such as testicular and lymphomatous cancers, treatment is palliative.

Benign	Malignant
Well circumscribed, often encapsulated	Invades surrounding tissue
Remains localized	Metastasizes via lymphatics and haematogenous routes
Slow growing (low mitotic rate)	Tends to have rapid rate of growth (high mitotic rate)
Damages surrounding tissue by pressure	Damages surrounding tissue by pressure, invasion and destruction
Well differentiated	Varying differentiation

Tumours can be divided broadly into three sites of origin: epithelial, mesenchymal and haemopoietic. Rarely, tumours can be of mixed origin. Over 80 % of tumours are epithelial in origin. Epithelial malignant tumours are generally named carcinomas and those of mesenchymal

Hospital Surgery: Foundations in Surgical Practice, ed. Omer Aziz, Sanjay Purkayastha and Paraskevas Paraskeva. Published by Cambridge University Press. © Cambridge University Press 2009.

origin, sarcomas. The table shows a classification of benign and malignant tumours according to site of origin.

■ Carcinoma in situ (CIS)

Tumours typically progress from normal cells to premalignant change, to cancer and then on to local invasion and metastatic spread. The premalignant stage is characterized by abnormal (dysplastic) cells that have not transgressed the basement membrane. If left, dysplastic cells may invade and progress to malignancy. Often carcinoma in situ (e.g. of cervix, CIS, or of breast ducts, DCIS) is actively treated to prevent progression to frank malignancy.

■ Grading

Tumours are graded by the histopathologist. This enables the surgeon and oncologist to stratify the tumour into prognostic groups to aid with tailoring of treatment according to risk of relapse. There are several ways to grade tumours. The most commonly used are the extent of differentiation and the rate of mitosis.

Benign tumours are well differentiated. They are composed of cells which closely resemble mature normal cells of the tissue of origin and are of uniform size and shape. Poorly differentiated tumours are characterized by pleomorphic cells (varying size and shape) and tend to have densely staining chromatin (hyperchromatic).

In general the growth rate of tumours correlates with their differentiation, thus malignant tumours tend to grow more rapidly than benign lesions, and undifferentiated (anaplastic) tumours tend to be very aggressive.

■ Staging

Along with tumour grading, the macroscopic size of the tumour and presence and extent of metastases are important factors to take into account when deciding treatment. A common staging system is the TNM which accounts for primary tumour size T, nodal metastases N (number and size) and presence or absence of distant metastases M. There is a TNM staging system for most cancers and these are discussed in other chapters. Patient fitness and co-morbidity also influence treatment decisions. Investigations such as CT scans, MRI and PET scans are used to clinically stage patients prior to treatment.

Tumour classification

Tumours of epithelial origin		
Tissue of origin	Benign	Malignant
Stratified squamous	Squamous papilloma	Squamous carcinoma
Glands or ducts	Adenoma Papilloma Cystadenoma	Adenocarcinoma Papillary carcinoma Cystadenocarcinoma
Neuroectoderm	Naevus	Melanoma
Renal epithelium	Renal tubule adenoma	Renal cell carcinoma
Liver cells	Liver cell adenoma	Hepatocellular carcinoma
Bile duct	Bile duct adenoma	Cholangiocarcinoma
Urothelium	Transitional cell papilloma	Transitional cell carcinoma
Placental epithelium	Hydatidform mole	Choriocarcinoma
Testicular epithelium (germ cells)	Seminoma	Embryonal carcinoma

Tumours of mesenchymal origin

Tissue of origin	Benign	Malignant
Connective tissue and derivatives	Fibroma Lipoma Osteoma	Fibrosarcoma Liposarcoma Osteosarcoma
Endothelial cells	Haemangioma	Angiosarcoma
Muscle	Leiomyoma Rhabdomyoma	Leiomyosarcoma Rhabdomyosarcoma (*cont.*)

Tissue of origin	Benign	Malignant
Mesothelium		Mesothelioma
Neural tissue	Neuroma	
		Glioma
		Astrocytoma
		Glioblastoma

Tumours of haemopoietic origin

Tissue of origin	Benign	Malignant
Lymphoid tissue		Lymphomas
Lymphocytes		Leukaemias Multiple Myeloma
Leucocytes		Leukaemias

Tumours of mixed origin

Tissue of origin	Benign	Malignant
Salivary gland	Pleomorphic adenoma	Malignant mixed salivary gland tumour
Gonadal embryonal	Mature teratoma	Immature teratoma

Principles of chemotherapy

EMMA J. ALEXANDER AND SUSAN CLEATOR

Chemotherapy is any pharmacological agent given with the intention of eradicating malignant cells, and can be given intravenously, orally and topically. It is the mainstay of treatment of germ cell tumours, lymphomas and leukaemias. It is also used with curative intent as an adjunct to surgery or radiotherapy (RTX) in many tumour types and with palliative intent in metastatic disease.

■ Systemic chemotherapy: definitions

Neoadjuvant: the use of chemotherapy prior to surgery or RTX to downstage tumour.

Adjuvant: the use of chemotherapy after surgery to eradicate micrometastases and improve overall survival.

Palliative: the use of chemotherapy to palliate symptoms and prolong the life of patients with metastatic disease.

■ Cytotoxic chemotherapy

Cytotoxic chemotherapy is relatively non-selective. It is not targeted to the tumour and damages normal cells as well as cancer cells. However, malignant cells are more sensitive to its effect because they do not have the same capacity for repair. Cytotoxic drugs predominately damage proliferating cells; malignant tumours are often rapidly growing and therefore susceptible to damage from cytotoxics. Rapidly proliferating normal tissues such as bone marrow and mucous membranes are also often affected, accounting for (some of) the common side-effects of myelosuppression and mucositis.

Hospital Surgery: Foundations in Surgical Practice, ed. Omer Aziz, Sanjay Purkayastha and Paraskevas Paraskeva. Published by Cambridge University Press. © Cambridge University Press 2009.

Cytotoxic chemotherapy drugs have a narrow therapeutic index. This means that the difference between maximum tolerated dose (MTD) and minimum effective dose (MED) tends to be small. Therefore great care is required when prescribing these drugs and patients need to be monitored carefully throughout treatment.

■ Mechanism of action of cytotoxics

Cytotoxics act at various stages of the cell cycle; different drugs work at different stages. The most common targets are:

- DNA repair – alkylating agents, e.g. cyclophosphamide.
- DNA synthesis – antimetabolites, e.g. 5-fluorouracil (5-FU), methotrexate.
- Mitosis – vinca alkaloids and taxanes, e.g. vincristine, docetaxel.

■ Combination chemotherapy

Cytotoxics are often used in different combinations to maximize cell kill and to try to overcome drug resistance. Combinations often include drugs with different mechanisms of action and non-overlapping in toxicity.

■ Assessing patients for chemotherapy

Due to the narrow therapeutic range of cytotoxic drugs, great care must be given in selecting the right patients for treatment and the right drugs to give them. Several factors need to be taken into consideration.

1. Performance status (PS) – this is a way of assessing the patient's fitness for palliative chemotherapy. There are several ways of scoring PS. Generally in the UK the ECOG classification is used (see below). Old age is not necessarily a disqualifier for chemotherapy. Generally chemotherapy is not given to patients of PS 3 or 4. Important exceptions to this would be curable tumours such as certain lymphomas.

2. Renal impairment – many chemotherapy agents or their metabolites are excreted in urine and may accumulate if there is renal impairment. Dose reductions need to be made and some drugs are best avoided even in mild renal impairment.
3. Liver impairment – many chemotherapy agents are metabolized in the liver or excreted in bile. If there is significant liver impairment some drugs may not be given.
4. Cardiac impairment – anthracyclines, e.g. doxorubicin, can cause a reduction in ejection fraction and monitoring may be necessary.
5. Bone marrow reserve – may be poor if patient has had prior radiotherapy or chemotherapy and dose adjustments may need to be made.
6. Infertility – some chemotherapy drugs may cause reduced fertility, infertility and early menopause. This may be more relevant for some patients than others.

■ Performance status: Eastern Cooperative Oncology Group (ECOG)

0 – fully active; able to carry out all activities without restriction
1 – restricted in physically strenuous activity; ambulatory and able to carry out light work
2 – ambulatory and able to carry out all self care but unable to carry out any work activities; up and about for more than 50 % of waking hours
3 – capable of only limited self care; confined to bed or chair 50 % or more of waking hours
4 – completely disabled; cannot carry out any self care; totally confined to bed or chair.

■ Common side-effects of chemotherapy

Chemotherapy side-effects are different for different drugs but may include nausea and vomiting, fatigue, mucositis, alopecia, diarrhoea, rash, allergic reactions, myelosuppression, peripheral neuropathy and renal impairment.

Febrile neutropaenia and neutropaenic sepsis is a life threatening complication of chemotherapy and a medical emergency. Neutropaenia = neutrophil count < 1.0. **Urgent action necessary**: fluid resuscitation, cultures of blood, sputum etc. and initiation of broad-spectrum antibiotics e.g. piperacillin/tazobactam and gentamicin. **Discussion with a senior member of the medical team is mandatory.**

Extravasation is chemotherapy leaking from a cannula into subcutaneous tissues. It can cause severe necrosis of skin and may require plastic surgery. Aspirate from cannula and seek urgent advice from oncology team.

■ Monitoring patients through treatment

The patient is seen prior to every administration of drug. Blood tests including FBC are performed before next prescription. Response to chemotherapy is assessed clinically or with imaging every 2–4 cycles (except for adjuvant treatment). Tumour markers in serum may be monitored e.g. CEA for colorectal, CA19-9 for pancreatic cancer. Monitoring of toxicity is mandatory.

■ Commonly used regimes

Certain types of cancer respond well to certain chemotherapy agents and therefore these drugs are referred to as active agents for that type of tumour.

- 5-FU-based chemotherapy combination for gastrointestinal cancers e.g. 5-FU and oxaliplatin (FOLFOX).
- Anthracycline-based in breast cancer e.g. doxorubicin and cyclophosphamide (AC).
- Gemcitabine in pancreatic carcinoma.
- Taxane or platinum-based alone or combination in ovarian and lung carcinoma e.g. paclitaxel or cisplatin.

■ New therapeutic targets

Many new drugs are under development in oncology. These newer drugs are often based on increased knowledge of tumour cell molecular biology.

- Kinase inhibitors – many tumours have abnormal intracellular signalling pathways, such as over activity of tyrosine kinases. Inhibiting these pathways can lead to tumour cell death e.g. imatinib (Glivec) which is active in chronic myeloid leukaemia (CML) and gastrointestinal stromal tumours (GISTs).
- Monoclonal antibodies – target specific over-expressed surface receptors e.g. HER 2 in some breast cancers – targeted by trastuzumab (Herceptin); CD20 in some lymphomas – targeted by rituximab; EGFR on colorectal tumours – targeted by cetuximab.
- Anti-angiogenic drugs – tumours often exhibit new vessel formation (neoangiogenesis) which is required for their growth. This is stimulated by growth factors e.g. VEGF which is targeted by the antibody bevacizumab (Avastin).

These novel targeted agents are not cytotoxics and therefore do not have the typical side-effects of chemotherapy.

Radiotherapy in cancer treatment

DANIELLE POWER

Radiotherapy remains a mainstay in the treatment of cancer. Comparison of the contribution towards cure by the major cancer treatment modalities shows that of those cured, 49 % are cured by surgery, 40 % by radiotherapy and 11 % by chemotherapy. Many more patients may benefit from radiotherapy to enhance quality of life through palliation of symptoms of recurrent or metastatic disease.

■ Definition

Radiotherapy is the use of ionizing radiation to treat disease. Ionizing radiation may be delivered by X-ray beams, beams of ionizing particles such as electrons, or by beta or gamma irradiation produced by the decay of radioactive isotopes.

■ Biological action of ionizing radiation

Ionizing radiation causes damage to cellular DNA both directly, and indirectly through toxic free radicals produced when radiation interacts with water within the cell. Rapidly proliferating cells are particularly sensitive to this damage. This leads to single and double DNA-strand breakage and unless repaired, causes reproductive death of the cell. Ionizing radiation can also cause DNA base mutation, and a risk of late carcinogenesis; an important consideration in the treatment of children, young adults and benign diseases with radiation.

Hospital Surgery: Foundations in Surgical Practice, ed. Omer Aziz, Sanjay Purkayastha and Paraskevas Paraskeva. Published by Cambridge University Press. © Cambridge University Press 2009.

External beam radiotherapy: X-rays, gamma-rays (clinically equivalent to X-rays but produced by radionuclide decay) or electrons emitted from an external source are incident on the skin and deposit energy either superficially or more deeply, depending on the characteristics of the beam. High-energy, penetrating therapeutic X-ray beams (and electrons) are typically produced by megavoltage linear accelerators. This complex equipment is located in radiotherapy departments, housed in bunkers to minimize radiation exposure to staff when the machine is activated.

Brachytherapy: radioactive sources are placed within body cavities or into tumours to produce a high dose of radiation locally, minimizing damage to normal healthy tissues. For example, intracavity treatment of gynaecological malignancies.

Radionuclides: certain radioactive isotopes are avidly taken up by tumour cells and cell death results from the emitted radiation locally with high specificity. For example, radioactive iodine (^{131}I) can be used to treat well-differentiated thyroid cancer, or strontium (^{89}Sr) for painful bone metastases. Although well tolerated, systemic radionuclide treatment involves radioprotection issues for patient's relatives and staff.

■ Radical radiotherapy

May have advantages over radical surgery as first-line treatment – see table below.

Indication	Examples of cancers where used
Organ preservation	Head and neck, brain tumours, anal cancer
Neoadjuvant treatment – to facilitate surgery	Locally advanced rectal cancer
Medically inoperable patients due to co-morbidities	Lung cancer, bladder cancer, oesophageal cancer
Patient choice due to differing toxicity profiles	Prostate cancer

■ Treatment planning and delivery

External beam radiotherapy aims to deliver a tumourcidal dose of radiation to a predefined tumour volume, while minimizing dose to normal tissues and 'critical' structures. *Radical treatments*: patients being prepared for radical treatment will undergo a series of steps to ensure the treatment is administered as safely and accurately as possible:

■ **Patient positioning and immobilization:** may involve an immobilization device e.g. a moulded plastic shell to fix head in a particular position for treatment of head and neck cancer.

■ **Localization of the tumour:** needs detailed clinical assessment and/or radiological investigations and an understanding of the likely route of cancer spread. Tumour volume may be defined just by examination e.g. skin cancer, or using a simulator which uses fluoroscopic X-ray images to help localize tumour, or more frequently with a CT-scanner linked to the radiotherapy planning system for detailed analysis of tumour position. Identification of the area to be treated is assisted by the use of indelible skin marks placed at the time of taking the localization X-ray or CT scan.

TUMOUR PLANNING

Involves designing the optimum arrangement of multiple radiation beams to deliver a radical treatment dose to the tumour, while avoiding structures around it, resulting in a plan for treatment. With CT planning, this is called *three-dimensional conformal radiotherapy planning (3D-CRT* (Figures 121 and 122)*)*. Margins are added to the tumour volume at the time of planning to account for microscopic or subclinical spread of disease e.g. nodal areas at risk, and an additional margin is added to take account of day-to-day variation in patient set up (which is why immobilization is crucial) or internal organ movements e.g. lung respiration in lung cancer. Techniques are developing to minimize these margins and to deliver the radiotherapy more accurately. For example, *intensity modulated radiation therapy (IMRT)* is a form of 3D-CRT that modifies the radiation by varying the intensity of each radiation beam, possibly allowing more dose to be delivered to the tumour, but not to normal tissues. This technique is currently evolving in UK radiotherapy departments, but is not yet standard care.

- **Verification:** once a plan has been developed, it is necessary to check that this can be translated effectively back to the patient in the defined treatment position. This is usually done on a treatment simulator, which reproduces exactly the movement of the treatment machine but produces a diagnostic X-ray or digital image to be checked.
- **Treatment:** Once the plan has been verified, treatment can proceed, but there are further checks undertaken on the treatment machine to ensure accuracy of dose delivery.

■ Treatment dose

The unit of radiation dose is the gray (Gy) and is a measure of absorbed energy (1 Gy = 1 J/Kg). Confusingly, neither the total number of treatments nor total dose given are a reflection of the biological dose received. There are three components to a biological radiation dose:

1. Total dose
2. Number of treatments (fractions)
3. Overall treatment time.

Examples of radical doses
60–70 Gy in 30 fractions
55 Gy in 20 fractions
40 Gy in 15 fractions

Examples of palliative doses
8 Gy in 1 fraction
20 Gy in 5 fractions
30 Gy in 10 fractions

■ Fractionation

Conventional fractionation for a radical treatment is 1.8–2 Gy per fraction for five days a week, the total dose being determined by tumour sensitivity, and tolerance of critical normal tissues in treatment area. *Hypofractionation* uses a larger dose per fraction, thereby decreasing the overall treatment time. *Hyperfractionation* uses a smaller dose per fraction (<1.8 Gy) and may treat to higher overall dose. *Accelerated fractionation* shortens the overall treatment time with standard or reduced dose per fraction. These are all possible mechanisms by which the therapeutic index of radiotherapy can be manipulated – trying to achieve the greatest chance of tumour kill, while minimizing long-term damage to normal tissues.

■ Side-effects of treatment

Acute effects: occurring during radiotherapy, usually after third week progressively, resolving after treatment. Common is a non-specific fatigue. Also specific local effects depending on area being treated. Due to temporary loss of cell division within an epithelial surface. *Late effects*: potentially most serious, as irreversible. Thought to be due to loss of 'reserve' stem cells and vascular changes. The intensity of acute toxicity with treatment does not necessarily predict for late effects and the use of large dose per fraction size increases risks of late effects. See table for examples.

Examples of possible sequelae of radical radiotherapy		
Anatomical site	Acute effects	Late effects
Skin	Erythema, dry or moist desquamation	Pigmentation, telangiectasia, subcutaneous fibrosis, rarely necrosis
Head and neck	Odynophagia, dysphagia, hoarseness, xerostomia	Dry mouth, thyroid dysfunction, cartilage necrosis, fistulae, dental decay, glue ear
Lungs/mediastinum	Odynophagia, dysphagia, hoarseness, cough, pneumonitis	Lung fibrosis, oesophageal stricture or fistula, dyspnoea or chronic cough
Abdomen/pelvis	Nausea and vomiting, pain, diarrhoea, urinary frequency, dysuria, nocturia, cytopaenia	Proctitis, sigmoiditis, stricture, contracted bladder and frequency or incontinence, infertility, impotency, liver or kidney damage
Brain	Earache, headache, dizziness, hair loss, erythema, glue ear	Hearing loss, damage to middle or inner ear, pituitary gland dysfunction, cataract, cognitive impairment

■ Palliative radiotherapy

Can be used for a variety of symptom issues related to relapsed or metastatic cancer. A single radiation beam arrangement is simple and quick to plan either clinically or typically using a treatment simulator to localize the treatment area e.g. bone metastasis, lung cancer. Sometimes the beam is opposed (180°) to treat at depth.

Examples of use of palliative radiotherapy	
Bone metastases	Relief of pain, post-surgical fixation
Pelvic cancers, gastric cancer	To stop bleeding
Cutaneous metastases	To prevent ulceration/bleeding
Cerebral metastases	To reduce steroid use

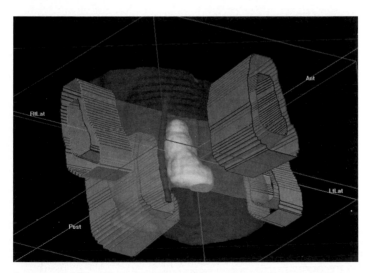

Figure 121

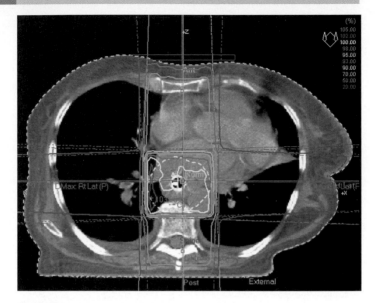

Figure 122

Palliative care

VENI EZHIL AND DANIELLE POWER

Definition: palliative care is defined as the active care of patients with active, progressive or advanced disease, often with a limited prognosis for whom control of pain, other symptoms, psychological, social and spiritual issues are paramount. The goal of palliative care is achievement of the best quality of life for patients and their families.

Principles of palliative care: main principles are to provide holistic, integrated care to patients and families. (1) Provide relief of pain and other symptoms. (2) Integrate the psychological and spiritual care. (3) Provide support to help patients live as actively as possible until death. (4) Help patient's families cope during the patient's illness and in their own bereavement. (5) Any patient may be referred with any diagnosis at any stage of disease.

Palliative care services in UK: there are four core service structures providing palliative care, including hospital support teams, community palliative care teams, specialist day care units, and specialist inpatient care mainly provided by hospices. Patients with any diagnosis may be referred to a specialist palliative care service at any stage of their illness. Referrals should be based on need not prognosis. Many national and local charities (for example Macmillan Cancer Relief, and Marie Curie) are the main providers of specialist palliative care services. A directory of services can be obtained fromwww.hospiceinformation.info.

■ Management of common symptoms

Pain: pain is experienced by the majority of patients, and is a major cause of morbidity, isolation and fear. Assessment and review of a patient's pain is important in achieving good pain control. The WHO

Hospital Surgery: Foundations in Surgical Practice, ed. Omer Aziz, Sanjay Purkayastha and Paraskevas Paraskeva. Published by Cambridge University Press. © Cambridge University Press 2009.

analgesic ladder provides a basic approach to the prescription of simple to opioid analgesia (see Pain control Chapter) with addition of adjuvant drugs to analgesics as required. It is important to use regular analgesia, with the appropriate breakthrough dose. **Special circumstances: bone pain** adjuvants include NSAIDs (if no contraindications), bisphosphonates (either iv or oral) as these inhibit bone resorption and have been shown to reduce need for analgesics and delay skeletal complication. **Neuropathic pain:** first line adjuvants include amitriptyline (10 mg increasing to 50 mg) or gabapentin (100 mg od increasing to 900 mg tds). Dexamethasone may be of help with nerve root or spinal cord compression. Second-line adjuvants and anaesthetic interventions should be confined to specialist pain or palliative care teams. **Visceral pain:** adjuvants include antispasmodics (colic), dexamethasone (liver capsule pain), interventional nerve blocks and others. **If the pain is not readily controlled, it is important to refer to a pain or palliative care specialist. Remember to prescribe anti-emetics and laxatives with weak or strong opioids.**

Syringe drivers: these are useful pocket-sized devices for delivering small volumes (can be high concentration) of drugs subcutaneously over a period of 24 hours. They can be used safely at home or in inpatient settings. Many drugs commonly used are not licensed for sc use and referral to specialist palliative care is vital. It is important to remember that it will take 12 hours before any significant effect will be delivered.

Nausea/vomiting: this is a common symptom, for example 50–60 % of patients with advanced cancer suffer with nausea or vomiting. Assessment of the cause(s) is vital in planning therapy. Choice of anti-emetics depends on the cause of vomiting/site of drug action. Like analgesia, it is important to treat regularly, by the appropriate route (oral, per rectum, iv, sc, etc.). First-line anti-emetics (except for chemotherapy and raised intra-cranial pressure) include metoclopramide or cyclizine. There is no evidence for superiority. Other anti-emetics should be used in discussion with palliative care teams.

Constipation: again a common symptom in most hospitalized, ill patients, exacerbated by dehydration, drugs (opioids, granisetron etc.)

and immobility. Anticipation of constipation, and pro-active treatment is important; for example laxatives should always be co-prescribed with opioids.

Management includes simple laxatives i.e. lactulose and senna or sodium docusate and Milpar, to more aggressive i.e. Movicol, osmotic laxatives (avoid spasmodics as this will increase colic), and in cancer patients only co-danthramer. Use suppositories (glycerine, Microlax, or phosphate enemas) in conjunction with orals. Spinal cord compression and paraplegia requires especially careful bowel control.

Anorexia and fatigue: these are increasingly common as diseases progress, especially cancers. It is important to maintain paced exercise to keep function, and to present small meals frequently. In some cancers with early presentation of anorexia, dexamethasone in small doses (4 mg od) or megestrol acetate 160 mg od may be helpful.

■ Other symptoms

Intestinal obstruction: generally uncommon but seen with increased frequency in patients with advanced or metastatic abdominal or pelvic malignancies. Causes include external compression by tumour, intraluminal occlusion by mass lesions, or motility disorder due to tumour infiltration of the mesentry or bowel wall. Management should be discussed between surgeons, oncologist and palliative care. Bowel obstruction secondary to advanced cancer is usually managed conservatively with iv fluids, analgesics and anti-emetics, preferably via subcutaneous syringe drivers. Nasogastric intubation is not usually required. Palliative surgery can be effective for symptom relief.

Depression.

Symptoms from pressure sores e.g. sacral and on feet need to be prevented, and if they occur managed with the tissue viability team and plastic surgeons if necessary.

Symptoms from contractures.

Practical procedures, investigations and operations

Urethral catheterization

IMRAN HAMID AND OMER AZIZ

This procedure involves the insertion of a latex, plastic or silicone catheter into the bladder via the urethral orifice. The contents of the bladder are collected in a drainage bag or urometer, allowing both specimen collection and measurement of urine output. This is an example of a closed passive drainage system.

Type	Indication
Foley	Uncomplicated catheterization and irrigation procedures
Coude	Useful for a hypertrophic prostate gland as it has an angled profile
Silastic	Suitable for long-term catheterization
Convene	For male patients. Prone to leakage. No invasive urethral element
Temporary	Monitoring urine output, relief of retention, and specimen collection
Intermittent/long-term	Self catheterization for neuropathic bladder (e.g. multiple sclerosis, diabetes, or spinal pathology), stroke, incontinence, palliative

The typical catheter size required is 14–16 French gauge (Fr).

■ Indications

- Monitoring urine output
- Relief of urinary retention
- Incontinence
- Empty bladder preoperatively

Hospital Surgery: Foundations in Surgical Practice, ed. Omer Aziz, Sanjay Purkayastha and Paraskevas Paraskeva. Published by Cambridge University Press. © Cambridge University Press 2009.

- Bladder irrigation
- Sterile specimen collection for microscopy, culture and sensitivity.

■ Contraindications

- Trauma/suspected urethral injury (e.g. pelvic fracture)
- Acute prostatitis.

■ Prepare your equipment trolley

- Catheterization pack: kidney bowl, gauze swabs, sterile drapes, cleaning solution dish
- Catheter: size 14 and 16 Fr, male or female length
- Drainage bag or urometer
- Specimen pot for MSU
- Sterile saline in a 10 ml syringe (check capacity of balloon in catheter)
- Normosol cleaning solution or equivalent
- Instagel lidocaine gel or equivalent
- Two pairs of sterile gloves
- Disposable apron.

■ Procedure

Explain procedure to the patient. If catheterizing a female patient request supervision from a suitable chaperone. Before exposing the patient ensure privacy, good lighting and position the patient in a supine position. For a female patient request her knees to be fully flexed with legs abducted (a.k.a. 'frog-leg' position). Wear a disposable apron, roll up sleeves, wash hands thoroughly and maintain a sterile field throughout. Stand to the right of the patient.

Cleaning: In the male patient use your left hand to retract the foreskin and hold the penis in position. This hand is now non-sterile. With your right hand clean the urethral orifice and glans with the sterile swabs and cleaning solution from the meatus towards the perineum. Place a drape over the penis and once again hold the penis with the left hand. In the female patient, use your non-dominant hand to spread the labia, while using your dominant hand to clean the introitus.

Analgesia: Instill local anaesthetic gel into urethral orifice while holding the penis perpendicular to the body. Wait for five minutes for the anaesthetic to take effect. Place a kidney bowl between the patient's legs.

Insertion male: while holding the penis perpendicular to the patient's body, insert the catheter into the urethral orifice. Use a consistent gentle pressure to feed the catheter. A subtle side-to-side twisting action may help. Ensure that the free end of the catheter is in the kidney bowl. If you feel resistance that cannot be passed, reposition the penis in a horizontal plane towards the patient's feet, and reapply gentle force. Urine may begin to flow, but continue to insert the catheter all the way into the bladder. Only inflate the balloon when urine is flowing, never before. Watch the patient's face as you inflate the balloon. Excessive discomfort may indicate that the balloon is still within the urethra. If catherization fails on two attempts, call for senior advice. **Never use undue force** as this may create a false passage (see Figure 123).

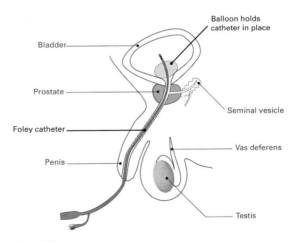

Figure 123

Insertion female: using a similar sterile technique as described above, locate the urethral meatus and insert a well-lubricated female-sized catheter.

Collection: use the specimen pot to collect a urine sample. Attach the catheter to the drainage bag or urometer.

■ Post-procedure considerations

- Return the foreskin to its original position. Failure to do so may cause *paraphimosis* (painful swelling and retraction of the foreskin). If this occurs, apply a cool-pack and call for senior help immediately. (See Paraphimosis Chapter.)
- Measure residual volume: note the volume and appearance of urine collected after 20 min. A large volume (>800 ml) of urine defines urinary retention. Also note the presence of blood and/or clots.
- As with any procedure, accurate documentation is mandatory. Record residual volume, procedure details, and name of chaperone. Inform ward staff of successful catheterization.
- Send a CSU (catheter stream urine).

■ Complications

- Infection
- Trauma
- Stricture formation
- Immobility.

Percutaneous suprapubic catheterization

PARASKEVAS PARASKEVA

■ Introduction

There are two main types of percutaneous suprapubic catheters used in practice: the Bonanno suprapubic catheter system and Stamey-type suprapubic catheter. These catheters differ in their methods of insertion as described below; however the indications and contraindications are the same.

■ Indications

- Failure to pass urethral catheter
- Urethral stricture
- False passage
- Surgeon choice
- Acute prostatitis
- Traumatic urethral disruption
- Peri-urethral abscess
- Long-term catheterization.

■ Contraindications

- Previous lower midline incision
- Non-distended bladder
- Coagulopathy
- Pregnancy
- Carcinoma of the bladder
- Pelvic irradiation.

Hospital Surgery: Foundations in Surgical Practice, ed. Omer Aziz, Sanjay Purkayastha and Paraskevas Paraskeva. Published by Cambridge University Press. © Cambridge University Press 2009.

■ Equipment

- Suprapubic catheter set of choice
- Urine drainage bag
- Sterile preparation
- Local anaesthetic
- Suture material.

■ Clinical examination

Confirm the presence of a bladder.

Inspect for scars.

If there is concern about the presence of a bladder an ultrasound scan can be performed or indeed used to guide the insertion.

Site of insertion of the suprapubic catheter is finger breadths above the symphysis pubis. If there is a previous midline scar, it is advocated that insertion should proceed under ultrasound guidance with the insertion site being 2–3 cm lateral to the incision (see Figure 124).

■ Technique: Bonanno

After fully informing the patient of the procedure and confirming the bladder on palpation, the patient is prepared and draped. Local anaesthetic is infiltrated into the skin and into the abdominal wall, and a small incision made in the skin.

The Bonanno catheter is prepared by straightening the catheter with the stylette *in situ* using a plastic sleeve. The sleeve is then removed, and the catheter inserted with a syringe on the end aspirating as it is inserted, always directed towards the pelvis. As the catheter is inserted the stylette is withdrawn. The flange of the catheter is sutured to the abdominal skin and the catheter connected to a drainage bag.

■ Technique: Stamey suprapubic catheter

- The method of insertion of this catheter is similar to the Bonanno catheter. Important differences in this technique are:

- A scalpel is used to make a small suprapubic incision to allow the insertion of a trocar and sheath into the bladder.
- When inserting the trocar, the aim is downwards toward the pelvis. Often there is a degree of resistance, hence a twisting motion may aid in entry to the bladder. Insertion is continued until urine flows freely from the sheath, entry into the bladder is also heralded by a decrease in resistance.
- Withdraw the trocar.
- Insert a standard Foley-type catheter into the sheath, then split the plastic sheath around the catheter to remove it. The balloon of the catheter is inflated with 10 ml of water. The catheter is secured with a drain suture and a dressing. It is then connected to a drainage bag.

■ Complications

- Bowel injury
- Leak from bladder
- Haemorrhage
- Infection
- Haematuria/clot retention
- Leakage around insertion site
- In a complicated or difficult insertion you must obtain a urology consult.

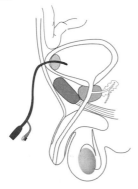

Figure 124

Vascular access

JOHANN EMMANUEL

Access to the venous system in its simplest form is indicated for fluid and medication administration; however central venous access has many more indications. Venous access can be divided into peripheral and central techniques.

■ Peripheral intravenous access

PERCUTANEOUS PERIPHERAL CANNULAE

Indications: fluid and medication administration.

Exceptions: potentially irritating solutions such as parenteral nutrition/ certain antibiotics and sclerosing chemotherapeutic agents.

Sites: dorsal veins on the hands and feet are the preferred location +/− anticubital fossa.

Sizes: cannulae are sized in steel wire gauge, 14G, 16G, 18G etc. The lower the number the bigger the cannula.

Insertion

Equipment: cannulae, alcohol swabs, adhesive dressing, tourniquet, gloves.

Finding a vein: apply tourniquet, gentle tapping over vein, clean area with swab.

Insert the cannula with bevel uppermost through skin and into vein. A flashback of blood will appear in the cannula chamber. Advance the needle another millimetre to ensure whole of bevel is within vein. Slide the plastic cannula over the needle into the vein. Remove the

Hospital Surgery: Foundations in Surgical Practice, ed. Omer Aziz, Sanjay Purkayastha and Paraskevas Paraskeva. Published by Cambridge University Press. © Cambridge University Press 2009.

tourniquet, and while pressing on the cannula tip remove the needle. Then either put the white cap provided onto the cannula or attach to giving set of fluids bag. Date the dressing and change cannula every 72 hours to reduce infection risk.

Secure with adhesive and dispose of needle in sharps bin.

- With larger cannulae inject local anaesthesia prior to insertion.
- For children apply local anaesthetic cream.

PERIPHERAL VENOUS CUTDOWN CATHETER

Indication: surgical technique when attempts at percutaneous (peripheral + central) techniques have failed.

Sites: saphenous vein/antecubital /femoral vein.

SAPHENOUS VEIN CUTDOWN

Insertion

Sterile procedure, local anaesthesetic infiltration.

Make a horizontal incision 1 cm anterior and superior to the medial malleolus. Isolate the vein with blunt dissection. Two silk sutures should be looped around the vein, the distal suture may be used to ligate the vein. With tension applied to the proximal suture loop, a venotomy is made with a blade, and a 22G cannula inserted and secured by tying the proximal suture loop. The incision can be sutured and an appropriate dressing applied.

INTRAOSSEOUS NEEDLE

The bone marrow contains non-collapsible veins.

Indications: emergency situations in children, where percutaneous attempts have failed. Simpler/preferred technique to cutdown access.

Site: proximal tibia, 1–3 cm below and medial to the tibial tuberosity; interosseous needle required.

Insertion (Figure 125)

Support the leg and apply enough pressure, after instilling local anaesthetic, to feel a 'give' through the periosteum. Then gentle twist to secure in place. Aspirate bone marrow and send to the lab, ensuring that it is labelled as bone marrow and not blood. Secure giving set and administer fluid.

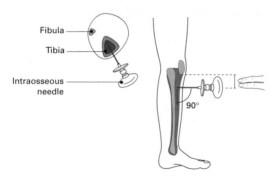

Figure 125 Interosseous access

■ Central venous access

CATHETER TYPES

Peripheral intravenous central cannula (PICC-line) – long catheter inserted peripherally into the brachial/axillary vein and advanced centrally.

Central venous line – single, double, triple and quadruple lumen. These represent the typical central line.

Silastic central venous catheters – Hickman (long-term use).

Implantable access port – Port-A-Cath etc. Catheter with port area placed subcutaneously.

Haemodialysis/filtration catheters – large-lumen catheters used for renal replacement therapy.

INDICATIONS FOR CENTRAL VENOUS LINE INSERTION

Haemodynamic monitoring
Parenteral nutrition
Chemotherapy
Haemodialysis/filtration
Administration of vasopressors
Pacing-wire insertion
Emergency access when peripheral circulation shut down
Drug administration (amiodarone/inotropes).

CONTRAINDICATIONS

There are no absolute, although coagulopathy may be considered a relative contraindication.

(See chapter on Central Line Insertion.)

Arterial cannulation

JOHANN EMMANUEL

■ Indications

- Continuous blood pressure monitoring
- Arterial blood gas analysis.

■ Complications

- Infection
- Thrombosis with distal ischaemia (*risk factors* are: size of catheter, multiple attempts, duration *in situ*, ischaemia, and pre-existing hypertension)
- False aneurysm.

■ Equipment

- Sterile drape and gloves
- Aseptic solution
- Local anaesthetic with needle and syringe
- Clear dressing
- Continuous flushing device
- 20 g Teflon cannula (e.g. Abbocath) and 2 ml syringe (plunger removed) or Seldinger arterial kit.

■ Sites

- *Radial artery*: accessible site, with good collateral flow. 10 % have either poor collateral flow or incomplete palmar arch, therefore

Hospital Surgery: Foundations in Surgical Practice, ed. Omer Aziz, Sanjay Purkayastha and Paraskevas Paraskeva. Published by Cambridge University Press. © Cambridge University Press 2009.

Allen's test (see Examination of the Vascular System Chapter) is used to confirm ulnar artery blood supply. Position for insertion of arterial line: hyper-extending the wrist with thumb abducted.

- *Brachial artery:* generally avoided, as if occluded, the collateral supply around the elbow may be insufficient.
- *Axillary artery:* generally avoided as difficult and uncomfortable for patient.
- *Femoral artery:* Higher infection risk.
- *Dorsalis pedis:* small calibre vessel, difficult cannulation.

■ Technique

Three techniques are commonly practiced:

1. **Direct cannulation: similar to peripheral intravenous access:**
   - Palpate the artery and its course.
   - Insert local anaesthetic subcutaneously.
   - Aseptic precautions.
   - Attach the 2 ml syringe to the cannula.
   - Insert as per an intravenous cannula (the 2 ml syringe acts as a reservoir for blood and confirms that the bevel is still within the artery).
   - Attach to continuous flushing device (see Figure 126).
   - Apply dressing to secure.
   - Discard sharps appropriately.
2. **Direct cannulation: transfixion technique:**
   - Differs to above technique only in that when blood is seen in the cannula, the cannula is advanced through the vessel (transfixes artery).
   - The needle is withdrawn slightly into the sheath before the whole cannula is withdrawn.
   - When blood appears in the syringe, advance the cannula, and then remove the needle fully.

3. **Seldinger technique:**
   - The artery is cannulated with a needle.
   - A guidewire is passed through and the arterial catheter is passed over the guidewire before it is removed.

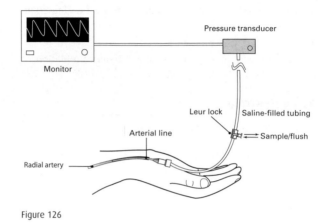

Figure 126

■ Additional points

- Following connection of the transducer, check the arterial tracing and ensure that there is a good dichrotic notch (the acute drop in arterial pressure pulse curves following the systolic peak), which is a good way of checking the line is in the correct place.
- Arterial lines are usually flushed with a heparin solution (e.g. Hepsal). Consult local hospital protocols.

Central line insertion

JOHANN EMMANUEL

In general cannulation of the internal jugular (IJV), subclavian (SCV) and femoral vein (FV) can be guided by anatomical landmarks; however guidelines produced by the UK National Institute for Clinical Excellence advise the use of ultrasound-guided techniques.

The Seldinger technique is most commonly performed, and consists of a guidewire inserted through a needle before the catheter is passed.

■ Equipment

- Sterile – gown, gloves, mask
- Central venous catheter pack
- Aseptic solution
- Local anaesthetic
- Blade
- Three-way taps
- Suture/clear dressing
- Pulse oximeter and cardiac monitor.

■ Technique for insertion

- Obtain consent.
- Proper positioning of patient will enhance success.
- Aseptic technique.
- Local anaesthetic infiltration (if patient awake).
- Flush the catheter with saline (all ports).

Hospital Surgery: Foundations in Surgical Practice, ed. Omer Aziz, Sanjay Purkayastha and Paraskevas Paraskeva. Published by Cambridge University Press. © Cambridge University Press 2009.

- A metal needle attached to a syringe is advanced subcutaneously towards the vessel while continuously aspirating, until venous blood is aspirated.
- Remove syringe and pass guidewire though needle. *If blood pulses out* this suggests an arterial puncture. In this case remove needle and apply pressure. *If resistance is encountered* remove the guidewire and re-insert the needle.
- Monitor for arrhythmias (if IJV or SCV): retract wire slightly if this occurs.
- Enlarge the skin puncture site with scalpel incision, and remove the needle, leaving the guidewire *in situ*.
- Pass the dilator over the guidewire to form a tract through subcutaneous tissue. The dilator only needs inserting a few centimetres; the vein does not need dilating.
- Remove the dilator, and thread the catheter over the wire ensuring that the end of the wire always protrudes for the catheter. This will prevent loss of the wire.
- Remove the wire, attach the three-way taps, aspirate and flush from all ports. Suture and apply dressing. Chest X-ray (IJV and SCV).

■ Ultrasound techniques

Current 'gold standard' for ensuring accurate line placement, but requires appropriate training prior to use. Can be used prior to insertion to confirm presence and position of vein or continuous scanning during insertion.

■ Landmark technique

INTERNAL JUGULAR VEIN

Several approaches have been described. The author uses the following, with the patient in Trendelenburg (head down) position:

1. Needle at apex of the triangle formed by the two heads of the sterno-cleidomastoid and the clavicle.

2. Needle inserted lateral to the palpated carotid artery at the mid-point of the anterior border of the sternocleidomastoid, aiming at the ipsilateral nipple.

SUBCLAVIAN VEIN

Position in the Trendelenburg position. An infraclavicular approach with a puncture site 2 cm inferior to the junction of the lateral 1/3 and medial 2/3 of the clavicle. The needle is advanced medially in the direction of the suprasternal notch, and guided posteriorly under the clavicle (see Figure 127).

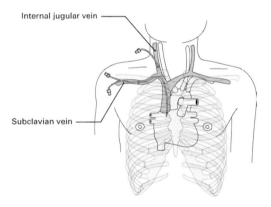

Internal jugular vein

Subclavian vein

Figure 127

FEMORAL VEIN

Position the patient in reverse Trendelenburg position. The femoral vein lies medial to the palpated femoral artery.

■ Complications

In general these can be divided into '*complications of line insertion*' and '*complications of the line itself*' (all of which can also be classified as *immediate, early* and *late*). Specific complications are:

- *Carotid artery puncture/cannulation* – use ultrasound/transduce needle prior to dilating.
- *Arrhythmias* – retract guidewire.
- *Pneumothorax/haemothorax* – high approach minimizes risk.
- *Chylothorax* (left-sided lines).
- *Air embolism* – ensure head down position/ensure taps capped off.
- *Thrombus formation*.
- *Infection* – incidence of local infection rises after five days. If unexplained pyrexia/WCC, change over guidewire, and send tip to microbiology. If positive result or local signs of infection, remove catheter.

Lumbar puncture

SHARLEET MAHAL AND OMER AZIZ

Definition: needle puncture of the spinal canal below the level of termination of the spinal cord (usually at L4–L5). Cerebrospinal fluid is sampled and pressure measured.

■ Indications

- Suspected subarachnoid haemorrhage (SAH) following CT scan.
- Suspected CNS infections.
- Therapeutic reduction of raised ICP (done following a CT scan *only in experienced neurosurgical hands due to risk of brain herniation*).
- CSF sampling for other conditions.

■ Contraindications

- Local skin infections over puncture site.
- Evidence of raised ICP on clinical exam (papilloedema) or on CT.
- Suspected spinal cord mass or intra-cranial mass lesion.
- Bleeding disturbance or warfarin therapy with INR >1.4.
- Spinal column deformities (may require fluoroscopic assistance).

■ Prepare the patient

- Explain procedure to the patient.
- Prepare lumbar puncture (LP) tray as follows:

Hospital Surgery: Foundations in Surgical Practice, ed. Omer Aziz, Sanjay Purkayastha and Paraskevas Paraskeva. Published by Cambridge University Press. © Cambridge University Press 2009.

- Spinal needle (Quinke type) 20G for children, 22G for adults.
- Antiseptic solution.
- Sterile drapes, gloves and gown.
- Disposable manometer.
- Three-way valve.
- Intravenous line connector and tube.
- Local anaesthetic – 5 ml of 1 % lidocaine.
- One fluoride and three plain CSF collection bottles.
- Expose the patient and place on their left side with their back perpendicular to the edge of the bed. Ask the patient to flex their knees and bring their chin down (the fetal position) which helps to widen the intervertebral spaces (see Figure 128).
- Palpate both iliac crests. A line in this plate goes through the L4 vertebra in the midline. Either the L4/L5 or L3/4 intervertebral space can be used for LP, and should be marked with a permanent marker (see Figure 128).
- Wear sterile gloves, gown and mask.

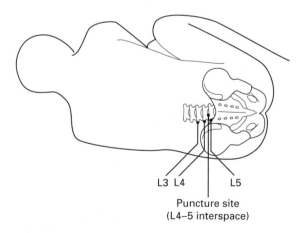

L3 L4   L5

Puncture site
(L4–5 interspace)

Figure 128

■ The LP procedure

- Clean and drape the area on the back taking care to cover both posterior iliac spines, up to L2 and down to the sacrum.
- Using a blue (23G) needle, infiltrate a few ml of 1% lidocaine under the skin and subcutaneous tissues at the marked site, carefully withdrawing before injecting.
- Position the spinal needle so that it is perpendicular to the skin at the desired site of insertion. Make sure the bevel of the needle is facing up and parallel to dural fibres to minimize trauma.
- Slowly advance needle horizontally, looking for three slight 'gives' as the needle first enters the spinal ligament, followed by the dura and finally the subarachnoid space. On withdrawing the stilette, CSF fluid should flow (see Figure 129).
- If bone is hit on advancing the needle, then withdraw and position below or above the spinal vertebra as appropriate. If necessary use the landmarks to orientate yourself and re-advance.

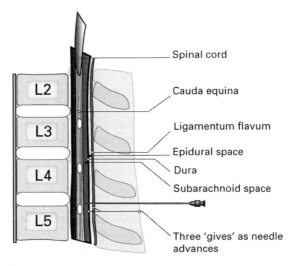

Figure 129

- Once the subarachnoid space is entered, attach the three-way stop-cock and manometer to measure and record ICP. This can be followed by CSF collection tubes (2 ml in each bottle).
- Place a plaster on the wound and ask patient to lie on their back for 60 min.
- Document procedure and findings in the medical notes.
- Send samples to the lab:
  - Microscopy, glucose, protein, culture, gram staining, and xanthochromia.
  - Other tests include cytology, virology, TB culture, fungal culture, serology and oligoclonal bands.

■ Interpretation

Normal findings in brackets.

- **Pressure** (5–20 cm CSF): >30 cm is virtually always indicative of raised ICP.
- **Colour** (clear): *red-stained* is suggestive of bleeding, *cloudy* suggests infection, and *frothy* suggests high-protein sample.
- **RBCs** (none): may be present in either a traumatic bloody tap (puncture of spinal venous plexus) or a subarachnoid haemorrhage. In the case of SAH, xanthochromia will be present in the supernatant fluid after spin down.
- **WBCs** (<5 per mm^2): if present then consider meningitis, encephalitis, inflammatory conditions and neoplastic meningitis.
- **Culture:** bacterial or fungal infection.
- **Protein** (5–45 mg/dl): a high protein content may be seen in meningitis, encephalitis, myelitis, tumours, inflammatory processes.
- **Glucose** (50–75 mg/dl): very low levels are seen in TB, fungal and neoplastic meningitis and mildly low levels in bacterial and some viral meningitis.

■ Complications

- **Headache** occurs in 15–30 % of cases. Dural leak can result in a low-pressure generalized headache accompanied by pre-syncope and nausea. The headache may be relieved by lying down, and aggravated by standing. In severe cases an epidural blood patch may be created using the patient's own venous blood. Smaller needles reduce chance of post-LP headache and patients should avoid codeine-based analgesia, using NSAIDs and paracetamol instead.
- **Meningitis** from bacteria introduced during procedure.
- **Nerve root trauma** (e.g. previous surgery in the area, scar tissue).
- **Haematoma** (e.g. patients on anticoagulation therapy).
- **Brain herniation** in the presence of increased intra-cranial pressure with brainstem compression.

Airway

JOHANN EMMANUEL

Artificial airways are used to maintain the patency of the airway, allowing an unobstructed passage between the mouth and the lungs. There are many such airways used by specialists that are beyond the scope of this chapter. The commonly used airways shall be described below.

These include: *tracheostomy, oropharyngeal/nasopharyngeal/laryngeal mask* airways and *endotracheal tubes.*

■ Oropharyngeal (Guedel) airway (Figure 130)

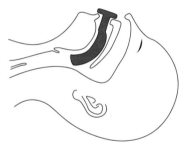

Figure 130 Guedel

Description: a plastic device inserted into the oropharynx to create airway between tongue and palate. This is a *non-definitive* airway.

Indications: airway maintenance in unconscious patients/without gag reflex.

Advantages: easy to insert/minimal training required. Less likely to cause trauma than nasopharyngeal airway.

Hospital Surgery: Foundations in Surgical Practice, ed. Omer Aziz, Sanjay Purkayastha and Paraskevas Paraskeva. Published by Cambridge University Press. © Cambridge University Press 2009.

Sizing: take airway and put flange at corner of mouth. Distal end should be at angle of jaw or the external auditory meatus.

Insertion: *adults* – insert with concavity facing upwards. Rotate 180 degrees as approaches posterior oropharynx. *Children* – insert with concavity downwards to avoid damaging soft palate/airway.

Complications: trauma to oral cavity during insertion, laryngospasm, vomiting in patients that are awake.

■ Nasopharyngeal airway (NPA) (Figure 131)

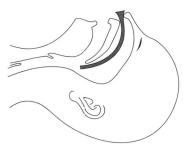

Figure 131 Nasopharyngeal

Description: a plastic tube inserted into the nostril and passed into the oropharynx to create an airway between tongue and palate. This is a *non-definitive* airway.

Indications: airway maintenance in semiconscious patient, and if placement of oropharyngeal airway is difficult.

Contraindications: base of skull fracture.

Advantages: easy to insert/minimal training required/better tolerated.

Sizing: diameter should easily fit through nostril, and is sized as the diameter of the patient's little finger. Length can be sized from tip of nose to tragus of ear.

Insertion: lubricate well with gel. Insert along floor of nostril perpendicular to face, keeping bevelled edge medially. If resistance occurs, withdraw and try other nostril. Often comes with a safety pin to insert on the distal flange to avoid aspiration by the patient.

Complications: nasal trauma. Contraindicated in patients with suspected base of skull fractures.

■ Laryngeal mask airway (Figure 132)

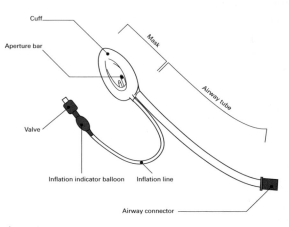

Figure 132

Description: laryngeal mask airways have an inflatable cuff that is inserted into the pharynx, but are *non-definitive airways* that do not prevent aspiration.

Indications: (1) General anaesthesia not requiring endotracheal intubation e.g. simple day-surgery cases; (2) Airway management in unconscious patients when endotracheal tube placement difficult. NB this however does not provide a definitive airway.

Advantages: simpler to insert. Requires some training to insert. No protection against gastric contents – unlike endotracheal tube.

Sizing:

Size 1 – neonates < 5 kg   Size 1.5 – child 5–10 kg   Size 2 – child 10–20 kg   Size 2.5 – child 20–30 kg   Size 3 – child/adult 30–50 kg   Size 4 – adult 50–70 kg   Size 5 – adult >70 kg.

Insertion: insert into the pharynx with the pointed end in the oesophagus and the distal opening over the laryngeal inlet. The mask is then inflated with air from a 20 ml syringe.

■ Endotracheal tube (Figure 133)

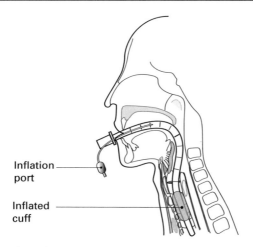

Inflation port

Inflated cuff

Figure 133

Description: endotracheal tubes are *definitive airways* as they provide a secure airway that allows oxygen delivery, ventilation and at the same time protects against passage of fluids (especially blood and gastric contents) to the lungs.

Indications:

1. Secure airway: protects lungs from gastric and upper airway contamination.
2. Ventilation.

Sizing:

Uncuffed tubes – children under eight years old
Adult female – 7.0–8.0 mm
Adult male – 8.0–9.0 mm

Insertion: is performed following pre-oxygenation of the patient. Supervised training required to undertake this procedure.

Complications: oesophageal/endobronchial intubation, trauma to mouth/oropharynx, physiological response to laryngoscopy, obstruction of tube.

■ Tracheostomy (Figure 134)

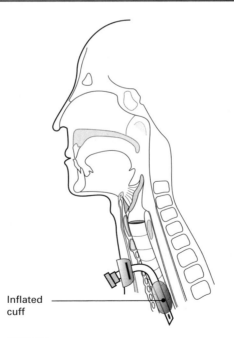

Inflated
cuff

Figure 134

Description: tracheostomies are *definitive airways* as they provide a secure airway that allows oxygen delivery directly into the trachea. These can be acute or chronic, and allow ventilation while protecting against passage of fluids (especially blood and gastric contents) to the lungs.

Indications: failed tracheal intubation, prolonged tracheal intubation, head and neck surgery, prevention of pulmonary aspiration.

Insertion: percutaneous/surgical technique that should only be undertaken by those with the appropriate training.

Complications: damage to surrounding structures (especially neurovascular and thyroid), haematoma, tracheal stenosis.

Chest drain insertion

ROS JACKLIN AND OMER AZIZ

■ Definition

A chest drain is a conduit for the removal of air or fluid from the pleural cavity. Three components are required: the chest drain itself, a container for collection (placed below the level of the chest) and a valve mechanism such as an underwater seal or Heimlich valve.

■ Indications

Pneumothorax (especially in ventilated patients)
Traumatic haemopneumothorax
Postoperative – e.g. thoracotomy, oesophagectomy, cardiac surgery
Large malignant pleural effusions
Empyema and complicated parapneumonic pleural effusion.

■ Pre-procedure considerations

- Obtain a pre-procedure chest X-ray except in the case of tension pneumothorax, and confirm site/side.
- Consider risks: correct any coagulopathy where possible, take care with differential diagnosis of pneumothorax and bullous disease.
- Drainage of a post-pneumonectomy space should only be carried out after consultation with a cardiothoracic surgeon.
- Explain the procedure and obtain patient consent.
- Consider premedication (opiate or benzodiazepine) if patient conscious.

Hospital Surgery: Foundations in Surgical Practice, ed. Omer Aziz, Sanjay Purkayastha and Paraskevas Paraskeva. Published by Cambridge University Press. © Cambridge University Press 2009.

- Consider image guidance if unable to aspirate free air/fluid with a needle.
- Prophylactic antibiotics e.g. a cephalosporin should be given in trauma cases.
- Prepare equipment including chest drain set, sterile preparation, local anaesthetic, underwater seal drain, silk suture, scalpel, dressings and pulse oximeter.

■ Procedure

- *Position the patient correctly* – either on a bed, hand behind head on the side of insertion to expose the axilla, upright leaning over a table with a pillow or in the lateral decubitus position. Patient should be on oxygen and have peripheral access.
- *Identify the site* – fifth intercostal space in the mid-axillary line, above the rib to avoid the neurovascular bundle. A 'safe triangle' for insertion is bordered by the anterior border of latissimus dorsi, the lateral border of pectoralis major and horizontal line superior to the nipple.
- *Aseptic technique.*
- *Local anaesthetic* – raise a dermal bleb prior to deeper infiltration of the intercostal muscles and pleura.
- *Make an incision just above and parallel to the rib.*
- *Blunt dissect* the subcutaneous tissue into the pleural cavity using Spencer Wells forceps or similar. The trocar should be discarded.
- *For a large chest drain, explore the track with a finger* to ensure there are no underlying organs that may be damaged at the time of insertion (smaller drains may be inserted using the Seldinger technique).
- *Place the tip of a small clamp in one of the drainage holes* and use it to guide the chest drain along the track and into the pleural space. If possible, the tip should be aimed apically to drain air and basally for fluid.
- *Secure the drain with a stay suture* (a strong suture material such as number 1 silk is appropriate), and place a second suture (e.g.

horizontal mattress type) suitable for closing a linear incision once the drain is removed (Figure 135).

■ *Connect to an underwater seal* (Figure 136).

■ Post-procedure considerations

■ Look for air bubbles or fluid evacuation and a respiratory swing in the fluid in the chest tube to ensure placement in the pleural space.

■ Clamping of a chest drain should normally be avoided in cases of pneumothorax due to the risk of tension pneumothorax. Drainage of a large pleural effusion should be controlled to prevent re-expansion pulmonary oedema.

■ Obtain a post-procedure chest X-ray.

■ Complications

■ There is no organ in the thoracic or abdominal cavity that has not been pierced by a chest drain.

■ **Early complications:** haemothorax, lung laceration, diaphragmatic/intra-abdominal damage, bowel injury in unrecognized diaphragmatic hernia, errors of tube placement – insertion too far, subcutaneous placement, displacement.

■ **Late complications:** drain blockage, retained haemothorax, empyema, pneumothorax post-removal.

■ Special considerations

Chest drain removal requires care. The patient should be asked to perform a Valsalva manoeuvre during removal to minimize the chance of pneumothorax. The drain should be removed briskly and firmly while an assistant ties the pre-placed closure suture and the site should then be quickly covered with an occlusive dressing.

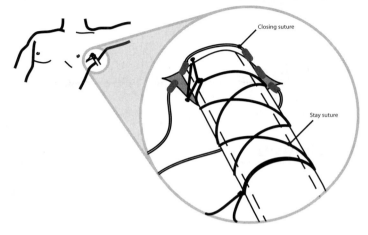

Figure 135 Example of stay and closing sutures

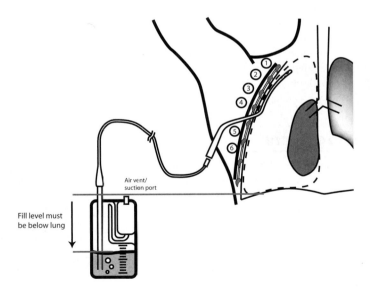

Figure 136 Chest drain attached to underwater seal bottle

Thoracocentesis

MOHAMMED SHAMIM RAHMAN AND OMER AZIZ

■ Definition

The clinical technique whereby fluid or air is removed from the pleural cavity (see also Chest drain insertion Chapter).

■ Indications

Emergency: in the acute situation where removal of fluid or air may prevent the restriction of normal ventilation and/or tamponade of the heart.

Diagnostic: sampling of fluid in the thoracic cavity for microscopy, culture, serology and cytology. The appearance of the fluid can allude to a diagnosis, for example milky fluid (chyle) aspirated from a 'chylothorax' implies rupture of the thoracic duct, while aspiration of blood from a 'haemothorax' is usually the result from penetrating chest injuries.

Therapeutic: when fluid continually accumulates despite medical therapy, repeated aspiration can provide symptomatic relief.

Radiographic: improving radiographs in areas which may otherwise be obscured by radio-opaque fluid in order to further aid diagnosis.

■ Procedure

Pre-medication with an intravenous anxiolytic (e.g. midazolam 1.5 mg), which should be given immediately before the procedure, or an intramuscular opioid given one hour before, keeping an antidote at hand.

Collect all the correct equipment prior to procedure. The following are recommended: antiseptic preparation solution, sterile gloves,

Hospital Surgery: Foundations in Surgical Practice, ed. Omer Aziz, Sanjay Purkayastha and Paraskevas Paraskeva. Published by Cambridge University Press. © Cambridge University Press 2009.

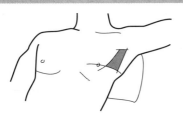

Figure 137 Positioning of patient for aspiration of air

gauze, sterile towels/drapes, 1–2 % lidocaine without epinephrine, 3–5 ml syringe and 18-gauge needle (for local anaesthesia), 22-gauge 3.5 cm needle, three-way stopcock, 50 ml syringe, 30 cm long large (16-gauge) catheter-through-needle intravenous placement system, appropriate containers for fluid for diagnostic tests, haemostat, adhesive dressing and an assistant as required.

Confirm the site of insertion both clinically and radiologically (unless in emergency when clinical suspicion is enough). Position of the patient depends on whether air or fluid is expected. For air, recline the patient at 30° supine placing their hand behind their head on the side of the lesion (Figure 137). For aspiration of fluid, seat the patient sideways on a chair with arms draped over a pillow (Figure 138). Clean the area thoroughly and apply the drape leaving enough room to enter the intercostal space. Infiltrate local anaesthetic into the superficial area. Attach a pulse-oximeter to the patient. Refill the syringe and attach the 22-gauge needle. Insert the needle **under** the desired area to touch the rib. Walk the needle off the top border of the rib until free and advance gently into the pleura. Advance the needle and inject small amounts of anaesthetic then aspirate. If no material returns, advance the needle again 0.5–1 cm. Repeat this until material or air is aspirated. Slowly retract the needle until it is just outside the pleural space and inject the remaining anaesthetic to provide good pleural anaesthesia, then remove the needle (Figure 138A). Remove the needle from the intravenous catheter system and attach the small syringe to the large needle, filled with local anaesthetic. Advance in the same way as before, into the pleural space

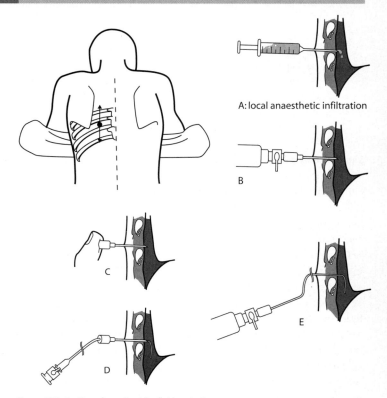

A: local anaesthetic infiltration

B

C

D

E

Figure 138 Seating of a patient for fluid aspiration

until matter is returned (Figure 138C). Remove the syringe while covering the inserted needle with a gloved finger with the patient holding his/her breath against a closed glottis (Figure 138D). Insert the catheter unit (without stylet) through the needle again with the patient holding the Valsalva manoeuvre (Figure 138E). Remove the needle over the catheter then attach the stop-cock to the catheter hub. Withdraw fluid using the large syringe. Specimens should be sent to the laboratory.

Cover the wound with the adhesive dressing on removal of the catheter unit.

■ Complications

As procedures are not without risk, consideration should be given as to whether or not the proposed benefits outweigh these risks. Specific to thoracocentesis, one should consent the patient for the benefits of the procedure, i.e. removal of fluid or air from the thorax, as well as outline the common risks. These include pain, the possibility of bleeding and a small risk of infection. There is also a risk of laceration of structures medial to the pleural space, such as the lungs and the pericardium.

Pericardiocentesis

MOHAMMED SHAMIM RAHMAN AND OMER AZIZ

This technique was introduced by Frank Schuh in 1840 and became the preferred treatment of pericardial effusions by the twentieth century. Prior to echocardiography a blind approach was used to access the pericardial sac, where serious complications were not uncommon.

Definition: The clinical technique of using a needle to withdraw fluid from the pericardial sac.

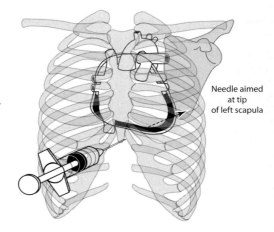

Needle aimed
at tip
of left scapula

Figure 139

■ Indications

Pericardial tamponade: except in those with myocardial rupture. *Therapeutic*: in those with a symptomatic pericardial effusion and in particular a large effusion, which may compress other thoracic

Hospital Surgery: Foundations in Surgical Practice, ed. Omer Aziz, Sanjay Purkayastha and Paraskevas Paraskeva. Published by Cambridge University Press. © Cambridge University Press 2009.

structures (trachea, lungs). *Diagnostic:* where an effusion is of unclear aetiology. *Biopsy:* of the pericardium.

■ Procedure

Pre-procedure considerations: obtain an echocardiogram to confirm the presence of an effusion. Pericardiocentesis need not be performed on those with small organized effusions, but on those with any of the following: large, symptomatic or severely decompensated effusions.

Collect the following equipment: direct current defibrillator, ECG machine or cardiac monitor, antiseptic preparation solution, gauze, draping towels/sheet, sterile gloves, syringes (10, 20 and 60 ml), 18–20 gauge cardiac needle, 1–2 % lidocaine without epinephrine, three-way stopcock, catheter-over-needle unit (16-gauge, at least 9 cm long) and appropriate tubes for culture of aspirate.

Position the patient at 30–45°. Shave the chest in men. The site of insertion of the needle can be either the infrasternal angle (left side of the xiphisternum and costal cartilage) directing the needle superiorly, posteriorly and slightly laterally (Figure 139).

Infiltrate local anaesthetic into the skin. Connect the needle with a three-way stopcock keeping the local anaesthetic needle attached to one port on the opposite side of the needle connection. Connect the transducer to the side port of the three-way stopcock and a sterile ECG recorder to the metal part of the needle. Insert the needle through the subxiphoid approach, pointing the needle toward the left shoulder. Advance the needle and syringe until the needle tip is posterior to the rib cage. The needle should be advanced toward the shoulder at an angle of 15–20° from the abdominal wall. While advancing the needle toward the pericardial space, aspirate the syringe and inject lidocaine for a better analgesic effect. Continue to advance the needle until fluid is aspirated in the syringe or the ECG monitor shows S-T elevation. Withdraw the needle slowly with negative pressure on the syringe if the ECG shows S-T elevation after clearing the needle with lidocaine. Re-insert the needle in a different direction very slowly until fluid is aspirated in the syringe.

When the needle tip is inside the pericardial space, a soft floppy-tip guidewire is passed through the needle. Wrap this guidewire around the heart. Remove the needle, and insert a soft catheter with multiple side holes over this wire. Remove the guidewire. Connect the catheter hub with the transducer and syringe with a three-way stopcock. Place the dressing, and secure the catheter to prevent displacement. Ensure that the catheter is flushed with 1–2 ml of fluid to prevent blockage. Either a pigtail or straight catheter can be used – the straight catheter having holes in its sides allowing further drainage and reducing the risk of blockage.

The catheter can be left *in situ* for up to 24 hours if so desired, draining passively. Negative suction should not be used.

In the immediate post-procedure period, the patient should be monitored and assessed for the following complications: hypotension, ventricular puncture, cardiac arrest, pulseless electrical activity, pneumothorax and liver laceration.

■ Complications

Laceration of coronary artery or vein, pericardial tamponade, acute left ventricular failure with pulmonary oedema, puncture or laceration of any cardiac chamber, bleeding, ventricular ectopic beats, atrial ectopic beats, arrhythmias, hypotension, pneumothorax and pulmonary oedema. Clearly the patient should be counselled for these complications prior to the procedure. The morbidity rate for two-dimensional pericardiocentesis is now 0–1 % with the mortality being close enough to 0 %.

For recurrent or persistent pericardial effusions a pericardial window may be indicated. Consult cardiothoracic team.

Nasogastric tubes

TIM BROWN AND PARASKEVAS PARASKEVA

A nasogastric (NG) tube provides a conduit into the gastrointestinal (GI) tract (Figure 140).

■ Indications

- *Drainage* of the GI tract.
- *Feeding* the GI tract, thereby bypassing the oesophageal sphincters.
- *Sampling* contents of upper GI tract.

■ Contraindications

- *Base of skull fracture* – if suspected a nasogastric tube is contraindicated because it may pass through a fractured cribriform plate to enter the brain. An orogastric tube is the conduit of choice in this instance.
- *Patients with an unsecured airway* – here a nasogastric tube may induce vomiting and lead to aspiration of gastric contents.
- *Facial fractures.*

■ Types

- *Ryles tube* – wide bore, used for short-term feeding or aspiration of gastric contents.
- *Fine-bore feeding tube* – not for aspiration of gastric contents as its thin soft rubber walls have a tendency to collapse with minimal suction.

Hospital Surgery: Foundations in Surgical Practice, ed. Omer Aziz, Sanjay Purkayastha and Paraskevas Paraskeva. Published by Cambridge University Press.
© Cambridge University Press 2009.

■ Insertion technique

Equipment required:

- Universal protection equipment
- Nasogastric tube (see above)
- Lubricant (KY jelly/2 % lidocaine gel)
- Adhesive tape
- Drainage bag
- A 50 ml bladder suction syringe
- Glass of water
- Bowl for gastric contents
- Stethoscope
- Litmus paper.

Procedure:

1. Explain procedure and gain consent (verbal or written) from patient.
2. Sit patient upright.
3. Measure the distance from nostril to trans-pyloric plane (midpoint of line from sternal notch to symphisis pubis) and mark on tubing.
4. Lubricate the end of the tube.
5. If patient has an intact swallowing reflex, ask him/her to hold a sip of water in their mouth until instructed to swallow. (This step should be omitted if the patient is incapable of a coordinated swallowing reflex.)
6. Pass tube upwards into the nostril and then push posteriorly towards the occiput to advance the tube through the nasal cavity and nasopharynx into the oropharynx.
7. If resistance is encountered, gentle rotation of the tube will aid its passage.
8. When the upper oesophageal sphincter is reached, ask the patient to swallow and push the tube into the oesophagus. Continue to advance the tube until the pre-marked level is reached.

9. Look into the patient's mouth to ensure that the tube has not become curled-up within the patient's nasopharynx/oropharynx.
10. At all times monitor the patient to ensure that the tube has not entered the trachea. (For example coughing, respiratory distress, saturation difficulties.)
11. Secure the tube with adhesive tape or holder that the manufacturer has provided with the tubing kit.
12. Connect to drainage bag.
13. Check position:
    a. Aspirate gastric contents using bladder syringe.
    b. Check pH of gastric contents for acidic fluid (NB patients on antacids or anti-ulcer medication may have a higher gastric pH than expected).
    c. Obtain a radiograph to ensure that the tube tip is within the stomach.
14. Document procedure in notes including method of position confirmation.

■ Tips

- If the tube has been in the fridge then the rubber walls become stiffer and will make insertion easier.
- Never push the tube with force as this may cause trauma, swelling and bleeding to occur. This will lead to failure of passage and will add difficulty to future attempts at placement by other members of your team.
- Never commence feeding through a tube whose placement has not been checked radiographically. 'NG feed pneumonia' is well documented.
- If a nasogastric tube is likely to be in place long term then consider placement of a percutaneous endoscopic gastrostomy (PEG), surgical gastrostomy, or jejunostomy. These techniques will all reduce discomfort and trauma to the upper GI and respiratory tracts.

■ Aspiration

As the tube passes to the pharynx, the gag reflex is strongly stimulated. This will cause retching and sometimes vomiting. If the patient has a very full upper GI tract (e.g. small-bowel obstruction) or uncoordinated swallowing (e.g. cerebrovascular event) then there is a real danger of aspiration of stomach contents. To prevent this, ensure that the patient is well positioned, good suction facilities are to hand, and help can be accessed without difficulty.

If there is any doubt about a patient's ability to protect their own airway then senior advice should be sought with a view to anaesthetic intervention.

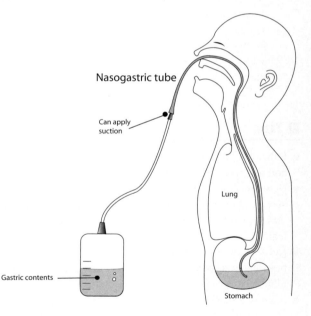

Figure 140

Abdominal paracentesis

PARASKEVAS PARASKEVA

■ Introduction

This procedure is the insertion of a drain into or aspiration of the peritoneal cavity. Drains can be inserted into the peritoneum in a trauma situation (diagnostic peritoneal lavage) and to manage renal failure (continuous ambulatory peritoneal dialysis). These will not be discussed here.

■ Indications

The indications for abdominal paracentesis are:

Therapeutic drainage of intra-abdominal fluid:
- Relief of abdominal distension
- Relief of pain
- Respiratory compromise.

Diagnostics on peritoneal fluid:
- Bacteriology
- Chemical pathology – protein content
- Cytology – suspected malignancy.

■ Contraindications

- Severely scarred abdomen
- Coagulopathy
- Bowel obstruction
- Pregnancy
- Infected skin at insertion site.

Hospital Surgery: Foundations in Surgical Practice, ed. Omer Aziz, Sanjay Purkayastha and Paraskevas Paraskeva. Published by Cambridge University Press. © Cambridge University Press 2009.

■ Equipment

- Either use a purpose-designed *paracentesis set*, or a *Bonanno* suprapubic catheterization set can be used.
- Drainage bag.
- Sterile preparation.
- Local anaesthetic.
- Suture material.
- Syringes and bottles for taking samples.

■ Technique

- The patient is placed in a supine position.
- The fluid/air interface is percussed out.
- The site is marked with a pen. Preferred sites of entry are shown in Figure 141. These are either of the lower quadrants (lateral to the rectus muscle), or below the umbilicus. Paracentesis site should not be at a site of prior incision and must not be infected.
- The patient is prepared and draped.
- The anaesthetic is injected into the skin and infiltrated down into the abdominal wall.
- Sampling: a 14-gauge needle with a syringe can be used to obtain peritoneal fluid.
- Therapeutic drainage: a *Bonanno catheter, CVP catheter* or *peritoneal dialysis catheter* are inserted using a stylette or a Seldinger technique.
- Samples are taken for cytology, chemical pathology and microbiology.
- The catheter is sutured in place and left on free drainage. Occasionally in massive ascites it is advisable to drain 2 litres at a time to avoid large haemodynamic shifts.
- If the catheter is not draining, check it is not blocked by flushing, if this has no effect the patient can be asked to change position to allow fluid to collect near the catheter. Alternatively the catheter will need to be manipulated to change the position.

- If there is concern as to the site of the fluid or if fluid has stopped draining from the catheter despite the above manoeuvres then an ultrasound scan of the abdomen is advised.

■ Complications

- Bacterial peritonitis
- Haemorrhage (especially inferior epigastric vessels)
- Bowel injury
- Bladder injury (avoid by inserting a urinary catheter to drain the bladder prior to insertion)
- Hypotension (prevent by giving colloid as a replacement)
- Persistent ascites leak.

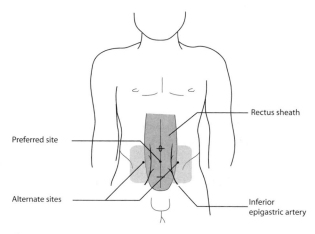

Figure 141

Diagnostic peritoneal lavage (DPL)

ZIAD ALYAN AND SANJAY PURKAYASTHA

■ Definition

DPL is an invasive diagnostic tool used in the assessment of abdominal trauma. The procedure is considered to be 98 % sensitive for intraperitoneal bleeding, in experienced hands. It should be undertaken by the surgical team attending to the patient as it may alter the physical signs present.

■ Indications

Investigating blunt abdominal trauma.

The investigation is useful in the following circumstances:

- Altered sensorium, head injury, patients under the influence of alcohol and/or elicit drugs.
- Altered sensation – spinal cord injury.
- Injury to nearby structures – ribs, pelvic fracture and spinal fracture.
- Equivocal findings subsequent to an abdominal examination.
- Lack of availability of ultrasound or CT scanners.
- In a patient not stable enough to be transferred to the CT scanner.

■ Contraindications

The absolute contraindication is the presence of indications for an emergency laparotomy.

Relative contraindications include morbid obesity, previous significant abdominal surgery, coagulopathy and pregnancy.

Hospital Surgery: Foundations in Surgical Practice, ed. Omer Aziz, Sanjay Purkayastha and Paraskevas Paraskeva. Published by Cambridge University Press. © Cambridge University Press 2009.

■ Procedure

There are two main methods: (1) Open technique. (2) Closed technique.

1. OPEN TECHNIQUE

- Decompress urinary bladder (catheterize patient).
- Decompress stomach (place a nasogastric tube).
- Surgically prepare the abdomen.
- Locally anaesthetize the site of insertion with lidocaine $+/-$ adrenaline, just inferior to the umbilicus.
- Vertically incise the skin and subcutaneous tissues.
- Lift the edges of the fascia with artery forceps. Incise the peritoneum.
- Insert a peritoneal lavage catheter.
- Connect a syringe and aspirate.
- If no frank blood is aspirated, instil 1 l of warmed normal saline or Hartmann's solution via tubing.
- Allow the fluid to mix by gently moving the abdomen. If this is contraindicated then allow fluid to remain for 5–10 minutes. Allow fluid to drain by placing bag below abdominal level.

Interpretation; a positive result is:

1. Frank blood.
2. Food, bile, or faecal matter visible.
3. $\geq 100\,000$ RBC/mm^3.
4. ≥ 500 WBC/mm^3.

2. CLOSED TECHNIQUE

The same general considerations and preparations are undertaken. At the same site as the open technique, a small incision made after local anaesthesia is infiltrated. The tubing is inserted using the Seldinger technique:

A cannula (usually a specific blunted cannula is available in DPL packs) is inserted in the incision and is used to penetrate the midline fascia in the abdominal wall. During insertion, a sudden give or 'pop' can be felt as the cannula passes through the fascia. Care must be taken not to insert the cannula too deeply and perforate the bowel. A flexible guidewire is passed through the cannula. The cannula is then removed and a catheter threaded over the guidewire. The guidewire is then removed. A syringe fitted on the catheter is used for aspiration.

The open technique is advocated by the authors as, although it takes longer, it is performed under direct vision and therefore has less potential for complications.

■ Complications

- ■ Haemorrhage (vascular injury)
- ■ Bowel injury
- ■ Bladder laceration
- ■ Wound infection.

There is a 1 % chance of major complications for both the open and closed techniques.

■ Other considerations

- ■ Both DPL and ultrasound scanning can screen for haemoperitoneum after blunt trauma. However, they cannot determine the source of the bleeding.
- ■ Laparotomy based solely on a positive DPL results in an unnecessary procedure in about a third of patients.
- ■ A negative lavage does not exclude a retroperitoneal injury, diaphragmatic injury or isolated perforations of the bowel.
- ■ The use of DPL is highly protocol driven and institution specific. The FAST scan and laparoscopy has replaced DPL in many institutions.

Rigid sigmoidoscopy

ROS JACKLIN AND PARASKEVAS PARASKEVA

■ Definition

Rigid sigmoidoscopy is a visual examination of the distal sigmoid colon and rectum using a rigid tube with a light source, called a sigmoidoscope. It consists of an outer hollow plastic or metal tube, an introducer which is withdrawn after the instrument has been inserted, and a light source. There is a hand pump connected by tubing so air can be insufflated to open up the bowel lumen ahead of the instrument.

■ Indications

Rigid sigmoidoscopy is indicated in the investigation of rectal bleeding. It can be used as a vehicle for biopsy of the rectum, for example in suspected inflammatory bowel disease or colorectal cancer. It can also facilitate decompression and reduction of sigmoid volvulus.

■ Procedure

1. PRE-PROCEDURE CONSIDERATIONS

- Ask the patient to evacuate the rectum, or clear it by administering glycerine suppositories or an enema prior to the procedure.
- Explain the procedure, including the reasons why you are doing it and the fact that it should cause only minor discomfort. Warn the patient they may experience the urge to defaecate or pass flatus during the procedure. Verbal consent is sufficient.
- Check your equipment, including light source.

Hospital Surgery: Foundations in Surgical Practice, ed. Omer Aziz, Sanjay Purkayastha and Paraskevas Paraskeva. Published by Cambridge University Press. © Cambridge University Press 2009.

- Position the patient correctly in the left lateral position, hips flexed and buttocks extending over the edge of the examination couch.
- Ensure adequate lighting.
- Inspect the perianal skin then perform a preliminary digital rectal examination to ensure nothing is blocking the rectum, followed by proctoscopy.

2. PROCEDURE

- Talk to the patient throughout, and place them in control – reassure them that you will stop if they are uncomfortable.
- Apply a generous quantity of lubricant to the sigmoidoscope, holding the introducer in place using your thumb.
- Instruct the patient to take deep breaths and introduce the sigmoidoscope the first few centimetres. After the tip has passed through the anal canal, aim posteriorly towards the sacrum.
- Attach the eyepiece, with the light source and air pump, and screw the viewing window closed (see Figure 142).
- Align the sigmoidoscope so that the rectal lumen is clearly visible. Use a swab to sweep away any faeces, blood or mucus obstructing your view.
- Periodically introduce air to open up the bowel lumen beyond the scope.
- Advance the instrument carefully, changing the direction of the scope as required to keep the lumen ahead visible. The rectosigmoid junction may be difficult to negotiate, but advance (without using force) to 18–22 cm if possible.
- Withdraw slowly, inspecting for mucosal lesions, including polyps and inflammation.
- Let the introduced air escape from the gut before removing the scope.

3. POST-PROCEDURE CONSIDERATIONS

- Warn the patient they may experience mild colicky discomfort after the procedure.

- Take care to check the re-usable portions of your equipment for contamination, and clean them thoroughly. Where possible use disposable tubing.

■ Complications

- It is possible to damage or even perforate the bowel wall with a rigid sigmoidoscope, so avoid the use of force.
- Bleeding or perforation can also occur at biopsy sites.

■ Special considerations

- Always have a chaperone in attendance when performing any intimate examination. It is advisable to document their presence, including the chaperone's name.
- Only the distal portion of the colon may be inspected using a rigid sigmoidoscope, so if symptoms are suspicious for colorectal cancer, further visualization of the colon is required.

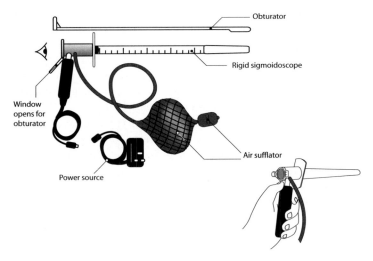

Figure 142 Equipment

Proctoscopy

ROS JACKLIN AND PARASKEVAS PARASKEVA

Definition: proctoscopy is a visual examination of the lower rectum and anal canal using a short rigid tube with a light source, called a proctoscope. Haemorrhoids may be treated by injection or banding, and biopsies may be taken without pain if the lesion is above the dentate line.

Indications: detection of diseases of the rectum or anus, or investigation of rectal bleeding.

■ Procedure

1. PRE-PROCEDURE CONSIDERATIONS

- Explain the procedure, including the reasons why you are doing it and the fact that it should cause only minor discomfort.
- Check your equipment including light source.
- Position the patient correctly in the left lateral position, hips flexed and buttocks extending over the edge of the examination couch.
- Ensure adequate lighting.
- Inspect the perianal skin for skin tags/lesions, fistula openings, fissures, perianal haematomas and rashes. Ask the patient to bear down and inspect for prolapse if symptoms are suggestive.
- Perform a preliminary digital rectal examination to ensure nothing is blocking the rectum. (If this is too tender for the patient to tolerate, do not proceed to proctoscopy. Suspect a fissure or anorectal abscess, treat appropriately and review the patient after treatment, or

Hospital Surgery: Foundations in Surgical Practice, ed. Omer Aziz, Sanjay Purkayastha and Paraskevas Paraskeva. Published by Cambridge University Press.
© Cambridge University Press 2009.

arrange an urgent examination under anaesthetic if you suspect sinister pathology.)

2. PROCEDURE

- Talk to the patient throughout, as their confidence and cooperation will be helpful.
- Apply a generous quantity of lubricant to the tip of the proctoscope, holding the handle with your fingers gripping the handle and your thumb holding the introducer in place to keep the two parts of the instrument assembled.
- Point the handle posteriorly.
- Instruct the patient to take deep breaths and introduce the proctoscope to its full length, aiming posteriorly towards the sacrum (Figure 143).
- Remove the introducer and attach the light source.
- Use a swab to sweep away any faeces, blood or mucus obstructing your view.
- Align the proctoscope so that the rectal lumen is clearly visible.
- Withdraw slowly, inspecting for mucosal lesions, including haemorrhoids, polyps or evidence of proctitis.
- Consider biopsy of any non-vascular lesions above the dentate line, and treatment of symptomatic haemorrhoids.

3. POST-PROCEDURE CONSIDERATIONS

- If haemorrhoids were visible and thought to be causing symptoms, they may be treated by injection (first degree) or banding (first or second degree).
- Discuss your planned treatment with the patient. See the table for a description of the technique.
- Warn the patient to expect some bleeding after the procedure, and some mild discomfort after banding.

Technique for injection	Technique for banding
Visualize the haemorrhoids clearly	Visualize the haemorrhoids clearly
Ensure the phenol is 5 % strength in oil (not 80 %)	Ask your assistant to load the banding machine with one band at a time
Insert the needle into the bulging part of each haemorrhoid in turn, above the dentate line	Hold the proctoscope with your left hand, and the suction tube of the banding machine in your right
You will feel a slight 'give' as the needle goes in. Slowly inject a few ml of oily phenol and the haemorrhoid should visibly balloon up	Position the tip of the tube over the upper part of the haemorrhoid, well above the dentate line, under direct vision
Do not continue to inject against resistance, or if you cannot see the haemorrhoid swell	Cover the side hole in the suction tube with your thumb so the haemorrhoid is drawn onto the tip
	'Fire' the band by pushing the outer sleeve on the bander forwards. The banded portion should form a spherical bulge. Reload and repeat on the next one

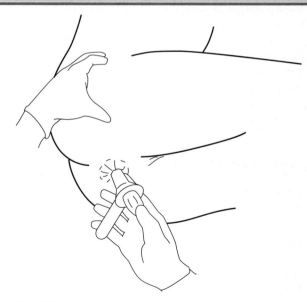

Figure 143

■ Complications

- Simple proctoscopy has few risks.
- Injection of haemorrhoids can result in prostatitis if the prostate is infiltrated with oily phenol, therefore take special care injecting anteriorly in men.
- Bleeding may occur after treatment of haemorrhoids. In addition, if a band is placed too low, incorporating tissue below the dentate line, the patient will experience considerable pain for several days.

■ Special considerations

- Always have a chaperone in attendance when performing any intimate examination. It is advisable to document their presence, including the chaperone's name.
- Remember that perianal conditions are common. Even in the presence of a local cause, rectal bleeding should still be investigated by visualization of the colon in patients with risk factors for colorectal cancer.

Oesophago-gastro-duodenoscopy (OGD)

SHAHID A. KHAN AND RUPERT NEGUS

■ Definition

OGD: visual examination of the upper gastrointestinal (GI) tract, from cricopharyngeus to the second part of the duodenum, using an endoscope (usually video-endoscope) (Figure 144).

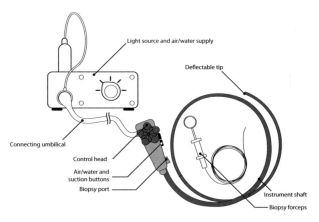

Figure 144

■ Indications

OGD may be used to investigate any symptoms referable to the upper GI tract. In addition to direct visualization, biopsies and brushings may be taken and various therapeutic manoeuvres performed using a dedicated channel that runs the length of the endoscope.

Hospital Surgery: Foundations in Surgical Practice, ed. Omer Aziz, Sanjay Purkayastha and Paraskevas Paraskeva. Published by Cambridge University Press. © Cambridge University Press 2009.

DIAGNOSTIC OGD

- Investigation of dyspepsia, dysphagia, anaemia (including duodenal biopsies for assessment of coeliac disease), suspected upper GI malignancy, upper GI haemorrhage (melaena/haematemesis) and abnormal barium studies.
- Screening for varices, Barrett's oesophagus, and postoperative surveillance of upper gastrointestinal cancer.
- Follow-up of gastric ulcers to assess for healing and malignancy.
- Occasionally used as an intraoperative aid for laparoscopic upper gastrointestinal surgery.

THERAPEUTIC OGD

- Upper GI bleeding:
  - Bleeding ulcers (duodenal and gastric) and other vascular malformations may be treated with a combination of direct adrenaline injection, heater probe application, clips and argon plasma coagulation.
  - Bleeding oesophageal varices are predominantly treated by banding and/or sclerotherapy; fundal gastric varices by glue therapy.
- Dilatation of strictures which may be secondary to benign disease (e.g. oesophagitis or caustic ingestion, Schatski ring, achalasia) or upper GI malignancy.
- Oesophageal stenting for dysphagia due to malignancy.
- Tumour debulking (e.g. via diathermy, local injection of toxic agents, laser photocoagulation, argon plasma coagulator, photocoagulation).
- Removal of foreign bodies and food bolus impaction.
- Removal of gastric polyps.
- Nutrition:
  - Insertion of percutaneous endoscopic gastrostomy (PEG) or jejunostomy (PEJ) feeding tubes e.g. in patients who cannot swallow due to stroke or other neurological conditions.
  - Placement of nasojejunal (NJ) feeding tubes e.g. in patients with acute pancreatitis.

■ Procedure (Figure 145)

PRE-PROCEDURE CONSIDERATIONS

- Ensure patient is stable enough to tolerate procedure and is cannulated.
- Biopsies, polypectomy and some therapeutic procedures may be contraindicated if the patient is on anticoagulation therapy or antiplatelet agents (check FBC and clotting pre-OGD, reverse coagulopathy if necessary and ensure blood and blood products are readily available in acute upper GI haemorrhage).
- Bacteraemia can occur during endoscopy, therefore administer antibiotic prophylaxis to high-risk patients, e.g. those with prosthetic heart valves or a history of endocarditis; check local or national (e.g. British National Formulary) microbiological guidelines.
- Patient must remain nil by mouth for at least six hours prior to OGD.

PROCEDURE STEPS

- Check that indications for OGD are appropriate.
- Ensure the patient understands why the procedure is necessary, the risks involved, and is able to give informed consent.
- For straightforward diagnostic OGDs, sedation is not usually required and pharyngeal anaesthesia with local anaesthetic spray is usually sufficient.
- At OGD, direct visualization of the oesophagus, stomach, duodenal bulb and second part of the duodenum is obtained. The gastric fundus is examined by retroflexion (J-manoeuvre).

POST-PROCEDURE CONSIDERATIONS

- Low threshold for suspicion of perforation if post-procedure neck or chest pain and/or surgical emphysema, especially following oesophageal dilation.
- See complications below.

■ Complications

- Over-sedation (reverse if necessary) leading to hypoxia or respiratory arrest.
- Allergic or idiosyncratic reaction to sedation or local anaesthetic (rare).
- Aspiration pneumonia, particularly with gastric outflow.
- Perforation can occur at any level of the upper GI tract, but is commoner in the pharynx and cervical oesophagus where the endoscope is passed blindly, particularly if the patient has a pharyngeal pouch. Perforation is rare in diagnostic OGD, but therapeutic manoeuvres carry increased risk, particularly dilation (1/1000 for benign oesophageal stenosis, up to 5 % for achalasia).
- Bleeding – rare in diagnostic OGD; more common after therapeutic procedures.
- Cardiac dysrhythmias, particularly in presence of hypoxia, but generally rare.

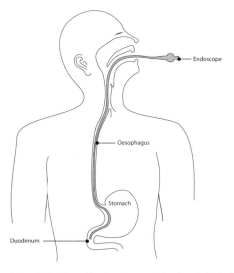

Figure 145 Schematic of endoscope being inserted into GI tract

Endoscopic retrograde cholangio-pancreatography (ERCP)

JONATHAN HOARE AND JULIAN TEARE

■ Definitions

Endoscopic retrograde cholangio-pancreatography (ERCP) is the passage of an endoscope to the second part of the duodenum allowing access to the major papilla, and the subsequent cannulation of the biliary and/or pancreatic ductal systems. These are opacified by injection of contrast media permitting their visualization and allowing for a variety of therapeutic interventions.

ERCP is a complex endoscopic procedure with a similar level of risk to some major operations; consequently it needs to be carefully planned. Since the advent of more advanced non-invasive imaging, i.e. magnetic resonance cholangio-pancreatography (MRCP) and endoscopic ultrasound, the majority of ERCPs performed are therapeutic rather than diagnostic. Pancreatic therapy and biliary manometry is usually only performed in specialist centres.

■ Indications

COMMON

- Removal of common bile duct stones prior to or after cholecystectomy.
- Diagnosis and stenting of biliary strictures; malignant (pancreatic cancer, cholangiocarcinoma) and benign (inflammatory, postoperative). Brushing the stricture can provide cytological samples.

Hospital Surgery: Foundations in Surgical Practice, ed. Omer Aziz, Sanjay Purkayastha and Paraskevas Paraskeva. Published by Cambridge University Press. © Cambridge University Press 2009.

OTHER

- Diagnosis of obstructive jaundice if other imaging inconclusive e.g. to confirm primary sclerosing cholangitis.
- Endoscopic therapy of postoperative biliary leaks i.e. by stenting.
- Severe gallstone pancreatitis, associated with biliary obstruction (early intervention with ERCP reduces morbidity and mortality).
- Investigation and treatment of recurrent acute pancreatitis e.g. by diagnosing and treating pancreatic duct stones and strictures.
- Diagnosis of 'sphincter of Oddi dysfunction' by biliary manometry.

■ Procedure

PRE-PROCEDURE CONSIDERATIONS

To keep your endoscopist happy, patients should be sent for ERCP with consent performed, a cannula in the **left** arm and a recent FBC and clotting screen clearly visible in the notes.

Anticoagulation

INR and platelet count should be documented as normal before the procedure. Frequently patients with obstructive jaundice have a prolonged INR which can be corrected with vitamin K.

As for other major procedures warfarin should be stopped and alternative anticoagulation instituted if necessary. There is no evidence that aspirin increases bleeding risk at sphincterotomy although most would like it stopped if possible. There is little evidence regarding clopidrogel but anecdotally it is felt to increase bleeding risk and should be stopped if possible. Consult local guidelines.

Antibiotics

With an obstructed biliary tree there is a significant risk of cholangitis following ERCP, hence such patients should be given prophylactic antibiotics (e.g. 750 mg oral ciprofloxacin 60–90 minutes before procedure or intravenous gentamicin/cephalosporin or ureidopenicillin immediately before). Those with a pancreatic pseudocyst should be treated similarly to prevent secondary infection.

There is a 6 % risk of bacteraemia at ERCP, double if the duct is obstructed. Antibiotic prophylaxis should be given to patients at high risk of endocarditis (same as for colonoscopy i.e. prosthetic heart valves, previous endocarditis, surgically constructed systemic-pulmonary shunt or conduit, synthetic vascular graft less than one year old, severe neutropaenia (neutrophils $< 1.0 \times 10^9$/litre)).

Consent and complications

Mortality associated with therapeutic ERCP is quoted at around 0.5 % in several large studies. Consent, ideally by the endoscopist, should follow a detailed explanation of the procedure to the patient.

Studies have shown that the majority of patients will have a rise in serum amylase post-procedure, with clinical pancreatitis occurring in approximately 5 %. The risk is increased in young females, and is particularly high in patients having biliary manometry (up to 20 % in some series). Pain occurs within a few hours of the procedure, and is usually self-limiting, but can be severe.

Significant bleeding can occur after biliary sphincterotomy in approximately 2 % of cases. If a patient has evidence of ongoing bleeding post-procedure they should be re-scoped by an experienced endoscopist. There are also the risks associated with any endoscopic procedure i.e. over sedation and perforation from passage of the scope.

■ Procedure

A 'side viewing' endoscope is passed to the second part of the duodenum and the major papilla localized. A catheter is then passed and duct cannulation attempted. Unless desired the pancreatic duct is avoided if possible to reduce the chance of pancreatitis. If the bile duct cannot be cannulated then a 'needle knife' can be used to cut into the bile duct through the wall of the duodenum, but this increases the chance of bleeding and perforation.

Once access is established a cholangiogram is obtained by the injection of contrast. Frequently a 'sphincterotomy' must be performed over a guidewire, dividing the muscular biliary sphincter by electrocautery, thereby widening the opening to the common bile duct. This allows the passage of instruments (e.g. balloon catheter or basket) to remove gallstones. A stent can usually be deployed across a stricture without a sphincterotomy. A final cholangiogram is taken to demonstrate the duct clear of stones or the stent correctly sited (Figure 146).

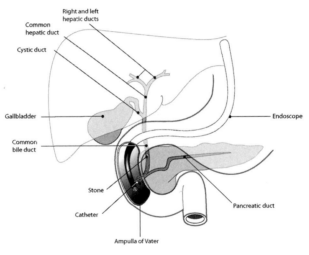

Figure 146

■ Post-procedure considerations

- The patient should be nil by mouth for six hours post-procedure and must be monitored for the development of complications. It can be difficult to distinguish retained air from pancreatitis initially. If there is any doubt the patient should be admitted, given an intravenous fluid infusion, and serial amylase measurements made. Most pancreatitis starts within one to six hours of the procedure.

■ Findings should be explained to the patient after sedation has worn off entirely, as the amnesic effect of benzodiazepines can persist for long after the patient is apparently awake.

■ The endoscopist/consultant should specify appropriate follow-up. In patients with gallstones laparoscopic cholecystectomy should be performed as soon as possible before another stone migrates from the gallbladder into the duct, running the risk of a 'retained stone' postoperatively.

Colonoscopy and flexible sigmoidoscopy

JONATHAN HOARE AND JULIAN TEARE

■ Definitions

The colonic mucosa is examined with and therapy delivered through, a flexible endoscope (also see Chapter on OGD). A limited examination of the sigmoid and descending colon, usually to the splenic flexure (approximately 60 cm with a straight scope), is termed 'flexible sigmoidoscopy'. With full 'bowel prep' and sufficient dexterity 'colonoscopy' can be performed when a scope is passed to the caecum, allowing access to the entire colonic mucosa, and the terminal ileum if necessary.

■ Indications

COLONOSCOPY

- Iron deficiency anaemia
- Blood in the stool or rectal bleeding
- Altered bowel habit (diarrhoea or constipation)
- Significant, unexplained weight loss, accompanied by gastrointestinal symptoms
- A family history of colon cancer
- A history of previous colon polyps or colon cancer
- Cancer screening in people with ulcerative colitis
- To assess inflammatory bowel disease
- Chronic, unexplained abdominal pain.

Hospital Surgery: Foundations in Surgical Practice, ed. Omer Aziz, Sanjay Purkayastha and Paraskevas Paraskeva. Published by Cambridge University Press. © Cambridge University Press 2009.

FLEXIBLE SIGMOIDOSCOPY

This is a limited examination and should not be performed when there is a significant chance of missing serious proximal pathology (50 % of all colon cancers are proximal to the splenic flexure), hence indications are limited. Senior advice/local guidelines should be sought if you are not sure which examination to book. The common indications are:

- Minimal bright red rectal bleeding
- As a screening test in asymptomatic people to detect colon polyps or colon cancer
- Persistent diarrhoea with no alarm symptoms e.g. in diagnostic work-up for irritable bowel syndrome
- After radiation treatment to the pelvis when a patient has lower gastrointestinal symptoms
- To assess inflammatory bowel disease.

■ Procedure

PRE-PROCEDURE CONSIDERATIONS

Bowel preparation

Colonoscopy: requires formal bowel preparation in order to empty the entire colon of faeces. Bowel preparation for inpatients is often poorly performed, preventing a thorough examination and frustrating the colonoscopist! An ideal 'prep' is shown below. The most commonly used cleansing solutions contain magnesium or phosphate ions, which act as osmotic laxatives (e.g. Picolax and Citramag). Because of the resultant fluid shifts and electrolyte load these should be used with caution in patients with cardiac or renal failure. The alternative is gastrointestinal lavage using balanced electrolyte solutions with polyethylene glycol (PEG) e.g. Klean-Prep. This is also useful if rapid bowel preparation is required in lower GI bleeding; however, patients find the large volume, 4 litres over 4–6 hours, and the resultant diarrhoea difficult.

Seven days before colonoscopy: stop iron tablets (a common omission; iron constipates and coats the mucosa with tarry stool). Consider if anticoagulants or antiplatelet therapy need to be stopped.

Four days before colonoscopy: stop constipating agents (codeine phosphate, Lomotil (co-phenotrope)).

Two days before colonoscopy: start 'low-residue diet' i.e. boiled/steamed fish, boiled chicken, egg, cheese, white bread, butter/margarine, rich tea biscuits, potato (no skin). Push oral fluids. PATIENT SHOULD NOT EAT HIGH-FIBRE FOODS such as red meat, pink fish, fruit, vegetables, cereals, salad, nuts, sweet corn, wholemeal bread etc.

Day before colonoscopy: good breakfast from the permitted list followed by fluid only until after the examination (small amount of milk allowed in tea/coffee) and 'bowel prep'. Intravenous saline can be administered, especially if the patient is elderly or unwell.

A typical regime is:	14.00	Senna granules or tablets	
	17.00	1 sachet Picolax	
	19.00	$\frac{1}{2}$ sachet Picolax	
Day of colonoscopy	06.00	if procedure a.m.	$\frac{1}{2}$ sachet Picolax
	10.00	if procedure p.m.	$\frac{1}{2}$ sachet Picolax.

Clear fluids can be continued until four hours before the procedure.

Flexible sigmoidoscopy: as in colonoscopy bowel preparation iron tablets should be stopped seven days before the procedure. A phosphate enema is administered approximately one hour before the procedure to empty the sigmoid and descending colon.

Anticoagulation

Warfarin: diagnostic procedures including standard biopsies are safe while patients are on warfarin (provided INR is not supratherapeutic). For therapeutic procedures including polypectomy and stricture dilation warfarin should be stopped as if for an operative procedure.

Aspirin or clopidogrel: aspirin and especially clopidrogel should be stopped seven days before a major therapeutic procedure. Small polyps, however, are probably safe to remove while the patient is on aspirin. If in doubt consult your own unit's policies.

Antibiotics

There is a 2–4 % risk of bacteraemia following a colonoscopy. It is recommended that patients at high risk of endocarditis be given antibiotic prophylaxis, i.e. prosthetic heart valves, previous endocarditis, surgically constructed systemic-pulmonary shunt or conduit, synthetic vascular graft less than one year old, severe neutropaenia (neutrophils $< 1.0 \times 10^9$/litre).

Consent

Should be taken only by individuals familiar with the procedure. Patients should be made aware that there is an approximate 1/1000 risk of a perforation associated with a standard colonoscopy and 1/300 risk of a significant bleed. Abdominal pain due to 'trapped wind' is relatively common (see Complications).

PROCEDURE

The modern way to perform colonoscopy is under only mild sedation, enabling the patient to easily change position, facilitating passage of the scope, and able to provide feedback to the endoscopist regarding pain experienced, thereby warning of potential trauma and subsequent perforation. Typical sedation would be 1.25–2.5 mg midazolam and 25 mg pethidine; further boluses given as necessary. Monitoring is by pulse oximetry. Colonoscopy can frequently be performed with no sedation or analgesia if necessary. Hyoscine (buscopan) (10–20 mg) is usually administered for its anti-cholinergic effect, preventing peristalsis.

Typically passage of the scope to the caecum takes 5–45 minutes depending on difficulty. There are few hard landmarks in the colon, the gold standard to confirm 'caecal intubation' being to pass the scope through the ileocaecal valve into the terminal ileum. The sudden change from colonic mucosa to small bowel mucosa and 'villi' provide documentary evidence of complete colonoscopy. If this is not possible then sighting the ileocaecal valve and/or the appendix orifice provide similar evidence.

During careful withdrawal of the scope is when most pathology is identified, biopsies taken and/or polyps removed. A complete examination should include retroflexion of the scope in the rectum to ensure distal pathology is not missed.

POST-PROCEDURE CONSIDERATIONS

Findings should be explained to the patient after sedation has worn off entirely, as the amnesic effect of benzodiazepines can persist for long after the patient is apparently awake.

Serious complications, i.e. perforation or bleeding, are more common when a complex procedure has been performed i.e. large polypectomy or stricture dilation. During colonoscopy air is blown through the scope to open the lumen and abdominal pain due to colonic distension is common.

Patients should be encouraged to pass wind; however, if they cannot a useful tip is to encourage them to adopt an 'all fours' prone position. This allows the sigmoid colon to fall forward facilitating passage of air and often providing great relief, although a little embarrassing! If pain does not settle then a perforation should be excluded. Both perforation and bleeding can present late (bleeding up to seven days and perforation up to three weeks). Bleeding tends to stop spontaneously and only supportive therapy is usually required.

Follow-up with review of histology should be arranged as necessary. A common source of confusion is appropriate surveillance intervals for screening colonoscopy following polypectomy. Repeat examinations should be performed at one, three or five years according to the algorithm given.

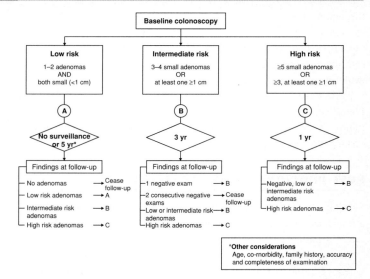

Algorithm: surveillance following adenoma removal. Adapted with permission from Atkins and Saunders, 'Surveillance guidelines after removal of colorectal adenomatous polyps' Gut 2002, 51

■ Alternatives to colonoscopy

It is important to consider alternatives before scheduling a colonoscopy as the procedure is not without risk and the bowel preparation can be difficult, especially for the immobile. For the investigation of iron deficiency anaemia in the elderly an abdominal CT with 'faecal tagging' (oral contrast the day prior to scanning) will pick up large lesions likely to cause anaemia, and has the advantage of not requiring bowel preparation, while giving additional information on other abdominal structures.

Barium enema requires bowel preparation but is less invasive than colonoscopy, although often still unpleasant for the patient. Many radiologists would argue that if a patient is not fit for colonoscopy, they are not fit for barium enema!

'*CT pneumocolon*': generating a 3D reconstruction of the colon, requires bowel preparation, but has been shown to be almost as sensitive as colonoscopy for polyp detection, and is a very good alternative if colonoscopy is impossible. It may have a future role in screening; however the large radiation dose is a disadvantage.

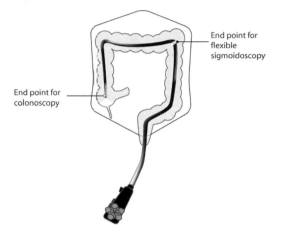

Figure 147 Extent of flexible sigmoidoscopy and colonoscopy

Local anaesthesia

SUSANNA WALKER

■ Definition

A local anaesthetic agent is a compound which produces temporary blockade of neuronal transmission when applied to a nerve axon.

■ Mechanism of action

- Local anaesthetics mainly block the function of sodium (Na^+) channels involved in membrane depolarization and propagation of action potentials.
- When a sufficient concentration of local anaesthetic is reached, and therefore an adequate number of Na^+ channels are blocked, depolarization does not occur in response to electrical stimulus as Na^+ influx is blocked. The blockade occurs from within the nerve axon.
- Local anaesthetics are weak, non-ionized bases formulated as protonated hydrochlorides, which enables them to be presented as a water-soluble preparation.
- After injection, the local anaesthetic exists as the non-ionized, lipid-soluble form (LA) and the ionized, water-soluble form (LAH^+). It is only the non-ionized, lipid-soluble form which can cross the nerve membrane, and block the Na^+ channel.

■ Pharmacokinetics

Proportions of non-ionized and ionized forms depend on the pKa of the local anaesthetic and the pH of the fluid in the tissue. *pKa is the pH at*

Hospital Surgery: Foundations in Surgical Practice, ed. Omer Aziz, Sanjay Purkayastha and Paraskevas Paraskeva. Published by Cambridge University Press. © Cambridge University Press 2009.

which a drug is 50 % ionized and 50 % non-ionized.

$LA + H^+ \leftrightarrow LAH^+$ $\qquad pH = pKa + \log 10 \; [LA]/[LAH^+].$

For basic drugs (proton acceptors), the lower the pH, the greater the proportion that exists in the ionized form. **While it is only the lipid-soluble, non-ionized drug which crosses the nerve membrane, it is the lipid-insoluble, ionized drug which is active.**

Using lidocaine as an example:

- pKa of lidocaine is 7.9.
- At standard body pH of 7.4, 24 % exists in the non-ionized form.
- This portion enters the nerve down its concentration gradient.
- Within the nerve axon, the standard pH is approximately 7.1. At this pH, a greater proportion exists in the ionized form (the active form). Therefore, of the LA that has passed into the nerve axon, approximately 80 % becomes ionized and active.
- The ionized (positively charged) drug is attracted to the negative charge of membrane proteins in the open Na^+ channels and blocks the channel, creating local anaesthesia.

■ Relating these principles to practice

1. ONSET OF ACTION

- With regards to basic drugs, the lower the pKa of the drug, the lower the degree of ionization at pH 7.4, and therefore greater percentage of non-ionized form and greater lipid solubility, leading to a more rapid onset of block. *This explains why lidocaine (pKa 7.9) has a faster onset of action than bupivacaine (pKa 8.1).*
- A drug with a higher pKa has an increased proportion of the drug in the ionized state at all levels of pH. Therefore, of the drug that has entered the nerve axon a greater percentage is in the active, ionized form. As a result, while onset of action is slower, offset of action is also slower. *This explains why bupivacaine has a longer length of action than lidocaine.*

- In areas of infection, such as abscesses, the pH of the tissue is lower than normal, therefore for each LA agent, a smaller proportion compared with normal is in the non-ionized, lipid-soluble form. *As a result local anaesthetic is less effective in infected tissues.*

2. POTENCY OF A LOCAL ANAESTHETIC IS RELATED TO LIPID SOLUBILITY

- Highly lipid-soluble compounds cross nerve membrane phospholipid bilayers more easily. Bupivacaine is more lipid-soluble and therefore approximately four times as potent as lidocaine. 0.25 % and 0.5 % bupivacaine are equivalent to 1 % and 2 % lidocaine.

3. DURATION OF ACTION IS ASSOCIATED WITH THE EXTENT OF PROTEIN BINDING

- *Extensive protein binding leads to a longer duration of action.* Bupivacaine and ropivacaine have a similar percentage of protein binding (95 %) and therefore a similar duration of action. Lidocaine, however, has only a 70 % protein binding, and therefore a much shorter duration of action.
- *Site of injection can affect duration of action.* Degree of vascularity of the site determines the speed at which local anaesthetic agent is absorbed systemically. Intercostal > epidural > brachial plexus > subcutaneous infiltration.

■ Maximum recommended doses

	Plain (mg/kg)	+ Adrenaline (mg/kg)
Lidocaine	3	7
Prilocaine	6	N/A
Bupivacaine	2	2
Ropivacaine	3.5	N/A

1 % lidocaine contains 10 mg/ml, 2 % lidocaine contains 20 mg/ml, 0.25 % bupivacaine contains 2.5 mg/ml etc.

■ Preparation additives

1. VASOCONSTRICTORS

- Most local anaesthetics cause a degree of vasodilation, so the addition of a vasoconstrictor increases the potency and duration of action by reducing the blood supply to the area. Usually adrenaline at maximum 5 μg/ml (1:200 000).
- May decrease systemic toxicity by decreasing rate of absorption, and minimize blood loss in highly vascular areas (e.g. suturing scalp lacerations). *Avoid using vasoconstrictors in end-arteries (digital or penile blocks) as ischaemia may ensue.*

2. ALKALIZATION

- Alkalization with sodium bicarbonate increases the speed of onset of a block by increasing the proportion of LA in the lipid-soluble phase at the time of injection. Rarely used, except in obstetric analgesia.

3. FORMULATIONS

- *EMLA cream* – eutectic mixture of local anaesthetic. An emulsion of 2.5 % lidocaine and 2.5 % prilocaine for topical anaesthesia. Apply 1 hr before procedure.
- *Ametop cream* – 4 % tetracaine gel. Also used for topical anaesthesia, but with faster onset than EMLA cream.

■ Local anaesthetic toxicity

A biphasic response occurs with **initial CNS excitation** due to selective inhibition of inhibitory cortical pathways. This is followed by **generalized CNS depression** at higher doses. Toxicity is related to factors such as the preparation and site of injection, but usually occurs after an accidental intravenous injection of a large dose of local anaesthetic. Signs and symptoms of toxicity start with **tingling of the tongue** and **lips**, progressing to **lightheadedness, tinnitus, slurred speech** and **restlessness**. With increasing levels, **convulsions** and then **coma** occur. Finally patients suffer from **apnoea, cardiac arrhythmias** and **ventricular arrest**. Management is primarily supportive and includes oxygen, airway control and anti-convulsants.

Regional nerve blocks

SUSANNA WALKER

■ Local infiltration technique

- Warn the patient about the initial needle pinprick followed by a burning sensation. The area will be anaesthetized but they will still be able to feel pressure.
- Inject local anaesthetic subcutaneously around a wound site, taking care to aspirate to avoid intravascular injection. Often best done with a thin needle (23G, blue).
- Some anaesthetic effect will occur within two minutes. Length of duration will depend on preparation used, but may last for 30–60 minutes with plain lidocaine.

■ Peripheral nerve blocks

1. HAEMATOMA BLOCK (Figure 148)

- This involves injection of local anaesthetic into a Colles' fracture haematoma, enabling manipulation of the fracture. This is often inadequate for successful manipulation of the fracture, and carries the risk of infection, having turned a closed fracture into an open fracture.
- It can only be performed in fractures less than 24 hours old as clot organization prevents the spread of anaesthetic.
- 15 ml of 1 % prilocaine should be used, or a lower dose according to weight.

Hospital Surgery: Foundations in Surgical Practice, ed. Omer Aziz, Sanjay Purkayastha and Paraskevas Paraskeva. Published by Cambridge University Press. © Cambridge University Press 2009.

■ Under full asepsis an orange (25G) needle should be inserted into the fracture haematoma. Gently aspirate blood to confirm the position of the needle, and then inject very slowly to minimize the risk of high blood levels leading to toxicity (see Figure 148).

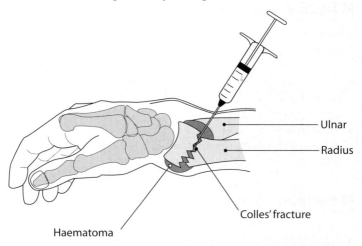

Ulnar

Radius

Colles' fracture

Haematoma

Figure 148

2. BIER'S BLOCK (Figure 149)

■ This is a block that used to be commonly performed in the A&E departments to enable reduction of Colles' fractures. The principle of the block is to inject a dose of local anaesthetic intravascularly into the arm to be operated on. The local anaesthetic is maintained within the arm by the use of an inflated tourniquet. However, it is now recognized that this technique carries a significant risk of toxicity, and so it is less commonly performed unless in an anaesthetic or operating theatre area of the hospital with staff present capable of treating local anaesthetic toxicity.

■ The block requires a special tourniquet apparatus which should be checked meticulously prior to use.

- Plain 0.5 % prilocaine should be used. This is because it is more rapidly metabolized than lidocaine or bupivacaine and therefore is less likely to lead to local anaesthetic toxicity. However, this should not be used in patients suffering from methaemoglobinaemia because of the metabolites produced.
- This procedure is also contraindicated in patients with severe hypertension, obesity, peripheral vascular disease and sickle-cell disease or trait. Caution should be taken in epileptic patients because of the risk of seizure with LA toxicity.
- The patient should be attached to full monitoring, should be starved, a preoperative assessment should have been made and full resuscitation equipment should be available and checked.
- The patient should have a cannula in both hands – the one to be blocked and the other arm in case of emergency.
- The arm to be blocked is elevated to attempt to exsanguinate, and then the tourniquet is inflated to 300 mmHg or at least 100 mmHg over systolic pressure. The tourniquet should be checked to ensure it is not leaking and the tourniquet time should be noted.
- The appropriate volume of 0.5 % prilocaine should be injected slowly. Adequacy of block can be tested after five minutes. If the block is inadequate, 10–15 ml of N-saline can be injected at this stage to increase the spread of the prilocaine.
- The tourniquet must remain inflated for at least 20 minutes after injection of the prilocaine to minimize systemic spread. The tourniquet should then be deflated slowly, while monitoring and observing the patient for any signs of toxicity. The tourniquet should be re-inflated if there are any signs of toxicity and the patient should be treated accordingly.
- The patient should be monitored for a further two hours for any delayed signs of toxicity.

Note: the use of Bier's blocks has been limited due to the need for an anaesthetist to be present.

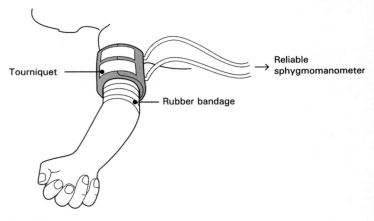

Tourniquet

Reliable
sphygmomanometer

Rubber bandage

Figure 149

3. RING BLOCK (Figure 150)

- This is often used for simple procedures on the fingers and toes.
- The technique aims to block the digital nerves which run on the medial and lateral sides of the fingers and toes.
- Use plain lidocaine, a 23G needle, and position the patient with the palm of the hand or sole of foot on a firm surface.
- Insert the needle on the lateral side of the digit to be blocked at the base of the digit, close to the webspace. The needle should angle slightly towards the midline. Continue to insert the needle until approaching the skin on the palmar surface. Aspirate to check position, then inject, and continue to inject while withdrawing the needle.
- Repeat this process on the medial side of the digit.
- Use a total of 2–4 ml of lidocaine in an adult.
- An additional injection subcutaneously across the base of the digit on the dorsum may be required for anaesthesia proximally.

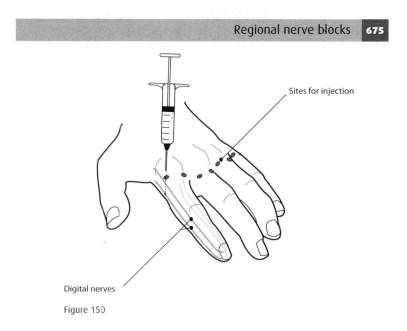

Sites for injection

Digital nerves

Figure 150

4. FEMORAL NERVE BLOCK (Figure 151)

- This is an excellent block to provide analgesia for patients with a fractured femur.
- The femoral nerve passes under the inguinal ligament and lies laterally to the femoral artery.
- The patient should be positioned supine, the inguinal ligament should be identified and the femoral artery palpated.
- The point of injection is 1 cm lateral and 1–2 cm distal to the femoral pulsation. The skin at this point should be thoroughly cleaned and anaesthetized with subcutaneous infiltration of lidocaine. Then a 22G needle should be inserted slowly, aiming slightly cephalad. A small pop may be felt as the needle passes through the fascia lata. A second pop may be felt as it enters the nerve sheath. The patient may report some paraesthesia; if this is severe withdraw the needle slightly prior to injection.

- Aspirate and then slowly inject approximately 15 ml of bupivacaine 0.5 %, according to patient's weight. A larger volume of a lower concentration local anaesthetic may be used e.g. 0.25 %. A further 5 ml may be injected subcutaneously laterally towards the anterior superior iliac spine. This will anaesthetize the lateral cutaneous nerve of the thigh.
- For a more accurate nerve blockade a nerve stimulator should be used to accurately identify placement of the needle in relation to the nerve.

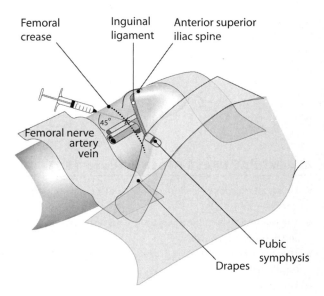

Figure 151

Sutures

TIM BROWN AND PARASKEVAS PARASKEVA

Purpose: to hold healing tissues in apposition until such time that fibro-blast and myofibroblast activity has restored natural tensile strength.

■ Ideal suture characteristics

- Sterile and resistant to infection.
- Causes minimal tissue reaction.
- Easy to handle and atraumatic to tissues.
- Holds knots securely.
- Stays strong until its purpose is complete and absorbs completely thereafter.

No single suture material fits this description. Different materials are used depending on the situation.

■ Suture size

Classification of suture size refers to the diameter of the strand. This is measured by 'zeroes'. The more 'zeroes' a strand has, the smaller it is i.e. 00 (2-0) is larger than 0000 (4-0). Strand diameter correlates to tensile strength.

Material classification and examples			
Natural			
Monofilament		Braided	
Absorbable	Non-absorbable	Absorbable	Non-absorbable
Poliglecaprone (Monocryl)	Stainless steel	Catgut	Silk
Polydioxanone (PDS)	Polypropylene (Prolene)	Polyglactin (Vicryl)	Polyamide (Nylon)

Hospital Surgery: Foundations in Surgical Practice, ed. Omer Aziz, Sanjay Purkayastha and Paraskevas Paraskeva. Published by Cambridge University Press. © Cambridge University Press 2009.

Rough guide to general usage and days before removal (guide only.)

Bowel:	3-0 Vicryl or PDS	
Vascular:		
Aorta:	2-0 Prolene	
Femoral:	4-0 Prolene	
Distal:	6-0 Prolene	
Skin (superficial):		
Face:	5-0 Monocryl/Nylon	ROS: 3-5 + steristrips
Torso + limb:	3-0/4-0 Vicryl/Monocryl/Nylon	ROS: 8-10
Scalp (full thickness):	1-0 Silk	ROS: 7
Abdominal wall:		
Linea alba:	0/1-0 PDS/Nylon	
Muscle layers:	2-0 Vicryl	
Hernia mesh sutures:	2-0 Prolene	
Tendons:	Ethibond (size dependent on tendon undergoing repair).	

(Note: ROS = Removal of Sutures)

■ Needles

Ideal needle qualities:

Smallest diameter possible

Easily handled

Sterile and non-allergenic

Sharp enough to go through intended tissue with minimal tissue damage

Identical needle and thread size, thereby minimizing tissue trauma while filling the needle tract completely.

■ Point types

1. Cutting: designed to go through dense tough tissue with minimal trauma.

2. Taper point (round needle): passes through tissue by stretching it to breaking point and not cutting. These are associated with higher localized tissue trauma, but useful for elastic tissues (e.g. peritoneum).
3. Blunt point: for pushing tissue away from needle rather than cutting it (e.g. liver needle).

■ Needle types

1. Straight: easily manipulated by hand. These are now falling from favour as they are thought to have higher incidences of needle stick injury.
2. Curved: sized by the circumference of circle (e.g. 1 cm). Has a moment and predictable tissue path. These require a supinating/pronating wrist action for optimal efficiency.

The needle should be held, with an appropriately sized needle holder, 1/3 of the way up from the junction of needle and suture material.

'No touch technique' involves no contact between surgeon and needle through the skillful use of forceps and needle holders. This is recommended to minimize needle stick injury.

For formal basic surgical technique training, it is recommended that trainees take the Basic Surgical Skills course that is organized and run by The Royal College of Surgeons.

See www.rcseng.ac.uk/education/courses/basic_surgical_skills.html/ for details.

Bowel anastomoses

TIM BROWN AND PARASKEVAS PARASKEVA

■ Anastomoses

Definition: the surgical connection of separate or severed tubular hollow organs to form a continuous channel (e.g. bowel to bowel, ureter to bowel, artery to artery).

■ Techniques

1. Hand-sewn
2. Stapled.

Currently there is no evidence to suggest that either is superior to the other, providing attention is paid to factors that influence successful healing of anastomoses.

■ Types of anastomosis (Figure 152)

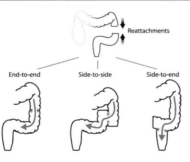

Figure 152

Hand-sewn bowel anastomoses use absorbable suture material (e.g. Vicryl, polydioxanone (PDS)) and aim to invert sutured edges. Sutures

Hospital Surgery: Foundations in Surgical Practice, ed. Omer Aziz, Sanjay Purkayastha and Paraskevas Paraskeva. Published by Cambridge University Press. © Cambridge University Press 2009.

can be interrupted or continuous. Previously, the two-layer technique was employed, when a full thickness suture layer was created, followed by a second seromuscular layer (see Figure 155) that buried the first suture line. Now, a single-layered anastomosis is advocated. This incorporates an **inversion** of the sero-submucosal layer, again using an absorbable material (e.g. Vicryl).

Vascular anastomoses use non-absorbable suture material (e.g. Prolene). Suturing is continuous in order to provide an equal distribution of tensile strength throughout the anastomotic line. As opposed to bowel anastomoses, vascular suturing aims to **evert** the anastomotic edges.

■ Stapling devices

These are commercially available disposable devices. They consist of a 'gun' that has a stapling mechanism and a cutting mechanism.

1. CIRCULAR STAPLING (e.g. CEEA CIRCULAR ENDOSCOPIC ANASTOMOTIC STAPLER)

For end–end anastomoses. Two ends of bowel are physically apposed within the staple gun. When fired, the gun forms two circular rows of staples joining the two bowel ends. Two 'doughnuts' of excess tissue are then cut with the gun's knife. When removed, the gun leaves behind a newly formed lumen with both previously cut ends in continuity. The 'doughnuts' should be checked to ensure there are complete rings of tissue (if not, it is likely that the anastomosis is not complete) and sent for histology to exclude disease process from the resection margins (see Figures 153 and 154).

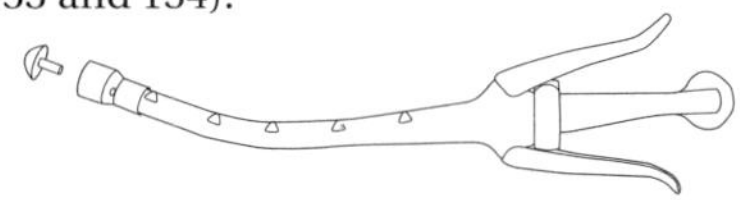

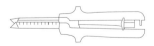

Figure 153 Circular stapler

Figure 154 Transverse stapler

2. LINEAR STAPLING (e.g. GIA, TA)

The linear stapling device is placed across the bowel to be divided. When fired, two rows of staples are formed. The device has a guillotine knife which is then activated by hand, cutting between the staple lines. In this way, the bowel has been divided and the cut surface closed securely.

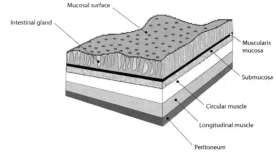

Mucosal surface

Intestinal gland

Muscularis mucosa

Submucosa

Circular muscle

Longitudinal muscle

Peritoneum

Figure 155 Layers of the bowel wall

Factors determining successful anastomosis

Operative factors	Patient factors
Adequate blood supply	Absence of:
Minimal foreign body reaction (NB absorbable suture)	Hypoxia
No sepsis around anastomosis	Jaundice
No haematoma at site of anastomosis	Uraemia
Tension-free join	Corticosteroids
No distal obstruction	Smoking
Anastomotic margins clear from disease	
Accurate alignment of tissue edges	

Skin grafts and flaps

MARIOS NICOLAOU AND PETER BUTLER

■ Skin grafts

DEFINITION

These are living or preserved tissue transfers from a donor to a recipient site *without* their blood supply. The first record of a successful skin graft in humans was credited to Sir Astley Cooper (1817) even though the technique of free skin grafting may have originated some 3000 years ago in India.

CLASSIFICATION

Can be divided into *autografts* (same person), *isografts* (genetically identical e.g. twins), *allografts* (same species) or *xenografts* (different species). Can be further classified into *split-thickness (SSG)* (epidermis with partial-thickness dermis), *full-thickness (FTSG)* (epidermis with entire dermis) and *composite* (composed of two or more tissues e.g. skin and fat). They are indicated in cases where there is lack of adjacent tissue for coverage and are the third option on the reconstructive ladder (see Figure 156). Choice of donor site is influenced by scar visibility and skin colour match.

GRAFT HEALING

Known as graft 'take' this has five phases: *adherence* [fibrin mediated] (immediately), serum *imbibition* [graft nourished from serum nutrients]

Hospital Surgery: Foundations in Surgical Practice, ed. Omer Aziz, Sanjay Purkayastha and Paraskevas Paraskeva. Published by Cambridge University Press. © Cambridge University Press 2009.

(1–2 days), *inosculation* [capillary re-anastomosis] (after 2 days), *revascularization* (3–7 days) and *remodelling* (weeks–months). Graft failure may arise because of: inadequate recipient site vascularization (avoid irradiated skin, exposed bone, cartilage or over-necrotic tissue), infection (especially β-haemolytic streptococci), fluid collection between the graft and the recipient surface (e.g. due to a haematoma or a seroma), shearing forces, co–morbidity (e.g. smoking, diabetes, vascular disease) and poor surgical technique (e.g. graft placed upside down). Other complications of skin grafting include skin colour mismatch and secondary contracture (especially with SSG).

SPLIT THICKNESS SKIN GRAFTS

These are usually harvested from the anterolateral thigh, although the buttocks, torso, upper inner arm and scalp can also be used.

Graft and donor site preparation

The traditional technique uses a Watson modification of the Humby knife set to approximately 0.5 mm blade clearance moved palindromically over the anaesthetized donor skin at an angle of 30–45°, exerting light pressure on the skin (see Figure 157). Liquid paraffin on the skin reduces unnecessary friction. Where available, an air-dermatome is used for the harvest. Meshing can be used to increase skin coverage (1:1.5); allows easier graft contouring, fluid drainage, but risks 'pebbled' appearance if stretched. Excess graft tissue can be stored for up to three weeks at 4 °C. The donor site is usually covered in alginate–based dressing (e.g. Kaltostat), soaked in a local anaesthetic (e.g. 0.25 % bupivacaine), secured with a crepe bandage or OpSite and left undisturbed for 14 days.

Grafting procedure

The graft is trimmed to match the defect and secured in place (shiny-side/dermis down) with an absorbable suture (e.g. 4-0 Vicryl) or staples. A non-adhesive dressing (e.g. Jelonet) is placed on the graft followed by a *bolster* dressing (saline-soaked cotton balls secured with 5-0 silk suture, see Figure 159) or foam (e.g. Lyofoam) and secured. The latter exerts uniform pressure on the graft, minimizes the risk of haematoma formation or direct trauma/shear and maintains a moist environment. The graft is inspected after 4–5 days (sooner if infection is suspected).

Advantages of SSGs

Can be used to resurface large wounds; donor site heals by re-epithelization; can be reharvested and can be done under local anaesthesia.

Disadvantages

Significant scarring and secondary contraction (avoid over joints), cosmetically unappealing, does not sweat or grow hair and the healed graft is very thin and can be unstable long term.

FULL THICKNESS SKIN GRAFTS

Usually harvested from thin skin, e.g. pre/post-auricular area, upper-eyelids, supraclavicular region, groin and antecubital fossae. Pre-planned tissue expansion can also be used to increase the size of the skin that can be harvested. This is the preferred type of grafting for facial defects.

Donor site and graft preparation

Donor site is marked using a correctly shaped and sized paper template. The graft is then scored, raised and the donor site primarily closed.

Grafting procedure

After defatting, the graft is sutured in place to cover the defect with interrupted non-absorbable sutures, e.g. 4-0 Prolene (see Figure 158).

A bolster dressing is then placed over the graft as described and the wound inspected after seven days.

Advantages

Better colour and skin texture match; presence of dermal appendages means that the graft can sweat, produce oils and grow hair; less scarring and improved cosmesis; less secondary contraction (used for defects over joints and on the hand).

Disadvantages

Require a well vascularized bed and have limited donor sites.

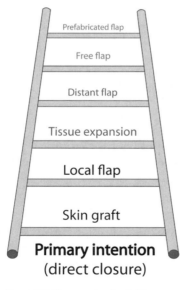

Figure 156 The reconstructive ladder

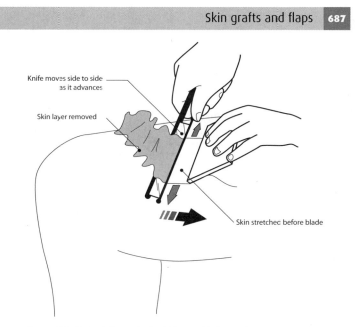

Knife moves side to side as it advances

Skin layer removed

Skin stretched before blade

Figure 157 The technique of split thickness skin harvesting

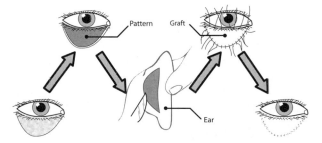

Pattern Graft

Ear

Figure 158 The technique of full thickness skin grafting

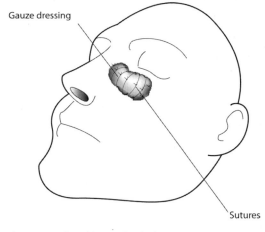

Gauze dressing

Sutures

Figure 159 Bolster (tie over dressing)

■ Skin flaps

DEFINITION

This is a segment of tissue used for reconstruction of a defect that maintains its own intravascular blood supply. The base of the flap is known as the *pedicle* and the unit of skin and tissue supplied by a source vessel is known as the *angiosome*. The first documented flap was performed by Sushruta (documented in his Hindu book Sushruta-Samhita) c. 600 BC who reconstructed nasal/earlobe defects using a pedicled cheek (or forehead) flap. Flaps can be classified according to their composition, vascularity and method of transfer (see Table).

COMMON TYPES

Z-plasty: this is a transposition flap that is especially useful for increasing tissue length in one direction (e.g. a contracture over a joint) or to change scar direction (e.g. an unsightly facial scar). The central limb of the 'z' is placed along the scar or line of contracture, whereas the distal limbs (which must have the same length) are at angles typically of 60° (30–90°) to the central limb (see Figure 161). The length gain in the direction of the central limb depends on the limb angle: 30° achieves 25 % length gain, 60° gets 75 % and 90° gets 120 %. Multiple z-plasties can also be applied in series.

Rhomboid flap: also known as the Limberg flap, this is a transposition flap used to close a rhombic–shaped defect (e.g. from a lesion on the temple). The flap is created by drawing a parallelogram with angles of 60 and 120 degrees. The short diagonal of the rhombus (see x in Figure 160) is then extended to a distance equal to its length and the flap is completed by drawing a line parallel to the nearest limb of the flap.

Bilobed flap: this is a rotational/transposition flap especially useful for defects on the nose and face. Two flaps are raised 45° degrees apart, the first flap is used to close the defect hence is designed to be equal to the width of the original defect and the second to fill in the defect created by the first flap. The second flap is constructed with an elliptical tip to facilitate side-to-side closure (see Figure 162).

Advancement flap: this flap is raised as a rectangle and undermined to allow movement over the defect. To facilitate the advancement, small triangles (known as *Burrow's triangles*) are made at the base of the flap (see Figure 163).

Distant flap: in these flaps, the donor and recipient sites are not in close proximity. Examples include cross-leg and groin flaps.

Free flap: this type of flap involves transplanting donor tissue with its feeding blood vessels (pedicle) from one part of the body to another. The donor blood vessels (artery and vein) are microvascularly re-anastomosed with size-matched recipient blood vessels to re-establish blood flow. Where possible nerves are also anastomosed. It is imperative that the donor tissue is able to survive on the dissected blood vessels. Several free-flap types exist although one of the more commonly performed ones is the transverse rectus abdominus myocutaneous (TRAM) flap used for breast reconstruction. Free flaps can also contain bone (fibular osteocutaneous free flap) and can be used for bony reconstruction of the mandible.

Tissue expansion: this method results in an increase of the surface of a tissue by the mechanical expansion of an implanted silastic balloon under it. The balloon can start to be inflated 2–3 weeks after implantation at a rate tolerated by the tissue and patient. The pressure exerted by the balloon on the tissue results in expansion (by the induction of epidermal mitosis). Several weeks/months are needed to achieve the desired tissue expansion. The extra skin can then be used locally or elsewhere.

Three classifications of flaps

Composition	Vascularity	Transfer
Cutaneous	Random-pattern	Rotation
Fasciocutaneous	(no dominant blood vessel)	Transposition
Musculocutaneous	Pedicled/axial	Advancement
Muscle	(dominant blood vessel)	Distant
Osteocutaneous	Reverse flow	Free
Omental/bowel	(distal blood supply)	

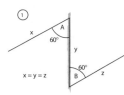
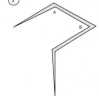
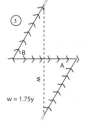

Figure 160 Rhomboid flap

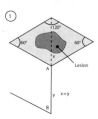
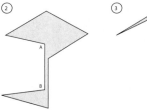
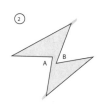

Figure 161 Z-plasty

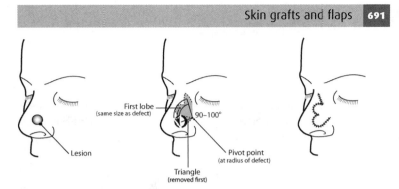

Figure 162 Bilobed flap

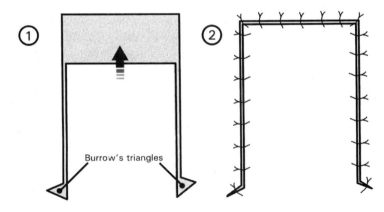

Figure 163 Advancement flap

Principles of laparoscopy

RACHEL MASSEY AND ARA DARZI

Laparoscopic surgery or minimal access surgery (MAS) is a rapidly advancing field within surgery and has the potential to greatly reduce the anatomical, physiological and pathological consequences of surgery to patients by having a positive impact on both postoperative pain and on length of inpatient stay. Many surgical and gynaecological procedures are now regularly performed using a laparoscopic approach. Below is a list of examples of the uses of therapeutic laparoscopy.

■ Scope of laparoscopic surgery

General surgery examples: diagnostic laparoscopy, appendicectomy, cholecystectomy, hernia repair, Nissen's fundoplication, repair of perforated duodenal ulcer, splenectomy, colectomy.

Gynaecology examples: oophrectomy, hysterectomy, tubal surgery, treatment of ectopic pregnancy, treatment of infertility.

Others: minimal access urology.

When deciding whether to perform a laparoscopic or open procedure there is rarely one method that is absolutely preferable over the other. It is always important to consider the fact that laparoscopic procedures may be technically more difficult, necessitate a higher level of experience and expertise, as well as requiring the availability of laparoscopic equipment and theatre staff familiar with the instruments. Without all of these factors the potential risks may outweigh any potential benefits.

Hospital Surgery: Foundations in Surgical Practice, ed. Omer Aziz, Sanjay Purkayastha and Paraskevas Paraskeva. Published by Cambridge University Press. © Cambridge University Press 2009.

■ Advantages and disadvantages of laparoscopy

Advantages	Disadvantages
Smaller incisions	Bleeding more difficult to control
Decreased rates of wound infection	Greater technical expertise
Earlier return to full activity	Specialist equipment required
Decreased exposure to body fluids with reduced contact with pathogens such as HIV and Hepatitis B and C	Increased incidence of iatrogenic damage when compared to open surgery e.g. bile duct injury in cholecystectomy
Better cosmesis	Higher intraoperative cost

In addition to considering the advantages and disadvantages of a laparoscopic procedure it is also very important to be aware that there are some absolute and relative contraindications to laparoscopy.

Absolute contraindications	Relative contraindications
Generalized peritonitis	Gross obesity
Intestinal obstruction – increased incidence of damage to bowel during insertion of ports	Pregnancy
Clotting abnormalities	Organomegaly
Liver cirrhosis	Abdominal aortic aneurysm
Uncontrolled shock	
Failure to tolerate general anaesthesia	

■ Basic equipment for laparoscopy (Figure 164)

(1) Monitor, (2) Light source, (3) Insufflator, (4) Camera, (5) Diathermy, (6) Suction and irrigation.

■ Establishing pneumoperitoneum

This can be hazardous, and careless port insertion can lead to injury of viscera such as the bowel, bladder or potentially the aorta or the vena cava.

There are open and closed methods of producing pneumoperitoneum:

OPEN (HASSON): KEY POINTS

- Generally preferred by surgeons.
- Considered safer – especially if there has been previous surgery.
- 1–2 cm infra-umbilical incision.
- Deepen to linea alba:
  - Incise linea alba between two stay sutures and open under direct vision.
  - Insert finger before introducing a blunt-tipped trocar to sweep away any adhesions.
  - Connect gas supply to establish pneumoperitoneum.

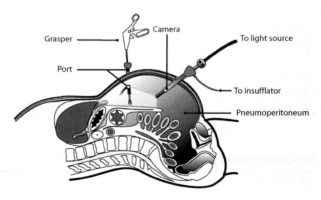

Figure 164 Laparoscopy

CLOSED (VERESS): KEY POINTS

- Most commonly used. Especially in gynaecology (Figure 165).
- Infra-umbilical skin incision.
- Grasp anterior abdominal wall with assistant and lift.
- Insert Veress needle perpendicular to abdominal wall until it penetrates the linea alba and peritoneum.
- A 'give' is felt indicating the peritoneal cavity has been entered.

With the Veress needle check:

- Mobility. Is the needle freely mobile?
- Fall of saline. Place a drop of saline on the Leuer connector of the Veress needle. It should fall freely if in the correct position as pressure within the abdomen is subatmospheric.
- Pressure: insufflate gas slowly – if the needle is within the peritoneal cavity the pressure should not rise significantly.

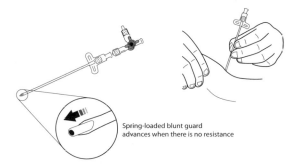

Spring-loaded blunt guard advances when there is no resistance

Figure 165 Veress needle

■ Postoperative considerations

1. Monitor all patients exactly as those who have had a laparotomy, with regular observations.

2. Remind patients that they may experience shoulder tip pain as a result of pneumoperitoneum stretching the peritoneum.
3. Encourage early mobilization.
4. Many patients can be discharged within 24 hours of a laparoscopic procedure and certain procedures (laparoscopic hernia repair and laparoscopic cholecystectomy) can be performed as day case surgery.

■ Complications of laparoscopic surgery and pneumoperitoneum

The complications of laparoscopic surgery can be broadly divided into four areas:

1. DURING INDUCTION OF PNEUMOPERITONEUM

■ Damage to viscus or vessels.
■ Misplacement of the gas.
■ Insufflation of the bowel lumen.
■ CO_2 embolus – which may lead to a metabolic acidosis.
■ Over-insufflation of the peritoneal cavity which may lead to cardiorespiratory problems.

2. AS A RESULT OF PORT PLACEMENT

■ Damage to underlying structures.
■ Haemorrhage – damage to underlying blood vessels – including in the abdominal wall.
■ Herniation through port sites.

3. DURING THE PROCEDURE

■ Diathermy-related injuries.
■ Unrecognized haemorrhage.

- Unrecognized division or ligation of structure – particularly in laparoscopic cholecystectomy, but a potential risk in all laparoscopic procedures.
- Visceral injuries.

4. PATIENT-RELATED COMPLICATIONS

- Ascites – may lead to leakage of fluid from port sites and lead to increased risk of postoperative port-site infection and herniation.
- Clotting abnormalities – increased rates of haemorrhage which may initially go unrecognized.
- Organomegaly – increased risk of organ damage.
- Obesity – can make operation technically more difficult.
- Malignant disease – potential risk of transfer of malignant cells to the skin via the port sites leading to skin secondaries.

■ Summary

Minimal access surgery is a rapidly expanding field with many routine surgical procedures now performed laparoscopically.

Laparoscopic procedures potentially offer the least anatomical, physiological and psychological trauma to the patient by reducing postoperative pain and length of hospital stay.

Some patients are not suitable for laparoscopic surgery as a result of a number of absolute or relative contraindications.

Complications of laparoscopic surgery may present differently to complications of open surgery and may not be apparent at the time of surgery.

Laparoscopic surgery generally requires a higher level of expertise and experience and may not be the best surgical option particularly in the emergency setting.

Patients who have had laparoscopic surgery should be monitored postoperatively exactly like those who have had open surgery.

Principles and safety of radiology

ANN ANSTEE AND MARC PELLING

■ Introduction

Interacting successfully with the radiology department is an important part of being a junior doctor. Arranging an investigation for a patient has three components:

1. **Requesting the investigation.** An encyclopaedic knowledge of radiology is not required; you may not be sure which investigation is best but you need to know your patient and understand the clinical question. If you are not sure what question is being asked, clarify this with a senior member of the team. If still in doubt discuss with a radiologist and if possible bring the notes and previous imaging with you.
2. **Pre- and post-investigation care.** Make sure that the patient is prepared for an investigation and it is safe for the patient to have the test. Inform the radiology department of any predisposing risk factors, for example if the patient has asthma, diabetes, is on metformin or has renal impairment. Also remember to warn the department if the patient has difficulties communicating, for example because of dementia, deafness or a language barrier.
3. **Find the result and document it in the notes.** There is no point in the patient undergoing an investigation unless the results are known and available.

■ Safety: in particular radiation

All procedures using ionizing radiation carry an associated risk of genetic damage and malignancy. The clinical benefit of the intended

Hospital Surgery: Foundations in Surgical Practice, ed. Omer Aziz, Sanjay Purkayastha and Paraskevas Paraskeva. Published by Cambridge University Press. © Cambridge University Press 2009.

Typical effective doses from diagnostic medical exposures

Radiographic examination	Typical effective dose in millisievert (mSv)	Equivalent number of chest X-rays	Approximate equivalent period of natural background radiation
Chest X-ray	0.02	1	3 days
Abdomen X-ray	0.7	35	4 months
Lumbar spine X-ray	1.0	50	5 months
IVU	2.4	120	14 months
Bone scan	4	200	1.8 years
CT abdomen/pelvis	10	500	4.5 years

investigation should outweigh this risk. Patients are increasingly aware of this and radiation dose can be discussed in terms of equivalent number of chest X-rays or approximate equivalent period of background radiation (See table above).

Pregnancy is a particular consideration; the last menstrual period of a female of childbearing age should be established and if there is any uncertainty about pregnancy status then the timing should be reviewed or another investigation considered. Ultrasound and MRI are radiation free.

■ Iodinated contrast media

These are widely used in radiological investigations e.g. CT scans, IVUs and angiograms. The administration of contrast is not without risk and the referring clinician should identify patients at risk of complications. Reactions after the administration of contrast media are well documented. These can be idiosyncratic, however risk factors for a reaction to contrast media include:

■ Previous generalized reaction to contrast medium.
■ Asthma – particularly if asthma is poorly controlled.
■ Allergy – multiple allergies or a severe allergy requiring medical treatment.

In these patients, the need to perform a contrast-enhanced study should be re-evaluated, an alternative investigation considered or the contrast study delayed until control of asthma is optimized. Close medical supervision and established iv access are advised during the study and for 30 minutes following iv contrast administration in these groups.

Contrast media nephrotoxicity is an important cause of hospital-acquired renal failure. Defined as an impairment in renal function (an increase in serum creatinine by >25 % or 44 mmol/l) occurring within three days of the administration of intravascular contrast medium and without an alternative aetiology. Contrast media have a direct toxic effect on the renal tubular cells and cause a reduction in renal perfusion resulting in renal impairment.

■ Risk factors

Raised serum creatinine levels, especially in patients with diabetic nephropathy, dehydration, congestive heart failure, age > 70 years, multiple myeloma and concurrent administration of nephrotoxic drugs e.g. non-steroidal anti-inflammatory drugs (NSAIDs) and aminoglycosides.

■ Preventative measures

- Consider alternative imaging techniques that do not require iodinated contrast medium.
- Ensure that the patient is adequately hydrated before and after the procedure.
- The smallest dose of contrast should be used.
- Low- or iso-osmolar contrast media should be used.
- Nephrotoxic drugs should be reviewed and stopped for at least 24 hours where clinically appropriate.
- Multiple studies using contrast media should be avoided within a short period of time.

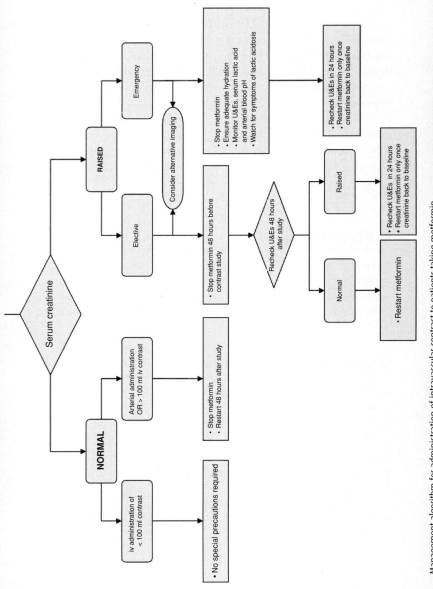

Management algorithm for administration of intravascular contrast to patients taking metformin

■ Contrast media and metformin-induced lactic acidosis

Metformin (a biguanide oral hypoglycaemic agent) is predominantly excreted via the kidneys. Any reduction in renal function, such as contrast medium nephrotoxicity, can lead to a decrease in renal elimination and precipitate a potentially fatal lactic acidosis in patients with pre-exisiting renal impairment. Intravascular contrast media should be administered with caution in this group.

■ Contrast media in pregnancy and breast feeding

No mutagenic or teratogenic effects have been described related to iodinated contrast media. However, neonatal thyroid function should be checked in the first week if iodinated contrast media has been given during pregnancy, as fetal/neonatal thyroid function may be depressed.

The potential risk of contrast medium being absorbed by a baby through breast milk after maternal contrast administration is considered too small to necessitate halting breast feeding.

■ Contrast media and isotope studies

Free iodide in contrast media is taken up by the thyroid gland; subsequent investigations and therapies that depend on the radiolabelled iodine being taken up by the thyroid can be impaired. A delay of two months after the administration of contrast media is needed before thyroid nuclear medicine studies or radioiodine treatment should be performed. MRI staging is advised in these patients. Intravascular contrast administration should be avoided in patients who are hyperthyroid.

X-rays

ANN ANSTEE AND MARC PELLING

■ Introduction

X-rays are transmitted through different parts of the body with varying intensity. The number of X-rays that are transmitted through a material depends on the atomic number and the density of that material. For example, bone has a higher atomic number and a greater density than air; fewer X-rays penetrate bone than the air-filled lungs. The plain radiograph is obtained when the emergent X-rays interact with a photosensitive plate.

Gas, fat, soft tissue/fluid, bone/calcification and non-organic radio-opaque materials/contrast can be differentiated on a plain radiograph.

■ Indications

'Making the Best Use of a Department of Clinical Radiology: Guidelines for Doctors' is a very useful reference. If in doubt, discuss the case with a radiologist.

Preoperative chest X-ray: not routinely performed. Consider if the patient is known to have cardiorespiratory disease, >60 years.

Preoperative cervical spine: not routinely performed. Consider in patients who are at risk of atlanto-axial instability, who may be at risk of subluxation at the time of intubation e.g. rheumatoid arthritis, Down's syndrome.

Hospital Surgery: Foundations in Surgical Practice, ed. Omer Aziz, Sanjay Purkayastha and Paraskevas Paraskeva. Published by Cambridge University Press. © Cambridge University Press 2009.

Post-procedure chest X-ray: to check the satisfactory position of tubes and lines:

- Nasogastric tube: tip should be seen within the stomach i.e. below the diaphragm; this should be confirmed before use.
- Endotracheal tube (ETT): flexion and extension of the neck can cause the tip of ETT to move by up to 5 cm; therefore the tip should be placed 5 cm above the carina. If seen within 2 cm of the carina then the likelihood of it passing into the right main bronchus is increased and the tube should be withdrawn.
- Tracheostomy tube: the tip should be seen centrally within the trachea at the level of T3.
- Central venous pressure lines: the tip of the line should be seen projected over the superior vena cava. Pneumothorax and mediastinal haematoma, the potential complications of line insertion, should be excluded.
- Pleural drains: check that all the side draining holes are seen within the chest. In a patient who is supine the tip of the tube is best placed anterior and superiorly for a pneumothorax or posterior and inferiorly for a pleural effusion.
- Swan-Ganz catheters: pulmonary artery flotation catheters are used to measure pulmonary artery wedge pressures as a reflection of left atrial pressure and should be seen projected over the right or left main pulmonary artery 5–8 cm distal to the bifurcation of the pulmonary trunk.

Post-operative chest X-ray: Not performed routinely. Consider if patient develops cardiac or respiratory symptoms.

Erect chest X-ray: This is used to detect sub-diaphragmatic air. In the acute setting this indicates a perforated viscus. The patient should be erect for **15 minutes** to maximize the sensitivity of the examination. Sub-diaphragmatic air is routinely seen post-surgically.

■ Chest X-ray

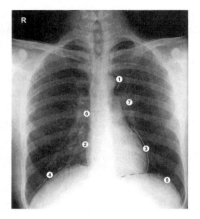

Figure 166 PA chest X-ray
1. Aortic knuckle, 2. Right atrium, 3. Left ventricle, 4. Right diaphragm,
5. Left diaphragm, 6. Right hilum, 7. Left hilum

REVIEWING THE CHEST X-RAY

ID: check the patient name and date of the study.

Orientation: check the side markers.

Projection: posteroanterior (PA) or anteroposterior (AP) film? The mediastinum is magnified on the AP film.

Position: is the patient erect or supine?

Rotation: are the medial ends of the clavicles equidistant from the spinous process of the vertebral body at that level?

Penetration: are the lower vertebral bodies just visible behind the heart?

Inspiration: is the anterior end of the sixth rib or the posterior end of the tenth rib above the diaphragm? Less than this suggests sub-optimal inspiration, more suggests hyperinflation.

Lungs: equal transradiency and volume, look for any patchy or focal lesions.

Diaphragm: the right is higher than the left; up to 3 cm difference is normal.

Heart: 1/3 of the heart is seen on the right side and 2/3 is seen on the left. The heart should not be greater than 50 % of the thoracic diameter on the PA film.

Mediastinal contour: identify the various anatomical structures comprising this image.

Hila: the left hilum is up to 2.5 cm higher than the right. A concave shape and vascular density should be seen.

Trachea: central position.

Soft tissues: are both breast shadows seen in females?

Bones: assess density; look for fractures and focal lucent or sclerotic lesions.

Review areas: apices, behind the heart, cardiophrenic angles, costophrenic angles, below the diaphragm.

■ Abdominal X-ray

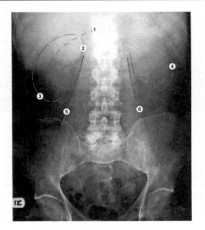

Figure 167 Abdominal X-ray
1. Inferior margin of the liver, 2. Gallbladder, 3. Right kidney, 4. Left kidney, 5. Lateral margin of right psoas muscle, 6. Lateral margin of left psoas muscle

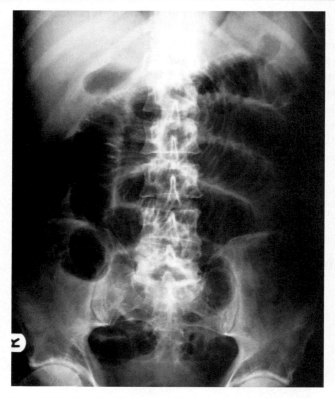

Figure 168 Multiple dilated loops of small bowel are seen centrally within the abdomen. Note that the valvulae conniventes extend across the bowel lumen

REVIEWING THE ABDOMINAL X-RAY

ID: check the patient name and date of the study.

Orientation: check the side markers.

Projection and position: supine, AP films are usual.

Small bowel: central location, the jejunum typically in the left upper abdomen with the ileum positioned in the lower right abdomen.

Valvulae conniventes (plicae circulares) are seen as complete rings extending across the small bowel. Gas/fluid levels are seen in normal small bowel; diameter of up to 3.5 cm.

Large bowel: is located peripherally and measures up to 9 cm at the caecum in the lower right abdomen and 5.5 cm at the transverse colon. Haustra are seen producing incomplete septations of the large bowel.

Renal tract: the renal outlines should be identified; normal renal size is 3.5 vertebral body heights. Inspect both kidneys, the course of the ureters and the bladder for renal tract calcification.

Gallstones: review the right upper quadrant; only 15 % of gallstones are visible on the plain film.

Soft tissues: look for the margin of the liver, spleen and psoas muscle.

Bones: assess density; look for fractures and focal lucent or sclerotic lesions.

Review areas: lung bases, hernial orifices; review paraumbilical region and obturator rings, look for surgical clips indicating previous surgery, abdominal calcification; review pancreas, aorta and exclude an appendicolith.

Contrast examinations

ANN ANSTEE AND MARC PELLING

Contrast agents such as iodine-based water-soluble contrast and barium are dense on X-ray and can be used to outline the GI and urinary tract. When using barium in the GI tract it is possible to then distend the organ with gas (low density contrast) to obtain a barium-coated (double contrast) examination, which provides finer mucosal detail.

■ Investigation of the gastrointestinal tract

With the increased availability of endoscopy services and the use of CT-based techniques like CT pneumocolon and 3D colonography, fewer fluoroscopic contrast examinations of the GI tract are performed. However, contrast examinations are dynamic and provide some functional information. Some very specific questions, such as the course of a fistula, are often best assessed fluoroscopically.

The successful and safe completion of contrast study of the GI tract depends on:

1. **Appropriate patient preparation.** See table overleaf for a summary of preparation procedures for the most common contrast studies of the GI tract. Local guidelines for appropriate antibiotic cover for patients at risk of developing endocarditis after rectal intubation should be confirmed with the microbiology department.

Hospital Surgery: Foundations in Surgical Practice, ed. Omer Aziz, Sanjay Purkayastha and Paraskevas Paraskeva. Published by Cambridge University Press. © Cambridge University Press 2009.

Guide to patient preparation for common contrast studies of the GI tract

Investigation	Patient preparation
Contrast swallow	None
Barium meal	Nil by mouth for 6 hours before
Barium follow-through	None
Small–bowel enema	Low-residue diet for 48 hours before; stop antispasmodic agents 24 hours before
Barium enema	Low-residue diet from 48 hours before; Picolax regime starting 24 hours before; clear liquids from evening before; antibiotic prophylaxis on the day of the procedure for patients at risk of developing endocarditis e.g. prosthetic heart valves, pulmonary shunts or rheumatic heart valves

2. **Adequate clinical information to ensure that the correct contrast medium and motility agent are used for a study.** For example, the use of barium in the setting of a suspected perforation is potentially fatal. See Table below. The GI effects of motility agents are unfortunately non-specific. A relevant history of the conditions listed in Table 131.3 is helpful.

Indications and contraindications of the commonly used GI tract contrast agents

Contrast medium	Indication	Contraindication
Barium sulphate	Provides the best mucosal detail	Perforation: 50 % mortality of intraperitoneal barium
Gastrografin	Suspected perforation	Risk of aspiration: may cause severe pulmonary oedema
Low osmolar contrast medium e.g. Omnipaque	Investigation of a patient at risk of aspiration	Iodine allergy

CASE STUDY

JS, a 58-year-old lady, had been following a smooth postoperative course after an anterior resection of a Dukes' B adenocarcinoma of the lower sigmoid. On day five she complained of abdominal distension associated with mild discomfort and spiked a temperature of 37.7 °C.

The consultant surgeon was concerned that the patient had developed an anastomotic breakdown and asked the team to arrange a contrast study to investigate this further.

Check list

■ **Suspected leak/perforation:** document this clearly on the request card so that a water-soluble or low osmolar contrast material is used. Remember barium used in this setting is potentially fatal.

■ **Allergy history:** document a history of iodine allergy or previous contrast reaction. See second table on previous page.

■ **Bowel preparation:** not required.

■ **Antibiotic prophylaxis:** as contrast will be instilled per rectum, document relevant endocarditis risk and ensure that the patient receives appropriate antibiotic cover.

■ **Adequate analgesia:** the patient may be required to turn to lie supine and prone. It may only be possible to perform an adequate examination if the patient is comfortable.

A Gastrografin enema confirmed the presence of an anastomotic leak.

Summary of pharmacological effects of GI tract motility agents used in radiology	
Motility agent	Relevant history
Buscopan (buty iscopolamine): antimuscarinic agent, smooth muscle relaxation	Glaucoma, tachycardia, myasthenia gravis, prostatic symptoms, paralytic ileus, pyloric stenosis
Glucagon: smooth muscle relaxation	Phaeochromocytoma, insulinoma, glucagonoma
Metoclopramide: dopamine antagonist, increases transit time	Acute dystonic reaction

■ Investigation of the urinary tract

Intravenous urogram or IVU. As iodinated contrast is excreted via the kidneys, obtaining X-rays of the renal area and abdomen at intervals after intravenous injection of contrast gives anatomical and functional information about the renal tract.

The limited IVU is one of the investigations frequently performed to investigate renal colic. A junior member of the surgical team is often asked to perform the intravenous injection of contrast 'out of hours'.

LIMITED IVU

1. Plain KUB radiograph: is a radiodense calculus seen? Reviewing the abdominal X-ray particular attention should be paid to the renal area, the line of the ureters and the pelvis/bladder.
2. Injection of intravenous contrast: remember to ask about:
   - Risk factors for a reaction to contrast media.
   - Risk factors for contrast media nephrotoxicity.
   - Metformin.

   See the section on contrast media, in the Principles and safety of radiology Chapter. Consider unenhanced CT or ultrasound if it is unsafe to proceed with the injection of contrast.
3. 20 minute post-micturition KUB: is there evidence of a delay in the passage of contrast or is an obstruction seen? A delayed 1 hour film may be needed.

Summary of investigation strategies in suspected ureteric colic		
Investigation	Advantages	Disadvantages
Unenhanced CT	High sensitivity and specificity; other causes of abdominal pain can be identified; contrast free	Increased radiation dose
Limited IVU	Lower radiation dose than CT; bedside interpretation	Intravenous contrast administration; other causes of abdominal pain are not identified
US	Indicated in pregnancy; no ionizing radiation or contrast	Less accurate than CT or IVU; radiologist/sonography input required

■ Digital subtraction angiography

This X-ray-based modality allows intravascular contrast to be seen more clearly as a mask image is taken before contrast is injected. As long as the patient remains in the same position this mask is subtracted from subsequent images to allow the vessel to be seen minus overlying bone and soft tissue.

PATIENT PREPARATION

- Informed consent obtained before sedation is given.
- Check clotting screen and usual contrast media risk factors.
- Establish whether the patient has a contraindication to use of a gastrointestinal motility agent.
- Check local guidelines for anti–coagulation and oral intake.

■ Examples of contrast study films (Figures 169–173)

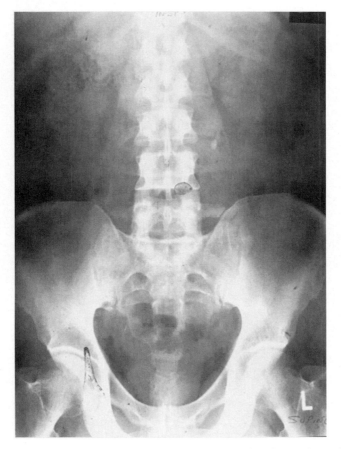

Figure 169 Control KUB (no contrast), showing a renal calculus inferior to the tip of the L3 transverse process on the left and subsequent IVU, with a dilated, pelvicalyceal system above the level of the same obstruction on the left side

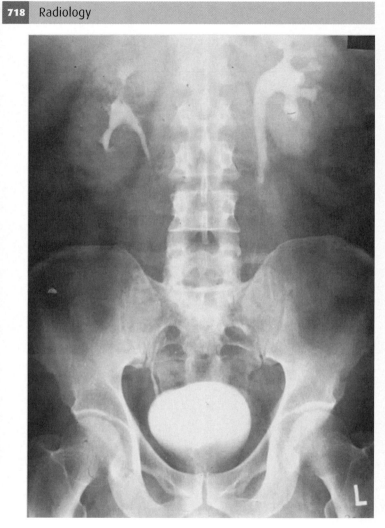

Figure 170 20 minute IVU

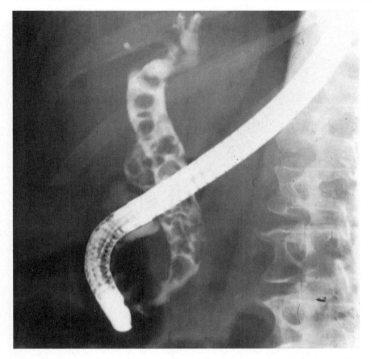

Figure 171 ERCP, showing multiple filling defects (gallstones) in a dilated common bile duct

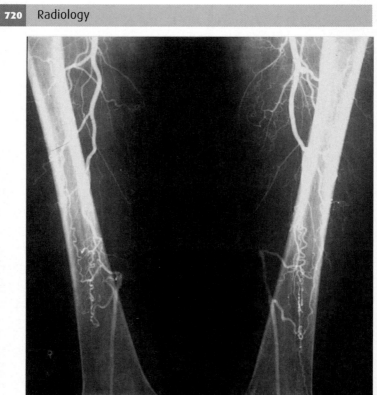

Figure 172 Angiogram (femoral): showing bilateral superficial femoral artery obstruction with the formation of multiple collateral vessels

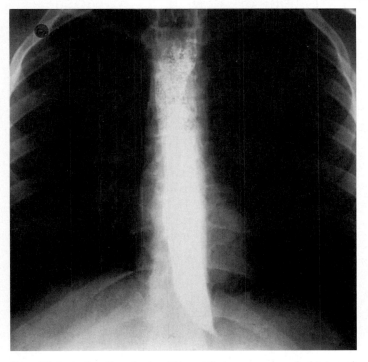

Figure 173 Contrast swallow: showing stricture at the lower oesophageal sphincter and a dilated oesophagus above this, containing particulate matter. The stricture has a characteristic bird's beak appearance and is suggestive of achalasia

Ultrasound

ANN ANSTEE AND MARC PELLING

Ultrasound images are produced when high frequency sound waves are reflected at tissue interfaces (Figure 174). These echoes are computed and an image produced in real time. Blood flow can also be demonstrated and analysed using Doppler.

There is no ionizing radiation so the technique is particularly useful in young or pregnant patients or where repeated examinations are required.

Ultrasound equipment is widely available. The machines are usually portable and the examination can be done at the bedside if necessary. High frequency sound waves are blocked by tissue-gas interfaces and it is not possible to scan through air-filled lung or gas-filled bowel.

Scan	Indication	Patient preparation
Upper abdomen	Biliary colic, acute cholecystitis, investigate solid organs of the upper abdomen	Nil by mouth for 6 hours
Renal tract	Renal failure, renal colic, haematuria	Full bladder. Catheter should be clamped at least 1 hour before the scan
Pelvis	Lower abdominal pain: to exclude gynaecological cause	Full bladder. Catheter should be clamped at least 1 hour before the scan
Appendicitis	Suspected appendicitis and to exclude a gynaecological cause	Full bladder. Catheter should be clamped at least 1 hour before the scan
Thorax	Tap/drain pleural effusion	Check Hb, platelets and clotting
Drain insertion or biopsy		Check Hb, platelets and clotting. NBM for 6 hours before a biopsy

Hospital Surgery: Foundations in Surgical Practice, ed. Omer Aziz, Sanjay Purkayastha and Paraskevas Paraskeva. Published by Cambridge University Press. © Cambridge University Press 2009.

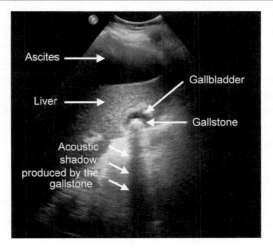

Figure 174 Ultrasound scan of the upper abdomen demonstrating (arrowed): ascites; liver; the thin-walled gallbladder distended by anechoic (black) bile. Gallstones are seen in this image; the larger (arrowed) is casting an acoustic shadow

For this reason it is helpful to fast patients prior to abdominal ultrasound. Abdominal ultrasound following endoscopy is particularly difficult because of bowel gas.

Ultrasound can also be used to guide procedures such as biopsies, drainages and to obtain venous access.

Appropriate patient preparation is essential.

■ FAST: focused abdominal sonography for trauma

Ultrasound may be used in the resuscitation suite by appropriately trained personnel, to try to identify abdominal trauma. FAST is a limited ultrasound examination directed at identifying the presence of free intraperitoneal or pericardial fluid. In the context of a trauma history, free fluid is usually due to haemorrhage and contributes to the assessment of the circulatory system. It is utilized to evaluate for free fluid in the following areas:

Perihepatic, perisplenic, pelvis, pericardium.

If positive, urgent surgical opinion with laparotomy or laparoscopy is indicated. If negative, maintain a high suspicion on clinical findings and repeat FAST or proceed to CT if stable. If not then again request an urgent surgical opinion.

Computed tomography (CT)

ANN ANSTEE AND MARC PELLING

As with plain radiographs, computed tomography (CT) exploits the fact that X-rays penetrate different tissues in the body by different amounts depending on their atomic number and density. A narrow fan of X-rays rotates around the patient and the emergent X-rays are detected by a ring of detectors. A technique called **filtered back projection** is used to reconstruct cross-sectional slices through the body.

Images are viewed on different window settings to maximize the detail seen within the tissues of interest.

Recent advances in CT, in particular multislice imaging, have expanded the role of this modality. Multislice CT is fast and provides high-resolution images, which can be reconstructed in any projection to provide a great deal of anatomical information. The speed of the examination is an advantage in many situations involving sick, confused or very young patients.

The main disadvantage with CT is the relatively high radiation dose and the need to administer intravenous contrast for the majority of studies.

A radiologist usually decides the scanning protocol and adequate clinical information is required for the correct protocol to be chosen.

■ Perforation of the gastrointestinal tract

The objective of a CT scan of the abdomen and pelvis in cases of suspected perforation is three fold: to detect the presence and level of the perforation with greater sensitivity than plain films and contrast studies, assess the underlying cause, and identify complications. The scan

Hospital Surgery: Foundations in Surgical Practice, ed. Omer Aziz, Sanjay Purkayastha and Paraskevas Paraskeva. Published by Cambridge University Press. © Cambridge University Press 2009.

should include the entire abdomen and pelvis; intravenous and water-soluble oral/rectal contrast should be administered in the absence of contraindications. The images should be viewed on a wide window setting.

The direct CT features of perforation are extraluminal free air or contrast and discontinuity of the bowel wall. Indirect features of perforation are an inflammatory reaction or abscess at the site of perforation. However, perforations arising at different locations have different imaging characteristics and these can indicate the level of the perforation even if it is not directly visualized.

Gastro-duodenal perforation typically causes a large volume of extraluminal air to be seen adjacent to the liver and stomach. In particular, air in the lesser sac and adjacent to the ligamentum teres are characteristic (Figure 175).

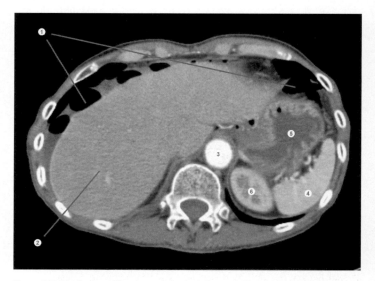

Figure 175 Distribution of free intra-abdominal air seen with a perforated duodenal ulcer: 1. Free intraperitoneal air, 2. Liver, 3. Aorta, 4. Spleen, 5. Stomach, 6. Left kidney

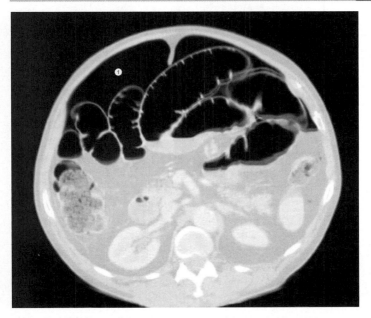

Figure 176 Distribution of free intra-abdominal air seen with a perforated caecum:
1. A large volume of free intraperitoneal air is seen

Small-bowel perforation is rare; the volume of extraluminal air is small and even at CT is detected in only 50 % of cases.

Large-bowel perforation may produce intra-or retroperitoneal air depending on the site of perforation. The volume of free air is typically large with perforation occurring secondary to bowel obstruction or endoscopic perforation, and small when occurring as a complication of diverticulitis (Figure 176).

Anastomotic breakdown typically occurs 7–10 days postoperatively when intra-abdominal free air is detected at CT routinely. In this group, the identification of a perforation is dependent on stable or increasing volume of free air or leakage of water-soluble contrast material.

■ Acute bowel ischaemia

Just as the clinical presentation of acute ischaemic bowel is varied and often non-specific, so too are the CT features of this condition. A CT scan should be obtained through the abdomen and pelvis, the exact protocol for this study is arrived at through discussion between the clinical team and the reporting radiologist to maximize the diagnostic accuracy of the scan. However, a patient with acute ischaemic bowel may be unable to drink water or oral contrast; co-existent renal failure may prevent the administration of iv contrast. The aim of the reporting radiologist is to (1) recognize the presence of ischaemic bowel, (2) identify the cause of ischaemia, and (3) identify complications.

CT features of acute bowel ischaemia include bowel wall thickening, dilation of the bowel, stranding of the mesenteric fat, ascites, alteration in bowel wall attenuation, alteration in bowel wall enhancement, pneumatosis (gas within the bowel wall) and gas within the mesenteric/portal veins. These features are non-specific, not uniformly present and depend on the cause, location, extent and severity of the ischaemia.

Causes of acute bowel ischaemia		
Cause of acute bowel ischaemia	Mechanism	Percentage of cases
Mesenteric arterial occlusion	Thrombosis, thromboembolism, aortic disease, vasculitis	60–70
Mesenteric venous occlusion	Infiltrative, neoplastic or inflammatory cause for thrombosis	
	Mechanical: bowel obstruction, over distension	5–10
Non-occlusive conditions	Hypotensive shock, pancreatitis, peritonitis radiotherapy, trauma	20–30

Figures 177 and 178: an 83-year-old man presented with a 10-day history of non-specific abdominal pain. On clinical examination he was noted to be in atrial fibrillation. CT scan of the abdomen and pelvis

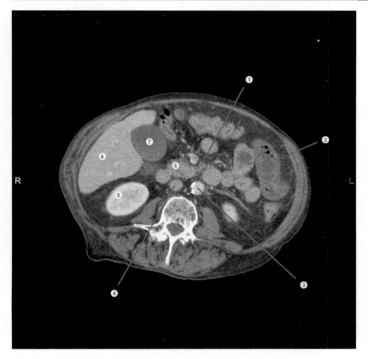

Figure 177 Axial image through the abdomen: 1. Thrombus within the superior mesenteric artery, 2. Thick walled small bowel (compare this with the normal bowel wall seen in Figure 176), 3. Aorta – calcification is seen in the atherosclerotic wall, 4. Inferior vena cava, 5. Right kidney, 6. Liver, 7. Gallbladder, 8. Pancreas

performed with dynamic intravenous contrast enhancement shows bowel wall thickening and alteration in bowel wall attenuation. A thrombus is seen within the superior mesenteric artery.

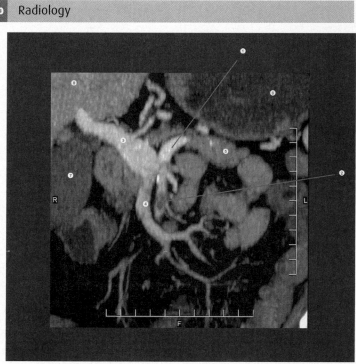

Figure 178 Coronal Multi-planar reformat (MPR) through the upper abdomen:
1. Superior mesenteric artery, 2. Thrombus within the superior mesenteric artery, 3.
Portal vein, 4. Superior mesenteric vein, 5. Pancreas, 6. Stomach, 7. Gallbladder, 8. Liver

Magnetic resonance imaging (MRI)

ANN ANSTEE AND MARC PELLING

Magnetic resonance imaging (MRI) is a cross-sectional imaging technique which allows excellent soft-tissue definition and has an extensive and expanding role in radiology. The examination is expensive and can be quite lengthy, depending on the number of sequences required. The bore of the magnet is quite narrow and claustrophobic patients are often not able to tolerate the examination. Small children and confused or demented patients may not be able to remain still and sometimes sedation is required. This needs to be pre-arranged with the MRI department and the anaesthetic team.

Although MRI does not use ionizing radiation there are other safety considerations arising from the use of the strong magnetic field; these should be considered in terms of electromagnetic and missile effects.

Both patients and staff are required to fill out a safety questionnaire before entering the scanner.

■ Contraindications to MRI

1. **Pacemaker/implantable defibrillator device:** deactivated by magnetic field; fatal.
2. **Intra-cranial aneurysm clips:** dislodge due to missile effect.
3. **Intra-ocular foreign body:** potential for injury resulting in impaired vision. Plain radiographs or CT scan with the patient looking up and down may be required to exclude an intra-ocular foreign body before a scan.
4. **Cochlear implants:** these devices are programmed by a magnet, and so subjecting the device to a large magnetic field will interfere with function and also risk dislodging mechanical parts; the potential

Hospital Surgery: Foundations in Surgical Practice, ed. Omer Aziz, Sanjay Purkayastha and Paraskevas Paraskeva. Published by Cambridge University Press. © Cambridge University Press 2009.

exists for a heating effect through the induction of a current in the cable.

5. **Pregnancy:** the effect of MRI on early pregnancy is unknown. Scans are therefore not performed during the first trimester.
6. **Prosthetic heart valves:** some older models of prosthetic valves are contraindicated, individual cases should be checked.

Other metallic objects may produce artefact but the patient will not be harmed by entering the scanner:

- Orthopaedic internal fixation devices
- Joint replacements
- Biliary stents
- Surgical clips and staples
- Previous coronary artery bypass grafting.

In the event of an arrest in an MRI scanner, the patient should be rapidly transferred outside the scan room for resuscitation.

Only MR-compatible oxygen cylinders are permitted within the scanning room.

Remove watches, swipe cards and loose metal objects that could be deactivated or be subject to a missile effect before entering the scan room.

MRI CONTRAST AGENTS

At the doses used in MRI, gadolinium is not regarded as having significant nephrotoxic effect. Gadolinium is not licensed for use in pregnancy. Breast feeding should be halted for an interval after the administration of gadolinium.

NEPHROGENIC SYSTEMIC FIBROSIS (NSF)

NSF is a tissue-based fibrotic reaction to some gadolinium-based contrast media (Gd-CM). A spectrum of disease has been reported ranging from a localized, non-progressive form to extensive fibrosis within the skin, subcutaneous tissues and internal organs, resulting in death in a proportion of cases. Risk factors for the development of NSF include severe renal impairment, CKD (chronic kidney disease) Stages 4 and 5 (GFR <30 ml/min), patients on haemodialysis and patients with reduced renal function who are awaiting liver transplantation. Patients with CKD Stage 3 (GFR 30–59 ml/min) and children under one year are at lower risk. These risk factors should be documented when requesting an MRI scan.

■ Magnetic resonance cholangio-pancreatography (MRCP) (Figure 179)

Indications include the investigation of cases of suspected duct calculi not seen on ultrasound. Consider MRCP after ultrasound in patients with painless obstructive jaundice to identify the cause of obstruction

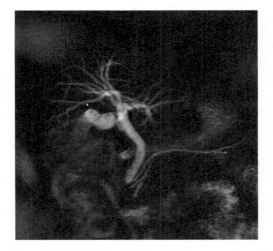

Figure 179 **MRCP:** this heavily T2-weighted sequence shows fluid as high signal (white). The intra- and extra-hepatic biliary tree is dilated, the common bile duct is distended and multiple filling defects representing stones are seen at its lower end. Gallstones are seen within the gallbladder. The pancreatic duct is not dilated

and define pattern of duct dilation. Preparation: nil by mouth four hours before investigation.

■ MR angiography

Non-invasive imaging technique providing excellent visualization of the vascular system.

■ Cord compression

MRI of the spinal cord should be considered in patients presenting with symptoms of acute cord compression.

■ MR colonography

One type of virtual colonoscopy that allows evaluation of colonic polyps and potential cancers. Bright and dark lumen MR colonography may be carried out; in bright lumen, the lumen of the colon is seen as white, and in dark lumen, the patients are given an oral contrast agent such as barium, which makes the lumen seem black. This latter technique has the advantage of better evaluation of smaller lesions, and distinguishes such pathology better from faeces coating the wall of the colon. MR colonography has the advantage of no ionizing radiation, however currently is not widely available. Its sensitivity and specificity have been shown to be similar to CT colonography.

SECTION 7
Clinical examination

History taking

REZA MIRNEZAMI AND OMER AZIZ

Clinical history taking is the most important part of making a clinical diagnosis of a patient's condition. As a skill, it develops with experience, so that ultimately it becomes comprehensive yet focused on making the diagnosis. Below is a guide to the components of clinical history taking that are important.

■ Patient details

Name, age, occupation.

■ Presenting complaint (PC)

In the patient's own words, the reason that has led to their presentation. Avoid using a diagnosis as the presenting complaint (e.g. use 'chest pain' as opposed to 'angina').

■ History of presenting complaint (HPC)

Explore each of the patient's *symptoms* in greater detail. For each symptom, explore the mode of onset, progression of the symptom, its severity, exacerbating and alleviating factors, associated symptoms, and any possible explanation the patient may give for its cause. Important components of the HPC are:

Pain: onset (sudden or gradual), site, character (sharp, dull, aching, burning, throbbing), radiation, intensity (out of 10), duration (constant versus waxing and waning), relieving factors, exacerbating factors

Hospital Surgery: Foundations in Surgical Practice, ed. Omer Aziz, Sanjay Purkayastha and Paraskevas Paraskeva. Published by Cambridge University Press. © Cambridge University Press 2009.

(eating, movements such as coughing, breathing), and associated symptoms. Two particularly important characters of pain that deserve mention are:

- *Peritonitis* – inflammation of the peritoneum causes this characteristic pain which is often sharp, and exacerbated by sudden movements such as coughing, and walking. Peritonism may be localized or generalized depending on the degree of inflammation.
- *The 'colics'* – these are pains produced by an obstruction of a hollow muscular viscus which continues to peristalse and contract despite the obstruction. They are severe, waxing and waning pains, and are often described by the patient as the worst kind of pain they have ever experienced (e.g. biliary colic and renal colic).

Vomiting: may also give important clues, particularly as to the site of bowel obstruction and the likely degrees of dehydration. How many times did the patient vomit? Is the patient vomiting spontaneously or only on ingestion of solids or liquids? What was the appearance of the vomitus? Was it associated with pain? What came first, the vomiting or the pain?

Fever: may be constant, or cyclical. The patient may be having 'temperature spikes'.

Change in bowel habit: if distinct should lead to the suspicion of colon cancer. Sinister features include alternating diarrhoea and constipation, a sudden change in bowel habit, associated rectal bleeding, and weight loss.

Bleeding: through any orifice requires close evaluation and should never be dismissed. *Haematemesis* may be fresh (bright red), dark (old clotted blood), or coffee-ground (slow gastric bleeding). Upper GI bleeds may be associated with melaena (the passage of dark, altered blood per rectum). *Rectal bleeding* may be bright red and coating the stool (suggesting a left-sided colonic or perianal cause) or dark and clotted blood mixed in with stool (suggesting a left-sided colonic cause).

■ Past medical history (PMH)

Enquire about any previous illnesses, accidents or operations. You will find that patients vary considerably in their ability to remember such details. A useful way to jog a forgetful patient's memory is to ask them about any previous hospital admissions. Try and ascertain the following:

- Acute illnesses, hospitalizations, and trauma
- Previous surgery
- Chronic diseases – hypertension, heart disease, diabetes, bleeding tendencies, asthma, arthritis and, in older patients, rheumatic fever.

■ Drug history (DH)

Any and all medications that the patient is currently taking. Also make a note of any medications that the patient has been taking until recently (for instance the patient may mention a recent course of antibiotics). For the surgical patient it is *particularly important* to find out if the patient is taking any of the following:

- Warfarin (should be stopped 3–4 days before surgery and if indicated, the patient should be heparinized during this preoperative period)
- Aspirin and clopidogrel (theoretical risk of bleeding and therefore some advocate that it should be stopped 7 days before surgery)
- Insulin (and oral hypoglycaemics)
- Steroids
- Oral contraceptive pill
- Monoamine oxidase inhibitors.

■ Allergies

It is very important to document carefully and convey to other medical staff looking after the patient. All allergies should be noted on a red wristband worn by the patient. Pay particular attention to antibiotics such as penicillin. If in doubt, consult a pharmacist.

■ Family history (FH)

Familial illnesses are often important clues (breast cancer, polyposis syndromes, MEN).

■ Social history (SH)

Ask about cigarette smoking and quantify in *pack years* (1 pack year = smoking 20 cigarettes a day for a year). Alcohol consumption (type of alcohol, drinking habit and number of units drunk per week). Marital status, sexual habits, life at home and recent foreign travel. Illicit drug use.

■ Systems review (SR)

To ensure that no aspect of the history has been overlooked. When starting off taking histories, it is important that this is as thorough as possible.

CARDIOVASCULAR SYSTEM

Chest pain; dyspnoea; paroxystrial nocturnal dyspnoea; ankle swelling; palpitations; dizziness; headaches; painful limbs; walking distance.

RESPIRATORY SYSTEM

Cough (productive/non-productive); haemoptysis; shortness of breath (SOB); wheeze.

GASTROINTESTINAL SYSTEM

Diet; appetite; any change in weight; abdominal pain; nausea and vomiting (N&V); flatulence and regurgitation; heartburn; haematemesis; indigestion; bowel habit; nature of stool; jaundice.

GENITOURINARY SYSTEM

Frequency; urgency; painful micturition; altered bladder control; loin pain; colour of urine; haematuria. In addition ask questions regarding sexual intercourse: dyspareunia; impotence, and in the female enquire regarding menstruation: regularity; frequency and duration of menses; painful (dysmenorrhoea).

NERVOUS SYSTEM

Headache; blackouts; dizziness or vertigo; paraesthesia; fits; memory disturbances; sensory disturbances (include vision, hearing and smell).

MUSCULOSKELETAL SYSTEM

Bone, joint or muscle pain; weakness; swollen joints; limitation of joint movements.

SKIN

Rash (if so, enquire regarding distribution, any associated symptoms e.g. itching, and any exposure to chemicals or cosmetics).

Abdominal examination

REZA MIRNEZAMI AND PARASKEVAS PARASKEVA

Follow a step-wise system: ***inspect, palpate, percuss*** and ***auscultate*** (in that order). To ensure that the abdominal examination is thorough and that nothing is overlooked, expose the patient from '*nipples to knees*'. In the clinical setting try to maintain the patient's dignity. Get the patient to relax – remember if the patient is tense, it will be difficult to feel anything within the abdomen. Ask the patient to lie down on the bed with the arms by the sides. Once you have ensured that the patient is suitably relaxed commence the examination.

1. *Inspection:*
   - Look for any general abnormalities, such as *cachexia*, frank *jaundice* or *pallor*.
   - Look for any obvious abdominal *swelling/distension* (Fat, Faeces, Flatus, Fluid, Fetus).
   - Look for *skin lesions* (e.g. spider naevi (liver disease), *pigmentation* (Addison's), tortuous veins (IVC obstruction), caput medusae (portal hypertension), striations (pregnancy/Cushing's).
   - Look for scars – do they correlate with the surgical history?
   - Check abdominal movements on breathing – does the patient appear to find this uncomfortable/painful? If so, this may be suggestive of peritonitis.
   - Check hands – clubbing, palmar erythema, leuconychia, Dupuytren's contracture, liver flap.
   - Check radial pulse – rate and rhythm.
   - Check face – dehydration, pallor of conjunctivae, jaundiced sclerae, telangiectasia, stomatitis.

Hospital Surgery: Foundations in Surgical Practice, ed. Omer Aziz, Sanjay Purkayastha and Paraskevas Paraskeva. Published by Cambridge University Press. © Cambridge University Press 2009.

- Gross inspection for hernias – ask the patient to lift their head off the pillow or cough. Look for incisional/paraumbilical/inguinal hernia.

2. *Palpation:*
   - Begin by palpating the areas you might otherwise overlook. Feel for supraclavicular lymphadenopathy (Virchow's node).
   - Now position yourself at the same height as the patient's abdomen. Ask the patient if they currently have any abdominal pain. If they answer positively, commence your examination distant to the site they report as being painful and work slowly towards that region.
   - Palpate the abdomen systematically over all the regions of the abdomen shown in Figure 180.

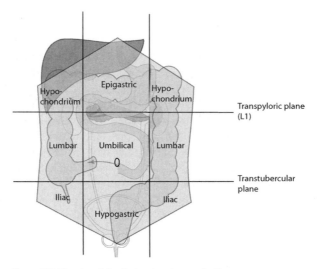

Figure 180 The nine abdominal regions in examination

- Assess the abdomen for any tenderness, rebound tenderness, guarding, rigidity or masses (note the site, approximate size, shape, consistency and mobility of any mass encountered on palpation) in the nine regions of the abdomen.

- Now repeat this, only palpate more deeply.
- Watch the patient's facial expression as this can give you valuable clues with regards to tenderness!
- Now palpate the normal solid abdominal viscera as highlighted below:
  a. Liver – start with your hand lying flat and transversely in the RIF. (Note: gross hepatomegaly can fill the entire abdomen!) Ask the patient to take a deep breath. If there is gross hepatomegaly then you may feel that lower edge of the liver against the radial aspect of your index finger as the liver descends with inspiration. If you feel nothing abnormal, repeat this with your hand positioned a little higher. Continue to do this until you have reached the costal margin.
  b. Spleen – start in the RIF. (Note – a very large spleen may extend across the abdomen into the RIF!) Ask the patient to take a deep breath. If you feel nothing abnormal, inch your hand upwards towards the left upper quadrant and repeat. Continue to do this until you have reached the costal margin.
  c. Kidneys – here the technique of bimanual palpation is used (Ballotting). For the right kidney place your left hand behind the patient's right loin and apply upward pressure. Now place your right hand on the right side of the abdomen. Now palpate deeply. Unless there is gross enlargement or the patient is extremely thin, the kidneys are usually impalpable.
  d. Uterus/bladder – these structures emerge from the hypogastrium. Assess their size in relation to distance from the symphysis pubis, or umbilicus.
- Palpate the abdominal aorta and note its calibre. In addition feel the femoral pulses on both sides.

3. *Percussion:*
   - Confirm organomegaly of solid viscera by percussion.
   - If you suspect the presence of ascites, confirm this by assessing for *shifting dullness*. Starting in the midline, percuss laterally until dullness is obtained. Then roll the patient away from this side.

Subsequent resonance on percussion confirms the presence of free fluid within the abdomen.

4. *Auscultation:*

- First listen for bowel sounds. With normal bowel, which contains a mixture of fluid and gas, you should hear low-pitched gurgling sounds every few seconds. The bowel sounds will be diminished in peritonitis or paralytic ileus and will be increased in cases of obstruction. Distension of the bowel secondary to mechanical intestinal obstruction leads to high-pitched, '*tinkling*' sounds.
- Next listen for systolic bruits over the aorta, and the femoral arteries.
- If you suspect pyloric obstruction, hold the patient at the hips and gently rock the abdomen from side to side, while auscultating over the epigastrium. Splashing sounds (a succussion splash) suggest that an intra-abdominal viscus, usually the stomach, is distended with fluid and gas.

5. *Groins:*

- Inspect and palpate for hernia and superficial inguinal lymph nodes.
- An inguinal hernia always lies supero-medial to a line drawn between the pubic tubercle and the anterior superior iliac spine, whereas a femoral hernia will lie infero-lateral to this line (the latter always lies medial to the femoral pulse).
- A reducible hernia may disappear with the patient lying flat and may require a cough to become visible.
- Pay particular attention to an irreducible, tender groin lump (this may be an incarcerated hernia which may require urgent surgery!)

6. *Genitalia:*

- In the male examine the testis for any swelling and/or tenderness and feel the cord. Any lumps occurring above them are going to be inguinal in origin; with beneath being scrotal. Look for any urethral discharge and penile abnormalities.
- In the female look for any vaginal discharge, and if necessary perform a vaginal examination.

7. *Rectal examination:*

- With a lubricated, gloved index finger perform the rectal examination, having first inspected for any visible external haemorrhoids, warts, fissures or skin tags.
- Assess for tenderness; note the anal tone and the presence of any masses. In the male assess the prostate for size, shape, consistency and symmetry, and in the female assess for cervical excitation.
- On withdrawing your finger note the presence of any blood, or mucus.

Examination of the respiratory system

REZA MIRNEZAMI AND OMER AZIZ

Ask the patient to remove his/her shirt/blouse and position the patient on the bed at an angle of approximately 45°. Once the patient is comfortable, commence the examination. Ensure that you have washed your hands and that they are at a temperature appropriate for palpation.

■ General inspection

- Look around the bed for sputum pot, peak flow metre and inhalers.
- Look for general abnormalities, such as *cachexia*, *pallor* and *cyanosis*.
- Is the patient on supplementary oxygen.
- Look for gross distension of the neck veins.
- Look for *scars* – do they correlate with the surgical history?
- Count *respiratory rate* noting dyspnoea, tachypnoea, laboured breathing, stridor or wheeze, or cough.
- Note the *breathing pattern* (e.g. *Cheyne-Stokes respiration*).
- Note chest shape. In normal subjects the AP diameter of the chest is less than the lateral diameter; in *hyperinflation* or '*barrel chest*' states – seen in states of chronic airflow limitation – the reverse may be true. Look for other chest wall deformities, for example *pectus excavatum* (funnel chest), or *pectus carinatum* (pigeon chest) where the sternum and costal cartilages project inwards and outwards, respectively.
- Look for any marked *kyphosis* or *scoliosis*.

Hospital Surgery: Foundations in Surgical Practice, ed. Omer Aziz, Sanjay Purkayastha and Paraskevas Paraskeva. Published by Cambridge University Press. © Cambridge University Press 2009.

■ Hands

- Inspect the hands looking for any *digital clubbing* (bronchial carcinoma, chronic pulmonary sepsis, cryptogenic fibrosing alveolitis, asbestosis), or *peripheral cyanosis*.
- Look for CO_2 retention tremor.

■ JVP

- With the patient lying supine at $45°$, assess the *jugular venous pressure* and the *jugular venous pulse form*. Remember the JVP may be raised in *cor pulmonale* (right heart failure due to lung disease).

■ Face

- Evert the lower eyelid and inspect the palpebral conjunctivae for *pallor*. Also look at the mouth and the tongue for signs of *central cyanosis*.

■ Palpation

- **Trachea** – feel for the position of the trachea to see if it is central. Do this by placing two fingers either side of the trachea and judge whether the distance between it and the sternocleidomastoid tendons on either side are equal.
- **Chest expansion** – place both hands on the anterior surface of the chest, with the fingers spread as far round the chest as possible, and bringing the thumbs together in the midline (but keep your thumbs off the chest wall). Ask the patient to take a deep breath in and then out. On inspiration your thumbs will separate. Ensure that both move equal distances away from the midline.
- **Radial pulse** – palpate the *radial pulse*, noting its *rate* and *rhythm* (remember that owing to its considerable distance from the heart the radial pulse is not a good pulse with which to assess pulse character). Also measure the *blood pressure* at this time. *Pulsus paradoxus* is a

drop in BP on inspiration. Minor drops can occur normally, but major drops can be associated with severe asthma, and a HR greater than 120/min and pulsus paradoxus in excess of 100 mmHg correlate with hypoxia, and are indicative of a severe attack.

■ **Carotid pulse** – palpate the *carotid pulse* and assess its *character*.

■ **Lymph nodes** – palpate for *cervical chain* and *supraclavicular lymph nodes* (the best way to do this is to stand *behind* the patient).

■ **Apex beat and chest wall** – palpate the chest and locate the *apex beat* (fifth left intercostal space, mid-clavicular line); assess its character. In the setting of pleurisy, or Tietze's syndrome (where there is inflammation of the costal cartilages) the patient may complain of chest wall tenderness on palpation.

■ **Tactile vocal fremitus** – with the palm of your hand placed on the chest, ask the patient to say '*99*'. Vocal fremitus refers to the *vibrations* you can feel on your hand as they do this. Compare this on both the front and back of the chest over the apical, middle and basal zones.

■ Percussion

■ Here the aim is to detect the *resonance* of the chest. Place your hand flat onto the patient's chest and spread the fingers. Tap, using the terminal phalanx of the middle finger of your other hand, onto the middle finger of the hand resting on the patient's chest. Do this on the front, back and sides (ensure you percuss over the *lateral zones* in the axillae) of the chest, over apical, middle and basal zones. Anteriorly percuss over the *lung apex* (middle third of the clavicle).

■ Auscultation

■ Ask the patient to sit up and take deep breaths in and out. Listen with the stethoscope over the front and back of the chest, covering the apical, middle and basal pulmonary zones. Compare each segment with that on the other side and note any differences in the quality of the breath sounds, and also listen for any *wheezes, crackles* (coarse or fine), and *pleural rubs* (see table). The sound of normal breathing is termed *vesicular breathing* and has a fine rustling quality.

Normal and pathological findings on respiratory examination

Tactile vocal fremitus	Percussion	Breath sounds
Normal – vibrations palpable	**Air in lungs** (emphysema) – resonance	**Normal** ('vesicular') – expiration shorter and softer than inspiration. No gap between phases
Consolidation – vibrations	**Air in the pleural cavity** (pneumothorax) – resonance	**Bronchial** – phases of equal length and quality (harsh and loud). Gap between phases
Pleural effusion/ pneumothorax – vibrations ↓/absent	**↓ air in lungs** (consolidation/collapse) – ↓ resonance	**Bronchovesicular** – phases of equal length but expiration is softer and smoother. No gap between two phases
Lung collapse – vibrations ↓/absent	**Fluid in the pleural cavity** (pleural effusion, haemothorax, empyema – 'stony dull' percussion note	**Asthmatic** – prolonged expiration, often with audible inspiratory and expiratory wheeze

Examination of the vascular system

REZA MIRNEZAMI AND OMER AZIZ

Always begin the examination by introducing yourself and ask the patient if they have any pain in the part of the body that you are about to examine. This avoids unnecessary patient discomfort.

■ Examination of the ischaemic arm

Exposure and positioning: expose and position the patient's arms and chest. Patient may be sitting or lying down.

INSPECTION

General inspection for:

- Signs of cardiovascular disease
- Respiratory rate (dyspnoea)
- Scars from previous cardiovascular surgery
- Pallor.

Inspect hands for:

- Nicotine-stained nails
- Clubbing
- Vasculitic lesions
- Finger pulp wasting
- Skin changes
- Colour (pallor, cyanosis).

Hospital Surgery: Foundations in Surgical Practice, ed. Omer Aziz, Sanjay Purkayastha and Paraskevas Paraskeva. Published by Cambridge University Press. © Cambridge University Press 2009.

PALPATION

- Feel the temperature of both arms with the back of your hands.
- Measure nail-bed capillary refill (normally <2 s).
- Feel *radial pulses* for rate, character, and rhythm. Look for *radio-radial delay* (coarctation of aorta) and a *collapsing pulse* (aortic regurgitation) by raising the patient's arm above the level of their shoulder. Apply mild traction on shoulder to see if radial pulse collapses (indicates a cervical rib).
- Feel *brachial pulse*.
- Feel for *axillary pulse* (if palpable may be abnormal).
- Feel for *subclavian pulse* in supraclavicular fossa (if palpable may be abnormal). Also you may feel a *cervical rib* here.
- Feel the *carotid pulses*.

AUSCULTATION

Listen for bruits over carotid and subclavian arteries.

COMPLETE THE EXAMINATION

By:

- Measuring the blood pressure in both arms
- Performing a full neurological examination
- Performing a full cardiovascular examination.

ALLEN'S TEST

- Occluding both radial and ulnar arteries by pressing tightly with your thumbs, ask the patient to make a fist five times. Watch the hands go pale.
- Release pressure on the ulnar artery while still occluding the radial, and watch the colour of the hand. If this goes pink, it suggests ulnar artery patency.

- Repeat the test but this time release the radial artery instead to assess its patency.

(Note: always performs Allen's test prior to a radial arterial line insertion or arterial blood gas sampling to avoid ischaemia.)

■ Examination of the ischaemic leg

Exposure and positioning: ask the patient to lie down. Both legs should be exposed, as should the abdomen up to the xiphisternum.

INSPECTION

General inspection of patient looking for signs of cardiovascular disease:

- Nicotine stained fingers
- Cholesterol xanthomata
- Scars in the abdomen and groins (AAA repair).

Inspection of both legs for:

- Pallor
- Venous guttering
- Discolouration
- Ulcers (look at pressure areas such as the heel and in between toes)
- Scars (popliteal fossa, and LSV harvest).

PALPATION

- Ask the patient if the leg is painful before examining it.
- Feel the temperature of the leg from the top down with back of the hands. Compare both sides.
- Measure capillary refill (<2 s is normal).
- Palpate the pulses (femoral, popliteal, posterior tibial, dorsalis pedis).
- Palpate for an AAA.

AUSCULTATION

Using a stethoscope, listen for bruits over the abdominal aorta, renal arteries, femoral arteries and superficial femoral artery at the adductor hiatus (Hunter's canal).

BUERGER'S TEST

- Ask the patient if either leg or hip is painful.
- With patient lying down, hold up both ankles to 60 degrees for two minutes. Normally legs should remain pink but pallor indicates peripheral vascular disease. The angle at which this occurs is *Buerger's angle*.
- Ask the patient to swing their legs over.
- Look for legs becoming engorged and purple, known as *reactive hyperaemia* (positive Buerger's test).

COMPLETE THE EXAMINATION

By:

- Measuring the *ankle brachial pressure index* (ABPI) – this is performed with a Doppler probe and a sphygmomanometer. The cuff is placed around the lower limb, and the Doppler probe used to determine the pressure at which the dorsalis pedis pulse becomes inaudible (ankle systolic blood pressure). The cuff is now placed on the upper arm and the Doppler probe used to determine the pressure at which the brachial pulse becomes inaudible (brachial systolic blood pressure). The ABPI is calculated by dividing the two:

$$\frac{\text{ankle systolic blood pressure}}{\text{brachial systolic blood pressure}}$$

- Neurological examination of the legs.
- Performing a full cardiovascular examination.

■ Examination of the abdominal aortic aneurysm

Exposure and positioning: ask the patient to lie down and expose the abdomen from nipples to knees. Both legs should also be exposed.

INSPECTION

General appearance and *hands* (as in examination of the ischaemic arm).
   Abdomen:

- Scars
- Distension
- Pulsatile epigastric mass.

PALPATION

Ask the patient if they have any pain in the abdomen.

- Perform superficial palpation in four quadrants.
- Feel for an obvious aortic aneurysm by gently placing a hand over epigastric region and noting pulsatility.
- Perform deeper palpation for the pulsatile mass.
- Place one hand either side of the pulsatile mass between the hands and demonstrate if it is expansile in nature.
- Feel for upper limit of the aneurysm (if you can get above it, this suggests it is infrarenal).
- Palpate for aneurysms over iliacs.
- Palpate the femoral and popliteal pulses.

AUSCULTATION

Listen for bruits over the:

- Abdominal aorta (above the umbilicus)
- Renal arteries

- Common iliac arteries
- Femoral arteries.

COMPLETE THE EXAMINATION

By:

- Examining the cardiovascular and peripheral vascular systems.

■ Examination of varicose veins

Exposure and positioning: ask the patient to stand up. Both legs should be exposed (ask them to hold up their gown).

INSPECTION

Inspect both sides from the front and back looking for:

- Visible dilated tortuous subcutaneous veins (in the distribution of the *long* and *short saphenous veins*)
- *Venous stars* (blue patches radiating from a single vein)
- *Gaiter area* venous insufficiency skin changes
- *Oedema*
- *Haemosiderin deposition*
- *Lipodermatosclerosis*
- *Eczema*
- *Ulceration*
- *Scars*
- *Limb hypertrophy* (Klippel-Trénaunay and Parkes-Weber syndromes).

PALPATION

- Ask the patient if they have any pain in the leg and then feel behind medial malleolus for pitting oedema.

- Feel for varicosities along the distribution of the long saphenous vein going through *key landmarks* (anterior to the medial malleolus → hand's breadth below patella → saphenofemoral junction (SFJ) medial to femoral pulse).
- At the SFJ feel for a saphena varix. Ask the patient to cough (an impulse will be present if the SFJ is grossly incompetent).
- Feel for varicosities along the distribution of the short saphenous vein going through *key landmarks* (posterior to lateral malleolus → popliteal fossa).

PERCUSSION: TAP TEST

- Place a hand on the medial side of the calf and another on the SFJ.
- Tap on the SFJ and if an impulse is felt distally this indicates incompetent valves below SFJ.

AUSCULTATION: DOPPLER TEST

- Place lubricated Doppler probe over the SFJ.
- Squeeze and release the calf listening for a single 'whoosh' as venous blood passes through the SFJ and a 'wop' as the competent SFJ closes preventing backflow of blood into the leg (normal result).

    In SFJ incompetence there is not only flow past the SFJ on squeezing the calf, but also backflow into the leg on relaxing it, producing a 'woosh' followed by a 'whoosh' sound.

TOURNIQUET (MODIFIED TRENDELENBURG) TEST

- Ask the patient to lie down and lift their leg up onto your shoulder.
- Empty the varicose veins by massaging them and once they are collapsed, place a tourniquet as high up in the thigh as possible.
- Ask the patient to stand up and observe.
- If the varicose veins recur, the incompetence (in perforator veins) is lower down.
- Repeat this with the tourniquet placed lower down.

COMPLETE THE EXAMINATION

By performing:

- Neurovascular examination of the leg
- Abdominal examination for any predisposing causes
- Obtaining a duplex scan of the leg to map out varicosities, and evaluate patency of the deep venous system.

The orthopaedic examination

REZA MIRNEZAMI AND PARASKEVAS PARASKEVA

The examination of any joint essentially involves three components:

■ General approach

LOOK – assess

- *Alignment* – is there any deformity or shortening; is there any unusual posturing of the joints and limbs at rest?
- *Joint contour* – are there any generalized or localized joint swellings? Are there any effusions?
- *Scars and sinuses* – are these from previous surgery or injury? Injury tends to produce an irregular scar, while a previous operation is suggested by a linear scar.
- *Skin.*
- *Muscle wasting.*

FEEL – assess

- *Skin temperature* – compare one side to the other. Is there any warmth or coldness (warmth is suggestive of inflammation)?
- *Swellings* – determine whether these are diffuse joint swellings or bony anomalies.
- *Tenderness.*
- *Measurements.*

MOVE – assess

- *Active* movement.
- *Passive* movement.

Hospital Surgery: Foundations in Surgical Practice, ed. Omer Aziz, Sanjay Purkayastha and Paraskevas Paraskeva. Published by Cambridge University Press. © Cambridge University Press 2009.

To complete the examination, measure relevant limb lengths, examine the joint above and below, perform a full neurovascular exam of the limb, assess the gait, and obtain two X-ray views of the joint in question.

■ Examination of the upper limb

Here we will consider the elbow and wrist regions.

ELBOW

LOOK – for

- **Deformities**:
  - **Cubitus varus** (or 'gunstock' deformity; this is most obvious with the elbow extended and the arms elevated, and is most commonly caused by malunion of a supracondylar fracture).
  - **Cubitus valgus** (common in non-union of a fracture of the lateral condyle).
  - **Olecranon bursitis** – the *olecranon bursa* occasionally becomes enlarged due to pressure or friction. When associated with pain is more commonly due to *infection, gout*, or *RA*.
  - **Swelling**.
  - **Loose bodies** – the commonest cause for a single loose body is *osteochondritis dissecans of the capitulum*. Multiple loose bodies may be seen in *osteoarthritis* or *synovial chondromatosis*.
  - **Scars**.

FEEL – for

- *Temperature* over the back of the joint.
- *Subcutaneous nodules*.
- *Synovial fluid* and/or *thickening*.
- *Tenderness*.
- *Hypersensitivity* or *thickening* of the ulnar nerve (it lies superficially behind the medial condyle, where it can easily be rolled under the fingers).
- Compare bony landmarks on either side. Is there a *discrepancy*?

MOVE

- Compare *active* and *passive* flexion and extension on both sides.
- Assess the radioulnar joints for pronation and supination. This is best achieved with the elbows tucked in to the sides and flexed at right angles.

WRIST

LOOK – for

- *Deformities*:
  - *Congenital* (radial club hand, where the infant is born with the wrist in marked radial deviation, and Madelung's deformity where the wrist is deviated forwards).
  - *Acquired* – various deformities may be seen after injury at the wrist. The deformity often seen in RA is radial deviation. The appearance of the wrist is usually normal in OA.
- *Ganglion* – painless lump, usually on the back of the wrist.
- *Swelling*.
- *Scars*.

FEEL – for

- *Temperature*.
- *Subcutaneous nodules*.
- *Tenderness*.
- *Synovial fluid* and/or *thickening*?
- Bony landmarks on either side. Compare – is there a *discrepancy*?

MOVE

- Compare *active* and *passive* palmar/dorsiflexion. The easiest way to assess this is to have the patient oppose palms (in the 'prayer' position).
- Now assess *active* and *passive* adduction and abduction movements at the wrist.

■ The *radiocarpal joint* is responsible for these movements. Now assess active and passive pronation and supination which relies on the inferior *radioulnar joint*.

■ Examination of the lower limb

Here we will consider the hip and knee regions.

HIP

LOOK – for
- *Deformities*.
- *Scars and sinuses*.
- *Muscle wasting*.
- *Swelling*.
- *The position of the limb*.

FEEL – for
- *Temperature*.
- *Soft tissue* and *bony contours*.
- *Tenderness*.
- Bony landmarks on either side. Compare – is there a *discrepancy*?
- *Limb length*; this can be gauged by positioning the patient flat on the couch with the anterior superior iliac spines at the same level. If there is any discrepancy in limb length, then this will be seen provided the pelvis is truly at right angles to the trunk and lower limbs. Establish whether there is true limb length discrepancy or if the discrepancy is only apparent.

MOVE
- Note that even a gross hip deformity can be obscured by movement of the pelvis; for instance a limitation of extension (causing a *fixed flexion deformity* of the affected side) can be masked if the patient arches the back into excessive *lordosis*. This potential for oversight

can be overcome by getting the patient to flex both hips to the limit simultaneously (thus preventing the lumbar lordosis); this is known as Thomas' test. Now holding one hip firmly in this position, gently lower the other limb. Thus you can assess the full range of both flexion and extension.

- In addition assess abduction (in this case fix the pelvis by placing one hip in full abduction, and then gently moving the other limb into abduction; this prevents the pelvis from tilting sideways – which can be misleading), adduction (ask the patient to cross one leg over the other; again watch the pelvis carefully), and medial and lateral rotation. To test rotation, position the patient with the hip and knee of the limb to be tested flexed to 90°; lift the leg by the ankle and gently rotate internally and externally.
- Trendelenburg test.

KNEE

LOOK – for

- *Deformities*:
  - 'Bow leg' (*genu varum*).
  - 'Knock knee' (*genu valgum*).
- *Scars and sinuses*.
- *Muscle wasting* (quadriceps).
- *Swelling/obvious joint effusion*.

FEEL – for

- *Temperature*.
- *Fluid* – there are two ways of assessing for this: (1) The *patellar tap* – compress the suprapatellar pouch with your left hand, and simultaneously with your right index finger push the patella sharply backwards. If the test is positive for fluid you can feel the patella striking the femur and bouncing off again. (2) The *bulge test* – empty the medial compartment by pressing firmly on that side of the joint. Now

lift your hand away and compress the lateral compartment sharply, a ripple will be seen on the emptied medial side if the test is positive. This is useful when you suspect that only a small amount of fluid is present.

- *Synovial thickening;* palpate around the joint margin.

MOVE

- Assess *active* and *passive* flexion and extension – while feeling for *crepitus* (which is a sign of patello-femoral degeneration).
- Rotation – with the knee flexed as far as it will go gently rotate the leg first internally and then externally.
- To assess the *medial* and *lateral knee ligaments* stress the knee carefully into valgus and varus. Do this with the knee first fully extended and then at 30° flexion. There is normally a slight degree of movement when the knee is flexed. Excessive movement suggests damage to the collateral ligament.
- Now assess the cruciate ligaments using the 'drawer test'; with both knees flexed at 90°, gently rock the upper end of the tibia backwards and forwards looking for any excessive anteroposterior glide. Excessive anterior glide suggests ACL laxity; conversely excessive posterior movement implies PCL laxity.
- Test the menisci, McMurry's test, Apley's grind.

■ Examination of the back

CERVICAL SPINE

LOOK – for

- *Deformities*:
  - *Torticollis.*
  - *'Cock-robin' posture* (lateral flexion due to cervical erosion secondary to RA).
  - *Hyperextension* (in ankylosing spondylitis).

FEEL – for

■ *Midline tenderness.*

MOVE

■ Assess active flexion, extension, lateral rotation and lateral flexion.

THORACIC SPINE

LOOK – for

■ *Deformities*:
  - ■ *Scoliosis* (lateral fixed deviation).
  - ■ *Kyphosis* (anterior facing concave curvature).
  - ■ *'Cock-robin' posture* (lateral flexion due to cervical erosion secondary to RA).
  - ■ *Hyperextension* (in ankylosing spondylitis).

FEEL

■ Palpate the *spinous processes* and the *interspinous ligaments*, noting any *tenderness* or the presence of any 'steps'.

MOVE

■ The thoracic spine is principally concerned with rotation, though a small degree of flexion, extension, and lateral flexion is also provided by this segment of the vertebral column.

LUMBOSACRAL SPINE

LOOK – for

■ *Deformities*:
  - ■ *Scoliosis* (lateral fixed deviation).
  - ■ *Lordosis* (posterior facing concave curvature).
  - ■ *Vestigial ribs* on the upper lumbar vertebrae.

FEEL

- Palpate the *spinous processes* and the *interspinous ligaments*, noting any *tenderness* or the presence of any 'steps'.

MOVE

- Assess active flexion, extension, lateral rotation and lateral flexion.

Examination of the cardiovascular system

REZA MIRNEZAMI AND OMER AZIZ

■ Exposure

Ask the patient to remove his/her shirt/blouse and position the patient on the bed at an angle of approximately 45° (to allow assessment of the jugular venous pressure and jugular venous pulse form). Also expose the legs and particularly ankles by rolling up trouser legs or removing trousers. Once the patient is comfortable, commence the examination. Ensure that you have washed your hands and that they are at a temperature appropriate for palpation.

■ General inspection – look for

- General abnormalities, such as *cachexia, pallor* (anaemia), *cyanosis* (central or peripheral), *malar flush* (red cheeks associated with mitral stenosis).
- *Dyspnoea* and/or *tachypnoea* at rest (left heart failure).
- Gross distension of the neck veins (cardiac tamponade/SVC obstruction).
- *Scars* indicating surgery. *Midline sternotomy, mini-sternotomy*, or *lateral thoracotomy* are the most common approaches. Also look for CVP line and chest drain scars.
- *Ankle oedema* (right heart failure).
- *Pacemaker/implantable cardiac defibrillator.*

■ Hands

- **Inspection** – look for digital *clubbing* (subacute bacterial endocarditis, or cyanotic congenital heart disease), *splinter haemorrhages*

Hospital Surgery: Foundations in Surgical Practice, ed. Omer Aziz, Sanjay Purkayastha and Paraskevas Paraskeva. Published by Cambridge University Press. © Cambridge University Press 2009.

(infective endocarditis), or *peripheral cyanosis*. *Janeway lesions* and *Osler's nodes* (infective endocarditis).

■ **Palpation** – take the patient's hand and assess the *temperature* (patients in heart failure are usually vasoconstricted, with the hands feeling cold); degree of *sweating* (in heart failure the hands may be overly sweaty owing to increased adrenaline secretion). Assess digital *capillary refill*.

■ **Radial pulse** – note *rate* (<50 = bradycardia, >100 = tachycardia) and *rhythm* (irregularly irregular in atrial fibrillation). Lift the patient's hand above their head and feel for a *collapsing pulse* (aortic regurgitation). Compare pulses in both arms if there is any suspicion of aortic arch dissection or coarctation.

■ Brachial pulses

■ Feel the brachial pulse.
■ Measure the patient's blood pressure.

■ Neck

■ **Jugular venous pressure** – with the patient lying supine at 45° and looking away from you, assess the *jugular venous pressure*. This should be no more than 3 cm above the sterna angle. Causes of raised JVP include right heart failure, congestive cardiac failure, and fluid overload. Palpate the liver to see if the JVP rises and assess JVP waveform.

■ **Carotid pulse** – palpate the *carotid pulse* lateral to the trachea. Be careful to palpate one pulse at a time. Assess its *character* (Water-hammer pulse of aortic regurgitation). Auscultate over the carotid arteries listening for *bruits*.

■ Face

■ **Inspection** – *sclera and subconjunctival pallor* (anaemia). Look at the mouth and the tongue for signs of *central cyanosis* (congenital cyanotic heart disease) and assess for poor dentition (risk factor for infective endocarditis).

■ Precordium

- **Inspection** – look more carefully for *scars*, or the presence of a *cardiac device* such as a pacemaker (though if not glaringly obvious this will become apparent on palpation). Assess the *pattern of breathing*. Look for any visible *abnormal pulsation*.
- **Palpation** – palpate the precordium and locate the *apex beat* (fifth left intercostal space, mid-clavicular line); assess its *character*. In addition feel for any *abnormal vibrations* or *thrills*.
- **Auscultation** – listen with a stethoscope over the mitral, tricuspid, pulmonary and aortic regions as shown in Figure 181. Note any

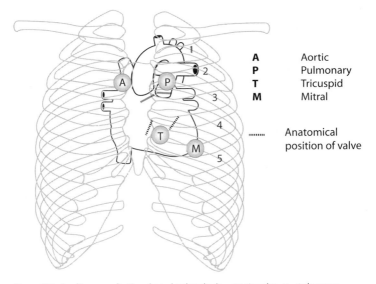

A	Aortic
P	Pulmonary
T	Tricuspid
M	Mitral
....	Anatomical position of valve

Figure 181 **Cardiac auscultation**; bony landmarks (A – Aortic valve; P – Pulmonary valve; T – Tricuspid valve; M – Mitral valve)

abnormalities such as murmurs. *Mitral diastolic murmurs* are best heard using the bell, with the patient rolled onto the left side. *Aortic diastolic murmurs* may be heard more easily with the patient sitting up, leaning forwards and holding his/her breath on expiration.

■ Lungs

- Ask the patient to sit forward and listen with a stethoscope over the lung bases, noting the presence of any *crepitations* indicating left-sided heart failure. Also look out for the signs of *pleural effusion*.

■ Sacral oedema

- **Inspection** – with the patient sitting forward, look for any obvious *sacral oedema*.
- **Palpation** – palpate the sacral region looking for *oedema* and *tenderness*.

■ Lower limb

- Inspect the lower limbs for *ankle oedema*.

Examination of the nervous system

REZA MIRNEZAMI AND OMER AZIZ

■ Speech

- Assess the three components of speech production (***phonation, articulation*** and ***language production***).
- You will already have heard the patient speak during the history-taking section. Are there any problems with *phonation*? (Dysphonia – reduced speech volume; aphonia – inability to produce sound.)
- Now assess *articulation* by asking the patient to repeat the following phrases – 'baby hippopotamus', 'West Register Street' and 'British Constitution'. Is there any dysarthria?
- Assess *language production* centres by (1) Listening to the patient's *spontaneous speech*, (2) Assessing *comprehension* by observing responses to simple commands (for example '*close your eyes*'), (3) Assessing the patient's ability to *identify* and *name* simple objects, for example a pen or watch, and (4) Assessing the ability of the patient to *repeat* sentences (for example '*no ifs, ands, or buts*'). Note whether there is an *expressive* dysphasia, or a *receptive* dysphasia.

■ Mental state and higher cerebral functions

- ***Consciousness*** – is the patient *alert, confused, obtunded, stuporous,* or *comatose*. Assess the level of consciousness more objectively using the *Glasgow coma scale*.
- ***Appearance and behaviour*** – assess the patient's general demeanour, physical appearance and responses to your questions during history taking. Also look for any obvious evidence of self-neglect, which can often be seen in advanced dementia.

Hospital Surgery: Foundations in Surgical Practice, ed. Omer Aziz, Sanjay Purkayastha and Paraskevas Paraskeva. Published by Cambridge University Press. © Cambridge University Press 2009.

- **Affect** – note the patient's *affect*.
- **Cognitive function** – assess by using the *mini-mental state examination*.
- **Dyspraxia and apraxia** – ask the patient to perform simple upper and lower limb tasks, for example for the upper limb, write a sentence, or do up his/her shoelaces).

■ The cranial nerves

- See table below.

Summary of the assessment of cranial nerves	
Olfactory nerve (I)	Use a characteristic-smelling object under each nostril to examine. Very rarely tested in the clinical setting unless the patient reports recent change in sense of smell
Optic nerve (II)	Assess colour vision and visual acuity. Also examine the fundi using an ophthalmoscope
Oculomotor (III), trochlear (IV) and abducens (VI) nerves	Examine the pupils (size, shape, symmetry, accommodation and light reflexes – direct and consensual), and examine eye movements
Trigeminal nerve (V)	**MOTOR** – look for wasting of the temporalis, and ask the patient to clench their teeth allowing you to feel the muscle bulk of the masseter; note any wasting **SENSORY** – test sensation to temperature, light touch and pin prick over the forehead, medial aspects of the cheeks and the chin (these areas correspond to the ophthalmic, maxillary and mandibular divisions of the trigeminal nerve)
Facial nerve (VII)	Inspect the face for any obvious asymmetry/palsy before assessing the muscles of facial expression ('blow out cheeks', 'shut your eyes tightly')
Vestibulocochlear nerve (VIII)	Perform Rinne's and Weber's tests to assess hearing
Glossopharyngeal (IX) and vagus (X) nerves	Assess the gag reflex. If there is a lesion the palate is seen to be pulled to the normal side on saying 'ah'
Accessory nerve (XI)	Assess strength in sternocleidomastoid and trapezius muscles
Hypoglossal nerve (XII)	Ask the patient to protrude the tongue (will deviate towards the side of a lesion)

■ The motor system

INSPECTION

- Note the patient's *posture*.
- Now ask the patient to hold both arms out in front of the body with the palms facing down. Ask the patient to now close his/her eyes and look for any downward *drifting* of the arms.
- Inspect for signs of *muscle wasting*.
- Inspect for any *fasciculations*.
- Note any *involuntary movements*, for instance resting tremor as seen in Parkinson's disease.

GAIT

- Observe the patient walking a short distance in the examination room and assess:
  - Can the patient walk unaided?
  - Can he/she walk in a straight line?
  - Does he/she demonstrate a normal arm swing?
  - Can he/she turn around with ease?
- Ask the patient to perform a *heel to toe* walk; note whether this causes the patient to veer to one side or the other.
- Additionally ask the patient to perform *Romberg's test*; this involves getting the patient to stand with feet together and eyes shut. If the patient is more unsteady with the eyes closed, then the test is positive.

TONE

- *Arms* – ensuring the patient is relaxed, take the arm and slowly flex and extend the elbow. Next, with the elbow flexed, hold the hand and pronate and supinate the forearm. Assess for any *interruption in the smoothness* of the movement indicative of increased tone.

- *Legs* – first with the patient lying flat on the examination couch gently rock the legs from side to side, holding at the knee. If tone is increased the foot and leg move together (normally the foot lags behind the leg). Also you can flex and extend the knee, with support at the upper leg and the foot.

- *Clonus* – involuntary muscular contractions due to sudden muscle stretching are a sign of upper motor neurone disease.

POWER

- In the upper limbs test for *shoulder abduction* (**C5** – deltoid), *elbow flexion* (**C5, C6** – biceps), *elbow extension* (**C7, C8** – triceps), *wrist extension* (**C6, C7** – wrist extensors), *finger extension* (**C7, C8** – finger extensors), *grip strength* (**C8, T1** – finger flexors), *thumb abduction* (**C8, T1, median** – abductor pollicis brevis), index finger abduction (**T1, ulnar** – dorsal interossei).

- In the lower limbs assess for power in *hip flexion* (**L1, L2** – iliopsoas), *hip extension* (**L5, S1** – gluteus maximus), *knee flexion* (**L5, S1** – hamstrings), *knee extension* (**L3, L4** – quadriceps), *ankle dorsiflexion* (**L4, L5** – tibialis anterior and long extensors), *plantar flexion* (**S1, S2** – gastrocnemius).

- For each of the above muscle groups power should be assessed and graded against *resistance* applied by the examiner. Grade the power in each group as shown in the table below.

The MRC scale for assessment of power	
Grade	Response
0	No movement
1	Flicker of muscle when patient tries to move
2	Movement, but not against gravity
3	Movement against gravity, but not against resistance
4	Movement against resistance, but not to full strength
5	Full strength (examiner cannot overcome the movement)

REFLEXES

- Tendon reflexes may be *increased, decreased* or *absent*. Test the tendon reflexes for supinator, triceps and biceps in the upper limb, and assess knee and ankle jerks in the lower limb.
- If you find a reflex appears to be absent, confirm this by *reinforcement*. Refer to the table below for annotation of reflexes.

Annotation of tendon reflexes	
Normal	+
Brisk	++
Very brisk, with associated clonus	+++
Absent	0
Present with reinforcement only (decreased)	±

COORDINATION

Assess:

- *Gait*.
- *Upper limb coordination:*
    - *Finger-nose test* – ask the patient to touch the tip of your index finger then touch the tip of their nose with their index finger. Get them to repeat this several times. Note the presence of any tremor or overshooting ('past-pointing').
    - Test for *dysdiadochokinesis* – ask the patient to alternately pronate his/her arm and correspondingly tap the palm and then the dorsum of the hand onto the palm of the other hand.
- *Lower limb co-ordination:*
    - *Heel-shin test* – ask the patient to place one heel on the knee of the other leg and slide the heel down the lower limb along the shin and down the dorsum of the foot. Lift the leg and repeat the movement several times.

■ The sensory system

- *Light touch* – with a wisp of cotton wool.
- *Proprioception* – move the distal interphalangeal joint of the index finger/big toe up and down. With the eyes shut ask the patient to indicate the direction of movement.
- *Vibration* – use a 128 Hz tuning fork. Place on the patient's chin. If he/she can feel the vibrations then place it now on the DIP joint of the index finger/big toe. If the patient cannot sense the vibrations move proximally to the nearest bony prominence and repeat.
- *Pin-prick* (nociception).
- *Two point discrimination* – a sensitive test for peripheral nerve injury.
- *Temperature*.

Appendices

Pathology reference ranges

SUKHMEET S. PANESAR

The interpretation of any clinical laboratory test involves an important concept in comparing the patient's results to the test's 'reference range.' This range is established by testing a large number of healthy people and observing what appears to be 'normal' for them. The results of this specific population of people are averaged and a range (± 2 standard deviations of the average) of normal values is established. This incorporates 95 % of the patients sampled. Some factors that influence these values are the patient's age, sex, diet, stress, anxiety and medications being taken.

Note: reference ranges are very institution dependent. These are a rough guide. Please consult your local guidelines.

Haematology	
Haemoglobin:	
♂	13.5–17.7 g/dl
♀	11.5–16.5 g/dl
Mean corpuscular haemoglobin (MCH)	27–32 pg
Mean corpuscular haemoglobin concentration (MCHC)	32–36 g/dl
Mean corpuscular volume (MCV)	80–96 fl
Packed cell volume (PCV):	
♂	0.40–0.54 l/l
♀	0.37–0.47 l/l
White blood count (WBC)	$4\text{–}11 \times 10^9/l$
Basophil granulocytes	$<0.01\text{–}0.1 \times 10^9/l$
Eosinophil granulocytes	$0.04\text{–}0.4 \times 10^9/l$
Lymphocytes	$1.5\text{–}4.0 \times 10^9/l$

Hospital Surgery: Foundations in Surgical Practice, ed. Omer Aziz, Sanjay Purkayastha and Paraskevas Paraskeva. Published by Cambridge University Press. © Cambridge University Press 2009.

Haematology	
Monocytes	$0.2–0.8 \times 10^9/l$
Neutrophils	$2.0–7.5 \times 10^9/l$
Total blood volume	60–80 ml/kg
Plasma volume	40–50 ml/kg
Platelet count	$150–400 \times 10^9/l$
Serum B_{12}	160–925 ng/l (150–675 pmol/l)
Serum folate	2.9–18 μg/l (3.6–63 nmol/l)
Red cell folate	149–640 μg/l
Red cell mass: ♂ ♀	 25–35 ml/kg 20–30 ml/kg
Reticulocyte count	0.5–2.5 % of red cells ($50–100 \times 10^9/l$)
Erythrocyte sedimentation rate (ESR)	<20 mm in 1 hour
Plasma viscosity	1.5–1.72 mPa/s

Coagulation	
Bleeding time (Ivy method)	3–9 min
Activated partial thromboplastin time (APTT)	21–33 s
Prothrombin time	12–16 s
International normalized ratio (INR)	1.0–1.3
D-dimer	<500 ng/ml

Arterial blood gases	
P_aCO_2	4.8–6.1 kPa (36–46 mmHg)
P_aO_2	10–13.3 kPa (75–100 mmHg)
$[H^+]$	35–45 nmol/l
pH	7.35–7.45
Bicarbonate	22–26 mmol/l

Biochemistry – serum and plasma	
Alanine aminotransferase (ALT)	5–40 U/l
Albumin	32–50 g/l
Alkaline phosphatase (ALP)	35–135 U/l
Amylase	25–125 U/L
Angiotensin-converting enzyme	10–70 U/l
Aspartate aminotransferase (AST)	12–40 U/l
α_1-antitrypsin	1 1–2.1 g/l
Bicarbonate	22–30 mmol/l
Bilirubin	<17 μmol/l (0.3–1.5 mg/dl)
Caeruloplasmin	0.20–0.61/l
Calcium	2.20–2.67 mmol/l (8.5–10.5 mg/dl)
Chloride	98–106 mmol/l
Complement: C3 C4	 0.75–1.65 g/l 0.20–0.60 g/l
Copper	11–20 μmol/l (100–200 mg/dl)
C-reactive protein	<10 mg/l
Creatinine	79–118 μmol/l (0.6–1.5 mg/dl)
Creatine kinase (CPK): ♂ ♀	 24–195 U/l 24–170 U/l
CK-MB fraction	<25 U/l (<60 % of total activity)
Ferritin: ♂ ♀	 20–260 μg/l 6–110 μg/l
Postmenopausal	12–230 μg/l

Biochemistry – serum and plasma	
α-fetoprotein	<10 kU/l
Glucose (fasting)	4.5–5.6 mmol/l (70–110 mg/dl)
Fructosamine	up to 285 μmol/l
γ-glutamyl transpeptidase (γGT):	
♂	11–58 U/l
♀	7–32 U/l
Glycosylated (glycated) haemoglobin (HbA$_{1c}$)	3.7–5.1 %
Hydroxybutyric dehydrogenase (HBD)	72–182 U/l
Immunoglobulins (11 years and over):	
IgA	0.8–4 g/l
IgG	5.5–16.5 g/l
IgM	0.4–2.0 g/l
Iron	13–32 μmol/l (50–150 μg/dl)
Iron binding capacity (total) (TIBC)	42–80 μmol/l (250–410 μg/dl)
Lactate dehydrogenase	240–480 U/l
Magnesium	0.7–1.1 mmol/l
β$_2$-microglobulin	1.0–3.0 mg/l
Osmolality	275–295 mOsm/kg
Phosphate	0.8–1.5 mmol/l
Potassium	3.5–5.0 mmol/l
Prostate-specific antigen (PSA)	up to 4.0 μg/l
Protein (total)	62–77 g/l
Sodium	135–146 mmol/l
Free T3 (Triiodothyronine)	3.0–5.5 pmol/l
Free T4 (Thyroxine)	9–19 pmol/l
Thyroid stimulating hormone (TSH)	0.4–4.0 mU/l (Euthyroid)
Urate	0.18–0.42 mmol/l (3.0–7.0 mg/dl)
Urea	2.5–6.7 mmol/l (8–25 mg/dl)
Vitamin A	0.5–2.01 μmol/l
Vitamin D:	
25-hydroxy	37–200 nmol/l (0.15–0.80 ng/l)
1,25-dihydroxy	60–108 pmol/l (0.24–0.45 pg/l)
Zinc	11–24 μmol/l

Lipids and lipoproteins	
Cholesterol	3.5–6.5 mmol/l (ideal <5.2 mmol/l)
HDL cholesterol:	
♂	0.8–1.8 mmol/l
♀	1.0–2.3 mmol/l
LDL cholesterol	<4.0 mmol/l
Lipids (total)	4.0–10.0 g/l
Lipoproteins:	
VLDL	0.128–0.645 mmol/l
LDL	1.55–4.4 mmol/l
HDL:	
♂	0.70–2.1 mmol/l
♀	0.50–1.70 mmol/l
Phospholipid	2.9–5.2 mmol/l
Triglycerides:	
♂	0.70–2.1 mmol/l
♀	0.50–1.70 mmol/l

Urine values	
Calcium	7.5 mmol/day or <300 mg/day
Copper	0.2–1.0 μmol/day
Creatinine	0.13–0.22 mmol/kg body weight/day
5-hydroxyindoleacetic acid (5-HIAA)	5–37 μmol/day; amounts in ♂ < ♀
Protein (quantitative)	<0.15 g/24 hours
Sodium	60–80 mmol/24 hours

Useful formulae

SUKHMEET S. PANESAR

■ 1. Anion gap

Is calculated as: $([Na^+] + [K^+]) - ([Cl^-] + [HCO_3^-])$, all units in mmol/l (Normal: 16 ± 4 mmol/l).

Increases in anion gap seen in:

- Diabetic ketoacidosis
- Uraemic acidosis
- Drug ingestion (e.g. salicylates)
- Lactic acidosis
- Hypokalaemia
- Hypocalcaemia
- Hypomagnesaemia
- Hyperalbuminaemia
- Laboratory error.

A decreased anion gap is less frequent but can be seen in:

- Hypoalbuminaemia
- Increased immunoglobulins (e.g. myeloma)
- Hyperkalaemia
- Hypercalcaemia
- Hypermagnesaemia
- Lithium therapy.

■ 2. Body mass index (BMI)

$BMI = Weight\ (kg)/Height\ (m)^2$.

Hospital Surgery: Foundations in Surgical Practice, ed. Omer Aziz, Sanjay Purkayastha and Paraskevas Paraskeva. Published by Cambridge University Press. © Cambridge University Press 2009.

- A BMI of ≤ 20 means the patient is underweight.
- 20–25 is desirable.
- 25–30 is overweight.
- >30 is obese.

■ 3. Body surface area (BSA)

- BSA $(m^2) = 0.20247 \times$ Height $(m)^{0.725} \times$ Weight (kg) – Dubois and Dubois method.
- BSA $(m^2) = ($Height (cm) $\times$ Weight (kg)$/3600)$ – Mosteller method.

■ 4. Cardiac output (CO) (Fick method)

$$CO \text{ (l/min)} = \frac{\text{(oxygen consumption)}}{((\text{difference mixed venous and arterial } O_2 \text{ content in blood in vol\%}) \times 10)}$$

The cardiac output can be estimated by dividing oxygen consumption by the difference in oxygen content between arterial and venous blood. The difference between the arterial and mixed venous blood oxygen concentration correlates with oxygen uptake per unit of blood as it flows through the lungs (Fick principle). The method is cumbersome due to the need to collect expired air and arterial blood gases.

Oxygen (O^2) content in blood $=$ (haemoglobin in g/dl)

$\times$ (1.34 ml O_2 per gram haemoglobin) $\times$ (% O_2 saturation),

where 1.34 ml per gram is the amount of oxygen that a gram of haemoglobin can carry if 100 % saturated. Oxygen consumption can be estimated by calculating the patient's BSA and multiplying by the basal oxygen consumption of 125 ml oxygen per square metre BSA.

■ 5. Cerebral perfusion pressure (CPP)

Defined as the difference between the mean arterial pressure (MAP) and the ICP.

CPP $=$ MAP $-$ ICP.

■ 6. Corrected calcium

Corrected calcium = measured $[Ca^{2+}]$ + {(40 − [albumin]) × 0.02}.

Corrected calcium concentration estimates the total concentration as if the albumin concentration was normal – usually taken as 40 g/l. A typical correction is that for every 1 g/l that the albumin concentration is below this mean, the calcium concentration is 0.02 mmol/l below what it would be if the albumin concentration was normal. However, in interpreting values, adequate consideration must be paid to other factors which may affect albumin binding, for example, other proteins in myeloma, individual variation, and cirrhosis.

■ 7. Corrected phenytoin

Corrected phenytoin = measured phenytoin level/
   [(albumin × 0.2) = 0.1].

Especially important in **hypoalbuminaemia**.

■ 8. Creatinine clearance (CrCl)

CrCl = (140 − age) × IBW/(serum Cr × 72) × (0.85 for females).
Estimated ideal body weight (IBW) in (kg):

Males: IBW = 50 kg + 2.3 kg for each inch over 5 feet.
Females: IBW = 45.5 kg + 2.3 kg for each inch over 5 feet.

■ 9. Daily electrolyte requirements

- Na = 2 mg/kg/24 hr.
- K = 0.5 mg/kg/24 hr.

■ 10. Daily fluid requirements (adult)

- 40 ml/kg/24 hours (70 kg male = 2.8 l per day).

■ 11. Daily fluid requirements (child)

- For first 10 kg of body weight = 100 ml/kg per 24 hours.
- For second 10 kg of body weight = 50 ml/kg per 24 hours.
- For every further kg of body weight thereafter = 20 ml/kg per 24 hours.

■ 12. Glomerular filtration rate (GFR)

Normal GFR is 120 ± 25 ml/min/1.73 m^2 (95th centiles).

Estimated GFR (ml/min/1.73 m^2) is calculated by the abbreviated modification of diet in renal disease (MDRD) equation:

$$\text{eGFR} = 32788 \times (\text{serum Cr}/88.4)^{-1.154} \times (\text{age})^{-0.203} \times (0.742 \text{ if female}) \times (1.210 \text{ if black}).$$

■ 13. Expected date of delivery (EDD)

EDD = Date of last menstrual period (LMP) – 3 months + 7 days + 1 year.

■ 14. Calculating heart rate from an ECG

HR = 300/(number of large squares between successive QRS r-waves).
Normal = 60–80 beats/minute.

■ 15. Henderson-Hasselbach equation

$\text{pH} = 6.1 + \log([\text{HCO}_3{}^-] / (0.03 \times \text{P}_a\text{CO}_2)).$

■ 16. Mean arterial pressure (MAP)

MAP $= \frac{1}{3}$ (systolic blood pressure (SBP) – diastolic blood pressure (DBP))
    + DBP.

■ 17. Serum osmolality

Serum osmolality $= (2 \times (Na + K)) + (BUN/2.8) + (glucose/18)$.
(Normal: 285–295 mOsm/kg.)

Statistics and critical review

SUKHMEET S. PANESAR AND THANOS ATHANASIOU

■ Definition

A branch of applied mathematics concerned with the collection and interpretation of quantitative data and the use of probability theory to estimate population parameters.

■ Basic terms

Mean: the sum of observations divided by the number of observations. For *normal* distributions, the mean is the better measure of central tendency as it does not fluctuate with the sample.

Median: the value which divides the observations into two equal halves when they are arranged in order of increasing value.

Mode: the most frequently occurring value in a distribution. It fluctuates with the sample and many distributions have more than one mode, hence it should not be used on its own.

Range: the difference between the largest and smallest values.

Percentiles: these divide a data set into 100 equally sized groups

Interquartile range: the difference between the 75th percentile and the 25th percentile.

Standard deviation (SD): can be regarded as being approximately equal to the average distance each individual lies away from the sample mean. 68 % of the data will lie between 1 SD on each side of a normal distribution. 95.4 % of the data will lie between 2 SDs and 99.7 % between 3SDs.

Variance: a measure of how spread out a distribution is. It is equivalent to the standard deviation squared.

Hospital Surgery: Foundations in Surgical Practice, ed. Omer Aziz, Sanjay Purkayastha and Paraskevas Paraskeva. Published by Cambridge University Press. © Cambridge University Press 2009.

Standard error of the mean (SE): the standard deviation of the subgroup gives a statistic that determines the spread of that subgroup. However, often it is useful to know how variable the means of a number of such subgroups would be so that the range over which the mean of the whole population lies can be assessed without actually taking measurements on the entire population. This is where the SE is used. It is equal to the SD divided by the square root of the number of observations.

Normal distribution: most continuous data can be graphically represented as having a *normal* or *Gaussian* or *bell-shaped* distribution (A). The distribution is fairly symmetric with the data more concentrated in the middle than around the tails. Asymmetrical data produce graphical representations which can be said to be *positively skewed* (tail stretches to the right; B) or *negatively skewed* (tail stretches to the left; C).

Types of data: *quantitative data* is numerical (e.g. blood pressure). *Qualitative data* has no obvious numerical relationship (e.g. gender).

Relative risk (RR): the incidence of a disease in the exposed group divided by the incidence of the disease in the unexposed group. The RR is used as a measure of aetiological strength. A value of 1.0 indicates that the incidence of disease in the exposed and the unexposed are identical. Therefore, the data show no association between the exposure and the disease. A value greater than 1.0 indicates a positive association or an increased risk among those exposed to a factor. Similarly, a relative risk less than 1.0 means there is an inverse association or a decreased risk among those exposed. This implies that the exposure is protective.

Attributable risk (AR): information on the relative risk alone does not provide the full picture of the association between exposure and disease. The *AR* is a measure of exposure effect that indicates on an absolute scale how much greater the frequency of disease in the exposed group is compared to the unexposed, assuming the relationship between exposure and disease is causal. It is the *difference* between the incidence in the two groups.

Odds ratio (OR): relative risk can be calculated from cohort studies, since the incidence of disease in the exposed and non-exposed is known. In *case-control studies*, however, the subjects are selected on the basis of their disease status (sample of subjects with a particular disease (cases) and sample of subjects without that disease (controls), not on the basis of exposure. Hence, it is not possible to calculate the incidence in the exposed and non-exposed individuals. It is, however, possible to calculate the *odds of exposure*. This is the number of people who have been exposed divided by the number of people who have not been exposed.

■ Basic concepts

Null hypothesis: the hypothesis statement that the researcher seeks to disprove.

Chance: the likelihood of a particular result occurring at random without necessarily describing a general trend.

Probability: a measure of the chance of getting a particular outcome.

Probability value (or p-value): the probability that an observed statistical difference in any particular sample has occurred by chance. If below the significance level (usually 5 %), then the null hypothesis is rejected.

Confidence intervals (CI): calculated for a measure of treatment effect and to show a range within which the true treatment effect is likely to lie. Confidence intervals are preferable to p-values, as they indicate the range of possible effect sizes compatible with the data. A confidence interval capturing the value reflecting 'no effect' represents a difference that is statistically non-significant (for a 95 % confidence interval, this is non-significance at the 5 % level). A narrow CI captures only a small range of effect sizes, and one can be quite confident that any effects far from this range have been ruled out by the study.

Power of a study: is the probability of correctly rejecting a false null hypothesis. It is used to calculate the sample size and depends on the following:

- Size of the difference in the outcomes being measured.
- Significance level chosen.
- Variance and standard deviation.
- Distribution of the population.

Tests of significance: these are used to assess the extent to which the observations from an experiment support or refute the null hypothesis. Parametric tests e.g. *t-tests* are used to analyse data that follow a normal distribution. Non-parametric tests are also called distribution-free tests and do not rely on the distribution of the data e.g. *the Mann-Whitney U test.*

Types of error: *Type 1* error (false positive) occurs when a study shows an effect which in reality does not exist. *Type 2* error (false negative) occurs when an effect was there but the study missed it.

Correlation: this is used to evaluate the degree to which two variables are related. To assess the strength of the linear relationship between the two variables, two methods are used:

- *Pearson product moment correlation* or *Pearson's correlation* – this ranges from $+1$ to -1. A correlation of $+1$ means that there is a perfect positive relationship between the two variables. A correlation of -1 means that as one variable increases, the other decreases proportionately. Scatter plots are useful in seeing how well the two variables correlate with each other.
- *Spearman rank correlation coefficient* or *Spearman's rho* – it differs from the above in that mathematical calculations are

done after assigning ranks to the numbers. Remember correlation does not always imply causation.

Prediction (regression): if two variables are related, one can predict a person's score on one variable from their score on the second variable with great accuracy. Assuming that the variables are linearly related, the prediction problem becomes one of finding the straight line that best fits the data. This line is called the regression line.

■ Common statistical tests

T-tests – should only be used on data that is normally distributed. Furthermore, they are only applicable to quantitative measurements which can be summarized by sample means and standard deviations. There are three types:

1. *One sample* – to compare a sample mean with a known or hypothesized value, and where only a single sample of data has been collected.
2. *Independent* – to compare the means of two independent samples, as well as measurements of the same variable that have been collected on two different samples of individuals.
3. *Dependent* – to compare the means of two samples of measurements taken on the same subjects or on matched pairs of subjects; repeated measurements of the same variable have been collected on two different occasions on the same individual, or a single set of measurements have been collected on subjects/experimental units that are matched in pairs.

Chi-squared tests – these are used in the analysis of categorical data.

■ Types of epidemiological studies

Ecological: use groups or populations as opposed to individuals as units of observation. They include studies of geographical differences and time trends in disease incidence and prevalence e.g. a study looking at the incidence of ulcerative colitis for people living at different latitudes.

Cross-sectional: describe the distribution of a disease in relation to person, place or time e.g. a study looking at the different reasons for people consulting their plastic surgeons in three different cities by using a cross-section of the individual populations in the three cities.

Case-control: a case group with disease is compared with a control group without disease, and the proportion of those exposed in each group is compared e.g. a study looking at the occurrence of stroke in those patients who underwent surgery.

Cohort study: subjects classified according to the presence or absence of exposure to one or more factors and followed for a specific time period to determine the development of disease. Can be *prospective* or *retrospective* e.g. dividing 200 000 patients into three cohorts: non-smoker, moderate and heavy smoker, and following them for 25 years to assess their cause of death.

Randomized controlled trial (RCT): two or more interventions are compared and participants are allocated to different groups in an unbiased way. It is the gold standard for evaluating the evidence from clinical research. Additional features include *single or double-blindedness* and/or *placebo-controlled.*

Systematic review: the systematic identification, appraisal, classification, and interpretation of evidence on a topic in question. This is then presented to the reader as a summary of the evidence to date.

Meta-analysis: a statistical method of combining the results of a number of different studies in order to provide a larger sample size for evaluation, and to produce a stronger conclusion than can be provided by any single study. Meta-analyses are attempted when previous studies were too small individually to achieve meaningful or statistically significant results. Because combining data from disparate groups is problematic, meta-analyses usually are considered more suggestive than definitive.

Levels of clinical evidence

Level	Rating	Details
1	* * * * *	Based on randomized-controlled trials (RCTs) (or meta-analysis and systematic reviews of such trials). Must be of adequate size to minimize false positives and false negatives
2	* * * *	Based on RCTs but of *inadequate* size. These may show positive results which are not statistically significant or may have a high rate of false positives and false negatives
3	* * *	Based on types of study design other than RCTs e.g. non-randomized controlled or cohort studies, case-controlled studies, case series or cross-sectional surveys
4	* *	Based on the widely accepted and published opinion of respected authorities, expert committees etc., as presented in consensus conference or guidelines
5	*	Based on the experience and knowledge of individuals on particular guidelines after peer discussion

■ Measurements of health

Crude mortality rate (CMR): the total number of deaths in a specified period, divided by the average total population during that period, multiplied by 100. The main advantage of using the CMR is that mortality can be expressed in a single figure. This is useful when comparing mortality within an area over a period of time. The main disadvantage is that it does not take into account that the chance of dying varies according to age, sex, race and socioeconomic class.

Life expectancy: defined as the average number of years an individual of a given age can be expected to live if current mortality trends continue. Helps assess the health status of a population.

Specific mortality rates: the number of deaths occurring in a subgroup of the population. To support this, there are age-specific and gender-specific mortality rates. These help to detect which parts of the community are most affected by mortality.

Standardized mortality ratio (SMR): the ratio of observed deaths to expected deaths expressed as a percentage.

■ Screening, audit and critical appraisal

Screening: this is the practice of investigating apparently healthy individuals with the object of detecting unrecognized disease or its precursors so that measures can be taken to prevent or delay the development of disease or improve prognosis. Screening tests are generally not diagnostic. These are usually cheap and simple, and aim to identify people at high risk of the condition. Further diagnostic tests are then done to confirm the diagnosis.

Incidence: this is the number of new cases of a disease within a specified time interval. It measures a change from a healthy state to a diseased state. Hence it can only be assessed using follow-up studies e.g. cohort studies.

Prevalence: this indicates the number of existing cases of the disease of interest in a population. As it is often measured at a particular point in time, it is called point prevalence.

	Disease +ve	Disease −ve	
Test +ve	a	b	All test +ve: a + b
Test −ve	c	d	All test −ve: c + d
	All disease +ve: a + c	All disease −ve: b + d	

Sensitivity of screening test: proportion of true positive results detected by the screening test $(\%) = a/(a + c)$.

Specificity of screening test: proportion of true negative results detected by the screening test $(\%) = d/(b + d)$.

Positive predictive (diagnostic) value (PPV): the proportion of test positive results which are true positive results $= a/(a + b)$.

Negative predictive (diagnostic) value (NPV): the proportion of test negative results which are true negative results $= d/(c + d)$.

The predictive value thus indicates the likelihood of a positive or negative screening test result meaning the presence or absence of the disease, respectively. There is always a trade-off between sensitivity and specificity; as one increases the other decreases (or, at best, remains unchanged).

Evidence based medicine (EBM): is the enhancement of a clinician's traditional skills in diagnosis, treatment, prevention and related areas through the systematic framing of relevant and answerable questions and the use of mathematical estimates of probability and risk.

Clinical audit: a quality improvement process that seeks to improve patient care and outcomes through systematic review of care against set criteria and the implementation of change. Aspects of the structure, processes, and outcomes of care are selected and systematically evaluated and where indicated, changes are implemented. Further monitoring is used to confirm improvement in healthcare delivery. The essential stages of the audit loop are shown in the figure.

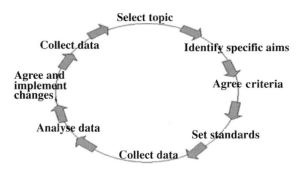

■ Critical appraisal of journals

Steps in reading a paper are as follows:

1. Identify the purpose of the study.
2. Assess the hypothesis that the authors are testing.
3. Evaluate the type of study design. The following terms may have been used:

Term	Meaning
Single blind	*Only* subjects do not know which treatment they get
Double blind	*Neither* subjects *nor* investigators know who is receiving what treatment
Cross-over	*Each* subject receives both the active treatment and control in random order, often separated by a *wash-out* period of no treatment
Placebo controlled	*Control* subjects receive a placebo which mimics the active treatment but has no clinical effect
Factorial design	A study that permits one to assess the effects both separately and combined of more than one independent variable on a given outcome

4. Decide whether the design of the study is appropriate for the research questions posed. Remember that all studies need not be randomized controlled trials.

Area being assessed	Preferred study
Causation	Cohort, case-controlled and maybe case reports
Screening	Cross-sectional survey
Diagnosis	Cross-sectional survey
Prognosis	Longitudinal cohort study
Therapy	RCT

5. Ask yourself the following questions:
   - Is the study original or similar to previously conducted research?
   - Who is the study about? How were the subjects recruited? What are the inclusion and exclusion criteria? Are the findings translatable into everyday treatment of patients?
   - Is a sensible study design used?
   - Is there any systematic bias?
   - Is the assessment blinded?
   - Are the statistical methods correct? Does the study have adequate power?
6. Interpret the results.
7. Apply the findings to the daily management of your patients.

Organ and tissue donation

MEI NORTLEY AND HELEN MANDEFIELD

There are two sources of organs for transplantation namely *cadaveric* or *live*. Cadaveric donors may be brainstem dead (*heart-beating*) donors or *non-heart-beating* donors (after cardiorespiratory arrest). Mode and location of death are major determinants of which organ or tissue may be donated. Organ donation tends to be mainly from an ICU setting, although occasionally from the emergency room as well. *Live* donors consent to donating a non-vital organ while otherwise well. *Commonly transplanted organs* include heart, lung, pancreas, liver, kidneys and small bowel. *Commonly transplanted tissue* includes eye tissue (corneas), heart valves, bone, menisci, tendons and skin.

■ Brainstem death

Acceptance of the concept of brainstem death has allowed donation from heart-beating donors. Of cadaveric transplants, heart-beating donors make up 80 % of the donor pool in the UK. 20 % of donors are non-heart beating. The diagnosis of brainstem death should be made by two doctors who have been registered for more than five years and are competent in the field. At least one of the doctors should be a consultant. Testing involves following set criteria, and repeating to remove the risk of observer error, although the time interval between tests is a matter of clinical judgement. Death is not pronounced until both sets of tests have been completed, and the legal time of death is that of the completion of the first set of tests.

Hospital Surgery: Foundations in Surgical Practice, ed. Omer Aziz, Sanjay Purkayastha and Paraskevas Paraskeva. Published by Cambridge University Press.
© Cambridge University Press 2009.

■ Legislation (2004 Human Tissue Act replacing the 1961 act)

Currently the UK holds an 'opt-in' policy on organ donation rather than 'opt-out'. The 2004 Human Tissue Act makes it lawful to take minimum steps to preserve organs while consent is sought from the next of kin. Consent is the fundamental principle underpinning the lawful removal and use of human organs and tissues from either the living or the deceased. Appropriate consent is defined as:

1. The deceased's wishes prior to his/her death.
2. Consent of a nominated representative.
3. Consent of a relative in a qualifying relationship e.g. spouse/partner, parents and siblings etc.

While the above information is a guide, codes of practice are being/have been developed to address this in more detail. The local '*donor transplant coordinator*' will be in a position to advise further.

■ Organ donor register

14.1 million people (approximately 24 % of UK population) have joined the NHS organ donor register (www.uktransplant.nhs.uk). Prior to any discussion about organ donation the NHS organ donor register must therefore be consulted. To refer a potential organ donor contact the local donor transplant coordinator via the hospital switchboard or intensive care department. The donor transplant coordinator will then access the register and be available to approach the potential donor's family.

■ Selection of donors

The absolute contraindications to organ donation include HIV and CJD infection. Donors are usually less than 80 years of age. Mode of death is most commonly a cerebrovascular event, fatal head injury or primary cerebral tumour. There must be no history of organ impairment with respect to the organ being considered. However it is important to remember that someone with chronic renal failure can, for example, be considered as a liver or thoracic organ donor. Donation can also be considered in donors with localized infections, including meningitis. Donation of a kidney can even be considered in a donor who had acute renal failure. Malignancy is also not always an absolute contraindication. Each case is different and the donor transplant coordinator will be able to advise on suitability.

■ Managing the potential organ donor

Prompt recognition of potential organ donors is vital. Where treatment is to be withdrawn and a patient is a potential 'non-heart-beating' donor the donor transplant coordinator must be alerted prior to withdrawal of treatment and cardiorespiratory arrest. Following brainstem death, organ protection and resuscitation of donors is paramount for graft survival in the recipient. Sequelae of brainstem death alone include hypothermia, drop in thyroid hormones, coagulopathies, diabetes insipidus and myocardial impairment. These must be managed promptly and meticulously after brainstem death testing, which is invariably within an ICU setting. Monitored parameters include:

- ECG monitoring
- Regular ABGs and pO_2 monitoring
- Urine output (optimally 1–2 ml/kg/hr)
- Invasive BP monitoring (arterial), aiming to maintain mean arterial pressure at 60–70 mmHg
- Maintenance of CVP $\geq$ 10 mmHg
- Temperature of 36 °C.

Factors in organ allocation

All patients who are waiting for organ transplants are registered on the UK Transplant National Transplant Database. In order to optimize chances of success, the best possible match for each patient is ensured by considering the following factors:

- Blood group
- Age
- Donor history
- Size matching of donor and recipient (e.g. small for size syndrome)
- Tissue typing for renal and pancreatic transplants – there are six HLA groups which are matched to the donors. These play a key role in the potential immune response to the graft.

Preparation of recipients

Regardless of organ, all potential recipients should have baseline investigations as follows:

- FBC, U&E, LFTs, glucose, lipid screen, coagulation screen.
- Septic screen – sputum, urine and blood MC&S.
- Hepatitis B, C, HIV, CMV, HSV, EBV,VDRL status.
- Tissue typing is performed for renal and pancreatic transplantation.
- Blood group compatibility without tissue typing is performed for heart and liver transplantation.
- Chest X-ray.
- Electrocardiogram.

Organ transplantation would be contraindicated in a recipient with:

- Multiorgan failure
- Active generalized sepsis
- Active malignancy
- Active peptic ulcer disease.

■ Future advances

Potentiation of non-heart-beating donors, xeno-transplantation and stem-cell research to produce tailor-made organs are wide ranging areas already being explored. Transplant surgery remains an exciting branch of medicine with much scope for further revolutionary pioneering.

Eponyms in surgery

SANJAY PURKAYASTHA

Eponymous: giving one's name to something, as to an institution or a clinical sign (from the Greek, 'epi' meaning to, and 'onoma' meaning name).

Achilles' tendon: the combined tendon of the gastrocnemius and soleus muscles of the leg. It joins the calf muscles to the calcaneum. From mythology it was the only part of Achilles' body that was still at risk after his mother had dipped him holding him by his heel into the river Styx.

Artery of Adamkiewicz: the largest of the medullary arteries which supply the spinal cord by anastomizing with the anterior spinal artery. Injury to this artery can result in ischaemia of the lower spinal cord – anterior spinal syndrome.

Adson's test: a test for thoracic outlet syndrome. The radial pulse is palpated and the patient's head turned to the opposite side of the arm being examined on deep inspiration. In the presence of compression of the thoracic outlet such as a cervical rib, the radial pulse will disappear.

Allen's test: tests the arterial supply to the hand which involves compression and release of radial and ulnar vessels and observation of colour change. Should be used prior to taking arterial blood gas samples from the radial artery or inserting an arterial line into this vessel.

Amyand's hernia: an inguinal hernia involving the appendix.

Amyrand's triangle: a diagrammatic triangular representation of the concentration of the constituents responsible for gallstone formation (bile salts, phospholipids and cholesterol).

Angle of Louis: the angle formed between the junction of the manubrium and the body of the sternum lies at the level of T4.

Hospital Surgery: Foundations in Surgical Practice, ed. Omer Aziz, Sanjay Purkayastha and Paraskevas Paraskeva. Published by Cambridge University Press. © Cambridge University Press 2009.

Baker's cyst: cysts in synovial membranes, especially of the knee joints, produced by synovial fluid escaping from a joint through a natural channel or through a hernial opening in the synovial membrane. Presents with mild aching and stiffness of knee or a swelling. May occur at any age, but more common in males 15 to 30 years of age.

Bankart's lesion: traumatic detachment of the glenoid labrum. This lesion is common after a traumatic anterior dislocation.

Barrett's oesophagus: a condition in which the oesophageal lining changes, becoming similar to the tissue that lines the stomach. A complication of gastro-oesophageal reflux disease resulting in squamous metaplasia.

Bennett's fracture: an intra-articular fracture of the base of the first metacarpal with involvement of the carpometacarpal joint.

Billroth I and II gastrectomy: removal of the pylorus with end to end anastomosis of the remaining stomach with the duodenum. In Billroth I the anastomosis is made directly to the duodenum, while in Billroth II the proximal duodenal remnant is closed and the gastric stump connected to the jejunum.

Boas' sign: hyperaesthesia of the skin overlying the inferior angle of the right scapula compared with that of the left. Seen in acute cholecystitis.

Boerhaave's syndrome: the spontaneous rupture of a non-diseased oesophagus, usually after vigorous vomiting. Associated with excessive alcohol ingestion.

Bowen's disease: carcinoma in situ of a squamous cell carcinoma type. Red velvety appearance.

Bochdalek's hernia: congenital diaphragmatic hernia due to failure of closure of the pleuroperitoneal hiatus, which allows protrusion of abdominal viscera into the chest. It is commoner on the left than on the right.

Brown-Séquard syndrome: hemisection of the spinal cord with the following neurological changes: paralysis, loss of position and vibration sense ipsilateral to the lesion, and ataxia; loss of nociception and temperature sensation contralateral to the lesion.

Bryant's triangle: an imaginary triangle of lines drawn on the body in fracture of the neck of the femur to determine upward displacement of the trochanter. This makes it easier to find pathological deviations in a number of deformities and conditions. It is especially used in diagnosing fractures of the neck of femur.

Calvé-Legg-Perthes disease/Perthes' disease: aseptic necrosis of the femoral head. Characterized by unilateral or bilateral avascular necrosis of the epiphysis of the head of the femur. The sporadic type is usually unilateral. It is commoner in boys, especially those aged 5–10 years.

Charcot's triad: the combination of jaundice, fever, usually with rigors, and abdominal pain (usually in the right upper quadrant). Classical presentation of cholangitis; if the presentation also includes shock and collapse it is known as Reynolds' pentad.

Chvostek's sign: tapping the face over the facial nerve (especially in front of the tragus of the ear) causes spasm of facial muscles, typically a twitch of the nose or lips. Seen in hypocalcaemia, tetany and sometimes in anxiety states.

Cloquet's nodes: small inguinal lymphatic nodes located in or next to the femoral canal.

Codman's triangle: a radiological sign of osteosarcoma: an incomplete triangular shadow between growing bone tumour and normal bone.

Colles' fascia: continuation of the inner layer of the superficial fascia (Scarpa's fascia) of the abdominal wall into the perineum.

Colles' fracture: fracture of the distal radius with dorsal displacement of the distal fragment.

Cooper's ligament: the pectineal ligament, a strong aponeurotic lateral continuation of the lacunar ligament along the pectineal line of the pubis.

Courvoisier's law: a palpable gallbladder in the presence of jaundice is unlikely to be due to gallstones. Typically caused by a malignant stricture obstructing the common bile duct. Causes include periampullary tumours and chronic pancreatitis.

Crohn's disease: a chronic inflammatory disease with symptoms variable according to anatomic location and amount of involvement. Can affect the GI tract anywhere from the mouth to anus, characterized by skip lesions, full thickness GI tract involvement, granulomata, and commonest in the terminal ileum.

Cullen's sign: periumbilical discolouration due to subcutaneous intraperitoneal haemorrhage. This may be caused by ruptured ectopic pregnancy or acute pancreatitis, for example.

Cushing's response: an acute increase of intra-cranial pressure, also causes compression of the cerebral blood vessels and cerebral ischaemia, producing an increase of systemic blood pressure over the vasomotor centre, with simultaneous reduction in heart rate and respiratory rate.

Dance's sign: empty right iliac fossa on clinical examination in patients (usually children) with ileocaecal intussusception.

De Quervain's thyroiditis: subacute, non-bacterial inflammation of the thyroid gland, often after a viral infection of respiratory tract.

Dercum's disease: a condition characterized by scattered areas of painful cutaneous nodules or lipomas. Development of the nodular, tender lipomas is gradual with localization largely to forearms and thighs. It occurs chiefly in menopausal obese women of middle age and may be familial.

Dieulafoy's lesion: a rare cause of recurrent gastrointestinal bleeding. A submucosal artery that runs too close under the intestinal mucosa and bleeds. Although this may occur throughout the GI tract, the commonest site is just below the oesophageal-gastric junction.

Doppler ultrasound: the Doppler-effect has made possible visualization of the flow in blood vessels, because ultrasonic sound is reflected from moving red blood cells. Velocity and the direction of the blood flow are shown on a monitor as a visible movement and in shifting colours.

Drummond's marginal artery: artery formed by the anastomosis between the ileocolic artery, middle colic artery, right and left colic arteries and sigmoidal artery. It is a continuous artery running along the inner perimeter of the large intestine from the ileocaecal junction to the rectum.

Dukes' classification: a staging system for colorectal cancer. The original Dukes' classification from 1932 described the staging of rectal carcinoma only, but can also be applied to carcinomas of the colon. It is divided into three simple stages, A to C. Stage D describes distant metastases and was added more recently.

Dupuytren's contracture: contracture of palmar fascia causing the ring and little fingers to flex into the palm so that they cannot be extended.

Ehlers-Danlos syndrome: disorder of connective tissue due to abnormal elastin characterized by hypermobility of joints, atrophic scar formation, loss of skin elasticity and easy bruising.

Erb's palsy: nerve lesion of brachial plexus, usually during childbirth, manifested as a flaccid paralysis of a group of muscles of shoulder and upper arm involving cervical roots of fourth, fifth, and sixth cranial nerves. The arm hangs by the side, internally rotated and flexed at the wrist. Normal movements are lost. This position is called 'waiter's tip' appearance.

Ewing's sarcoma: a primary tumour in the bone that may occur in any bone but is most prevalent in the diaphyses (shafts) of the long bones of the lower limbs.

Fitz-Hugh-Curtis syndrome: peritonitis of the upper abdomen in patients with a history of pelvic or sexually transmitted infections, often seen in women during gonococcic pelvic inflammatory disease or chlamydial infection. Common clinical features consist of sudden onset of sharp pain in the right upper quadrant of the abdomen, fever, nausea and vomiting. The pain is pleuritic in nature and may be referred to the right shoulder. In advanced stages, there may be adhesions that look like violin strings between the liver and the abdominal wall.

Fox's sign: a sign in haemorrhagic pancreatitis. There is ecchymosis of the inguinal ligament due to blood tracking from the retroperitoneum and collecting at the inguinal ligament.

Frey's syndrome: warmth and sweating over the cheeks on eating or thinking about food, or brought on by eating foods that produce a strong salivation stimulus. It may follow damage in the parotid region by trauma, mumps, infection or surgery. It is thought that autonomous fibres to salivary glands become connected to the sweat glands when they regenerate after any damage which originally caused their association to be interrupted.

Gerota's fascia: the connective tissue capsule of the kidney.

Grey Turner's sign: local areas of bruising around the flank due to extravasation of blood. It is a clinical sign seen after 2–3 days in acute haemorrhagic pancreatitis and other causes of retroperitoneal haemorrhage.

Guyon's canal: a small superficial tunnel-like structure at the base of the hypothenar eminence bounded by the flexor retinaculum and flexor carpi ulnaris. The canal transmits blood vessels and the ulnar nerve from the forearm to the hand.

Hartmann's procedure: the lower part of the sigmoid or the upper part of the rectum is resected. The bowel is then divided in the region of the descending colon. After the intervening segment of bowel has been removed, the proximal end of the descending colon is brought to the surface, as in the performance of an end colostomy. The proximal end of the distal segment is stapled or sutured closed and left in place leaving a blind rectal pouch. Now more commonly used for emergency procedures where the left colon/rectum has to be resected, e.g. perforated sigmoid diverticular disease.

Heineke-Mikulicz pyloroplasty: pyloroplasty of the stomach, performed to widen the outlet of the stomach and to make it non-functional. A short longitudinal incision is made through all layers of the pylorus and closed transversely.

Hasselbach's triangle: the triangular space bounded by the inguinal ligament, the exterior border of rectus muscle, and the inferior epigastric vessels. Hernias that protrude through this triangle are direct and those that protrude lateral to the inferior epigastric vessels are indirect.

Hilton's law: the nerve trunk supplying a joint also supplies the overlying skin and the muscles that move the joint.

Hunter's canal: the adductor canal, the space in the middle third of the thigh that gives passage to the femoral vessels and saphenous nerve.

Killian's dehiscence: triangular area in the wall of the pharynx between the oblique fibres of the inferior constrictor muscle, and the transverse fibres of the cricopharyngeus muscle, through which a pharyngeal pouch may occur.

Klippel-Trénaunay syndrome: a congenital vascular condition including varicose veins that usually involve the legs, buttocks, abdomen and lower trunk. Vascular anomalies may be present at birth or may appear in infancy. As the child grows the involved limb may hypertrophy and various veins may appear. There is often mild mental retardation.

Kocher's incision: oblique abdominal incision paralleling the thoracic cage on the right side of the abdomen for open cholecystectomy.

Krukenberg tumour: a malignant tumour of the ovary, usually bilateral, with fibromyxomatous stroma and scattered mucin-secreting signet cells. They are now known to be most frequently secondary to malignancies of the gastrointestinal tract, that have spread transcoelomically.

Le Fort's classification: classification of fractures of the face, Le Fort I, II and III. These increase in severity and add risk to maintaining an adequate airway.

Leriche's syndrome: a condition usually affecting young males, caused by atheromatous involvement or occlusion of the abdominal aorta by a thrombus just above the site of its bifurcation. The main symptoms are inability to maintain penile erection, fatigue in the lower limbs, cramps in the calf area, ischaemic pain of intermittent bilateral claudication; absent or diminished femoral pulses, pallor and coldness of the feet and legs. Onset usually between 30 and 40 years of age.

Leydig's tumour: a rare and usually benign hormone-producing tumour in the testicle, originating from Leydig interstitial cells or similar cells in the ovary. They produce androgens and oestrogens, causing virilization in women.

Lisfranc's amputation: partial amputation of the foot at the tarsometatarsal joint, with the sole being preserved to make the flap.

Littre's hernia: hernial protrusion of an intestinal diverticulum. More common in men and on the right side. When strangulation occurs: pain, fever, while small-bowel obstruction symptoms and signs are delayed. Example is a hernia sac containing a Meckel's diverticulum.

Luschka's foramen: the foramen of the fourth ventricle of the brain. One of the two lateral openings draining the fourth ventricle into the subarachnoid space.

Mallory-Weiss tear: severe, painless and sometimes fatal haemorrhage from the upper gastrointestinal tract due to a tear in the mucosa of the oesophagus or gastro-esophageal junction, usually preceded by severe vomiting.

Marjolin's ulcer: a squamous carcinoma which develops in a chronic scar such as a long-standing ulcer.

Maydl's hernia: hernia with strangulation of the intestine in the hernia sac, the loops of the intestines forming a 'W' shape.

McBurney's point: a guide to the position of the appendix. This point is 2/3 of the distance between the umbilicus and the right anterior superior iliac spine.

Meckel's diverticulum: a true diverticulum of the ileum derived from the unobliterated vitello-intestinal duct. It is a congenital sac or blind pouch, about 6 to 10 cm long, commonly found in the terminal ileum approximately 60 cm from the ileo-caecal valve. It may cause complications such as perforation, haemorrhage from peptic ulceration, intussusception or intestinal obstruction, or present as acute appendicitis.

Mirizzi's syndrome: a partial obstruction of the common bile duct secondary to an impacted gallstone in the cystic duct or infundibulum of the gallbladder. Four types are described. Type 1 has no fistula between the gallbladder and the CBD. Types II–IV do involve fistulae here.

Murphy's sign: a sign of inflammation of the gallbladder. When the gallbladder is palpated by pressing two fingers on the right upper quadrant, at the tip of the ninth costal cartilage at the mid-clavicular line, deep inspiration causes pain and there is inability to take a deep breath because the gallbladder is forced down to touch the fingers. Only positive when the test is negative on the left.

Nelaton's line: a line drawn from the anterior superior spine to the ischial tuberosity. In cases of dislocation of the hip, the tip of the greater trochanter of the femur is above this line.

The canal of Nuck: a pouch of peritoneum which extends into the inguinal canal and then labia majora in women. In women it accompanies the round ligament and is usually obliterated. This is analogous to the processus vaginalis in men.

Sphincter of Oddi: The muscle fibres around the opening of the common bile duct into the duodenum at the papilla of Vater.

Osler-Weber-Rendu syndrome: A familial syndrome characterized by multiple telangiectasia of the skin, and of the oral, nasal and gastrointestinal mucous membranes. They may ulcerate and bleed. Epistaxis and gastrointestinal haemorrhages are common features.

Paget's diseases:

1. Of the bone: chronic inflammation of bones, resulting in thickening and softening of bones, and the bowing of long bones. Manifests in middle-aged and elderly patients. Commoner in men, but more severe in women. There is an increased risk of osteosarcoma.
2. Of the nipple: a form of breast cancer. Starting as an eczematous condition around the areola. Characterized by large cells with a clear cytoplasm (Paget's cells) combined with a deeper carcinoma. Middle-aged women are most frequently affected.
3. Abscess: an abscess that forms around the residue of a former abscess after apparent cure.

Pancoast's tumour: a syndrome characterized by a malignant neoplasm of the cervical area, with destructive lesions of the thorax inlet and involvement of the brachial plexus and cervical sympathetic nerves. There may be pain in the shoulder radiating toward the axilla and along the ulnar aspect of the muscles of the hand. Atrophy of hand and arm muscles supplied by the ulnar nerve and Horner's syndrome may be apparent.

Perthes disease: disorder characterized by unilateral or bilateral aseptic necrosis of the emphysis of the head of the femur.

Peutz-Jeghers syndrome: a condition characterized by gastrointestinal polyposis associated with benign adenomatous (hamartomatous) tumours and mucocutaneous pigmentation consisting of discrete brown macules peri-orally. Anaemia due to bleeding from the intestinal polyps is a common finding. Malignancy supervenes in the polyps in a minority of affected persons.

Peyronie's disease: hardening of the corpora cavernosa of the penis caused by scar tissue, that replaces the normal elastic tissue of the tunica and forms in the wall of the tissue that surrounds the corpus cavernosum. This causes distortion and curvature of the penis, and, at times, inability to achieve an erection.

Pfannensteil's incision: a transverse, gently curved incision through the external sheath of the rectus muscles, about 2.5 cm above the pubic bone, commonly used for C-sections and access to the pelvis.

Phalen's test: a manoeuvre done to check for carpal tunnel pathology. The wrists are held in flexion for 60 seconds or less (if the patient begins to experience symptoms earlier) and the test is positive if it causes a reproduction of the patients symptoms (due to increased pressure in the tunnel caused by wrist flexion).

Plummer's disease: hyperthyroidism with a nodular goitre due to Plummer's adenoma. Prevalent in females; onset after 40 years of age.

Plummer-Vinson syndrome: characterized by an iron-deficiency anaemia, atrophic changes in the buccal, glossopharyngeal, and oesophageal mucous membranes (webs), koilonycha (spoon-shaped finger nails), and dysphagia.

Conditions named after Percival Pott:

1. **Pott's aneurysm: arteriovenous aneurysm** in which blood flows from an artery directly into a vein without going through a connecting sac.
2. **Pott's cancer/disease** of the scrotum: coal tar-induced cancer of the skin, particularly localized to the scrotum.
3. **Pott's disease of the spine:** usually of tuberculous origin, characterized by softening and collapse of the vertebrae, often resulting in kyphosis, a hunchback deformity (Pott's curvature). Occasionally, the

spinal nerves are affected, and a rigid paralysis (Pott's paraplegia) may result. Often infection spreads to paravertebral tissues giving rise to paravertebral abscesses.

4. **Pott's puffy tumour:** circumscribed oedema of the scalp associated with underlying osteomyelitis of the skull.

5. **Pott's fracture:** fracture of one or both bones just above the ankle. Fracture of the lower end of the fibula and medial malleolus of the tibia with rupture of the internal lateral ligament of the ankle, caused by outward and backward displacement of the leg while the foot is fixed.

Poupart's ligament a.k.a. inguinal ligament: a fibrous band forming the thickened lower border of the aponeurosis of the external oblique muscle between the anterosuperior spine of the ilium and the pubic tubercle.

Pringle's manoeuvre: is a surgical manoeuvre used in some abdominal operations. The bloodflow through the hepatic artery and portal vein are compressed either digitally or with a clamp on the hepatic pedicle in the free edge of the lesser omentum and thus helping to control bleeding from, for example, the liver.

Queyrat's erythroplasia: a chronic precancerous condition presenting with circumscribed red velvety lesion at the mucocutaneous junction of the mouth, vulva, penis or prepuce. Not seen on the glans penis of circumsized men. Like Bowen's disease, Queyrat's erythroplasia is considered as a variant of carcinoma in situ.

Raynaud's disease: peripheral vascular disorder of unknown aetiology characterized by abnormal vasoconstriction of the extremities upon exposure to cold or emotional stress. Other causes include excessive smoking or mechanical factors such as cervical rib. Symptoms include intermittent attacks of pallor or cyanosis of the digits (usually fingers) associated with cold or emotional disturbance, pallor or cyanosis that is bilateral or symmetrical, normal radial and ulnar pulse. No evidence of occlusive disease is present; gangrene may occur but is limited to the skin of the tips of the digits. The process is reversed by warming, but during the warming there may be intense flushing of the skin with pain and oedema. It is found most frequently in females between the ages of 18 and 30.

Richter's hernia: strangulated hernia in which only a part of the wall of the gut is involved.

Riedel's disease: a rare form of chronic inflammation of the thyroid, characterized by fibrosis of the thyroid, interfering with production of thyroid hormones and local compression. Attacks of suffocation due to compression of the trachea are the usual presenting symptoms. The thyroid becomes enlarged and forms a woody mass of scar tissue that may be confused with malignancy of the thyroid. Associated with retroperitoneal fibrosis.

Rovsing's sign: used in the diagnosis of appendicitis. It is said to be present when palpating on the abdomen in the left iliac fossa elicits greater pain in the right iliac fossa than in the left.

Santorini's duct: the accessory duct of the pancreas, a small duct draining a part of the head of the pancreas into the minor duodenal papilla.

Scarpa's fascia: deep layer of superficial abdominal fascia around edge of the subcutaneous inguinal ring.

Sister Mary Joseph's nodule: a hard mass or nodule which can be seen or felt deep in the subcutaneous tissue around the umbilicus. Sometimes present when pelvic or gastrointestinal tumours have metastasized.

Sjögren's syndrome: an autoimmune disease characterized by the occurrence of xerostomia, rhinitis sicca, parotitis, keratoconjunctivitis sicca, a dry mouth, dry skin, decreased sweating, dryness and crusting of the nasal passages and associated Raynaud's syndrome. Commoner in post-menopausal women (80–90 %). Connective tissue changes include a rheumatoid type of polyarthritis.

Smith's fracture: a flexion and compression fracture of the lower end of the radius, with forward displacement of the lower fragment (opposite of a Colles' fracture).

Spencer Wells forceps: haemostatic forceps. A type of artery forceps.

Sudeck's dystrophy: a variant of the reflex sympathetic dystrophy syndrome, with acute atrophy of bones, commonly of the carpal or tarsal bones, following a minor injury such as sprain. It is characterized by a burning pain that is exacerbated by emotional stress. Prevalent in the elderly and in women.

Swan-Ganz catheter: a thin, flexible, flow-directed catheter with a terminal inflatable balloon. It is inserted through the right atrium and ventricle into the pulmonary artery. The balloon is then inflated sufficiently to block the flow of blood from the right heart to the lung. This allows the back pressure in the pulmonary artery distal to the balloon to be recorded. This pressure reflects the pressure transmitted back from the left atrium.

Syme's amputation: an amputation at the ankle with removal of the malleoli and formation of a heel flap. The significant outcome of Syme's technique, in respect to prostheses, was that the patient had a foundation to walk on instead of cutting off the entire leg.

Thomas' splint: consists of a proximal ring that fits around the upper leg and to which two long rigid slender steel rods are attached. These extend down to another smaller ring distal to the foot. This splint has proved of especial value in the treatment of fractured femur.

Trendelenburg's position: position in which the patient is on an elevated and inclined plane, usually about 45°, with the head down and legs and feet over the edge of the table.

Trendelenburg's sign: a gait adopted by someone with an absent or weakened hip abductor mechanism. During the step, instead of the pelvis being raised on the side of the lifted foot, it drops. Thus it is seen as the patient's pelvis tilting towards the lifted foot, with much flexion needed at the knee on the affected side in order for the foot to clear the ground. The lesion is on the contralateral side to the sagging hip. A positive Trendelenburg sign is found in: subluxation or dislocation of the hip, abductor weakness, shortening of the femoral neck, any painful hip disorder. Remember – the sound side sags.

Trousseau's sign: carpal spasms and paraesthesia produced by pressure upon nerves and vessels of the upper arm sufficient to stop the circulation. The result is a sudden contraction of the fingers and hand into the so-called obstetrician's hand. It is indicative of latent tetany.

Turcot's syndrome: a rare, hereditary syndrome, characterized by brain tumours associated with colonic adenomatous polyposis. Other features include Café-au-lait spots, cutaneous port wine stain, diarrhoea, as well as focal nodular hyperplasia. Inheritance is autosomal recessive.

Volkmann's contracture: ischaemic flexion (muscle) contracture due to external pressure causing irreversible necrosis of the tissue in question, usually seen in the hand and resulting in claw hand. It usually results from impaired circulation following an elbow injury or improper application of a tourniquet.

von Hippel-Lindau syndrome: syndrome characterized by angiomata of the retina, haemangioblastoma of the cerebellum and walls of the fourth ventricle, commonly associated with polycystic lesions of the kidney and pancreas. Inheritance is autosomal dominant with variable clinical expression.

Waldeyer's ring: a ring of lymphoid tissue that encircles the nasopharynx and oropharynx. It is formed by the lymphatic tissue of the pharynx, the palatine tonsil and the lingual tonsil, as well as other collections of lymph tissue in the area.

Warthin's tumour: benign salivary gland tumour with lymphoid tissue covered by epithelium. Found almost exclusively in the parotid glands, where it occurs bilaterally, and is more common in men than in women.

Index